Risk Stratification of Thyroid Nodule: From Ultrasound Features to TIRADS

Risk Stratification of Thyroid Nodule: From Ultrasound Features to TIRADS

Editor

Pierpaolo Trimboli

MDPI • Basel • Beijing • Wuhan • Barcelona • Belgrade • Manchester • Tokyo • Cluj • Tianjin

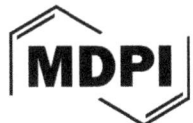

Editor
Pierpaolo Trimboli
Endocrinology
Università della Svizzera Italiana
(USI)
Viganello
Switzerland

Editorial Office
MDPI
St. Alban-Anlage 66
4052 Basel, Switzerland

This is a reprint of articles from the Special Issue published online in the open access journal *Cancers* (ISSN 2072-6694) (available at: www.mdpi.com/journal/cancers/special_issues/risk_stratification_of_thyroid_nodule).

For citation purposes, cite each article independently as indicated on the article page online and as indicated below:

LastName, A.A.; LastName, B.B.; LastName, C.C. Article Title. *Journal Name* **Year**, *Volume Number*, Page Range.

ISBN 978-3-0365-3760-3 (Hbk)
ISBN 978-3-0365-3759-7 (PDF)

© 2022 by the authors. Articles in this book are Open Access and distributed under the Creative Commons Attribution (CC BY) license, which allows users to download, copy and build upon published articles, as long as the author and publisher are properly credited, which ensures maximum dissemination and a wider impact of our publications.

The book as a whole is distributed by MDPI under the terms and conditions of the Creative Commons license CC BY-NC-ND.

Contents

Pierpaolo Trimboli
Ultrasound: The Extension of Our Hands to Improve the Management of Thyroid Patients
Reprinted from: *Cancers* **2021**, *13*, 567, doi:10.3390/cancers13030567 1

Teresa Rago and Paolo Vitti
Risk Stratification of Thyroid Nodules: From Ultrasound Features to TIRADS
Reprinted from: *Cancers* **2022**, *14*, 717, doi:10.3390/cancers14030717 3

Nina Malika Popova, Maija Radzina, Peteris Prieditis, Mara Liepa, Madara Rauda and Kaspars Stepanovs
Impact of the Hypoechogenicity Criteria on Thyroid Nodule Malignancy Risk Stratification Performance by Different TIRADS Systems
Reprinted from: *Cancers* **2021**, *13*, 5581, doi:10.3390/cancers13215581 15

Maija Radzina, Madara Ratniece, Davis Simanis Putrins, Laura Saule and Vito Cantisani
Performance of Contrast-Enhanced Ultrasound in Thyroid Nodules: Review of Current State and Future Perspectives
Reprinted from: *Cancers* **2021**, *13*, 5469, doi:10.3390/cancers13215469 31

Lorenzo Scappaticcio, Maria Ida Maiorino, Sergio Iorio, Giovanni Docimo, Miriam Longo and Anna Grandone et al.
Exploring the Performance of Ultrasound Risk Stratification Systems in Thyroid Nodules of Pediatric Patients
Reprinted from: *Cancers* **2021**, *13*, 5304, doi:10.3390/cancers13215304 51

Dorota Słowińska-Klencka, Mariusz Klencki, Martyna Wojtaszek-Nowicka, Kamila Wysocka-Konieczna, Ewa Woźniak-Oseła and Bożena Popowicz
Validation of Four Thyroid Ultrasound Risk Stratification Systems in Patients with Hashimoto's Thyroiditis; Impact of Changes in the Threshold for Nodule's Shape Criterion
Reprinted from: *Cancers* **2021**, *13*, 4900, doi:10.3390/cancers13194900 65

Fabiano Bini, Andrada Pica, Laura Azzimonti, Alessandro Giusti, Lorenzo Ruinelli and Franco Marinozzi et al.
Artificial Intelligence in Thyroid Field—A Comprehensive Review
Reprinted from: *Cancers* **2021**, *13*, 4740, doi:10.3390/cancers13194740 81

Arnoldo Piccardo, Francesco Fiz, Gianluca Bottoni, Camilla De Luca, Michela Massollo and Ugo Catrambone et al.
Facing Thyroid Nodules in Paediatric Patients Previously Treated with Radiotherapy for Non-Thyroidal Cancers: Are Adult Ultrasound Risk Stratification Systems Reliable?
Reprinted from: *Cancers* **2021**, *13*, 4692, doi:10.3390/cancers13184692 99

Philipp Seifert, Simone Schenke, Michael Zimny, Alexander Stahl, Michael Grunert and Burkhard Klemenz et al.
Diagnostic Performance of Kwak, EU, ACR, and Korean TIRADS as Well as ATA Guidelines for the Ultrasound Risk Stratification of Non-Autonomously Functioning Thyroid Nodules in a Region with Long History of Iodine Deficiency: A German Multicenter Trial
Reprinted from: *Cancers* **2021**, *13*, 4467, doi:10.3390/cancers13174467 109

Gilles Russ, Pierpaolo Trimboli and Camille Buffet
The New Era of TIRADSs to Stratify the Risk of Malignancy of Thyroid Nodules: Strengths, Weaknesses and Pitfalls
Reprinted from: *Cancers* **2021**, *13*, 4316, doi:10.3390/cancers13174316 123

Esther Diana Rossi, Liron Pantanowitz, Marco Raffaelli and Guido Fadda
Overview of the Ultrasound Classification Systems in the Field of Thyroid Cytology
Reprinted from: *Cancers* **2021**, *13*, 3133, doi:10.3390/cancers13133133 145

Stella Bernardi, Andrea Palermo, Rosario Francesco Grasso, Bruno Fabris, Fulvio Stacul and Roberto Cesareo
Current Status and Challenges of US-Guided Radiofrequency Ablation of Thyroid Nodules in the Long Term: A Systematic Review
Reprinted from: *Cancers* **2021**, *13*, 2746, doi:10.3390/cancers13112746 157

Sae Rom Chung, Jung Hwan Baek, Young Jun Choi, Tae-Yon Sung, Dong Eun Song and Tae Yong Kim et al.
Diagnostic Algorithm for Metastatic Lymph Nodes of Differentiated Thyroid Carcinoma
Reprinted from: *Cancers* **2021**, *13*, 1338, doi:10.3390/cancers13061338 175

Martyna Borowczyk, Kosma Woliński, Barbara Wieckowska, Elżbieta Jodłowska-Siewert, Ewelina Szczepanek-Parulska and Frederik A. Verburg et al.
Sonographic Features Differentiating Follicular Thyroid Cancer from Follicular Adenoma–A Meta-Analysis
Reprinted from: *Cancers* **2021**, *13*, 938, doi:10.3390/cancers13050938 187

Pierpaolo Trimboli
Advancements in Ultrasound and Ultrasound-Based Risk Stratification Systems for the Assessment of Thyroid Nodule
Reprinted from: *Cancers* **2022**, *14*, 1668, doi:10.3390/cancers14071668 203

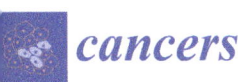

Editorial

Ultrasound: The Extension of Our Hands to Improve the Management of Thyroid Patients

Pierpaolo Trimboli [1,2]

[1] Clinic for Endocrinology and Diabetology, Lugano Regional Hospital, Ente Ospedaliero Cantonale, 6900 Lugano, Switzerland; pierpaolo.trimboli@eoc.ch
[2] Faculty of Biomedical Sciences, Università della Svizzera Italiana (USI), 6900 Lugano, Switzerland

Citation: Trimboli, P. Ultrasound: The Extension of Our Hands to Improve the Management of Thyroid Patients. *Cancers* **2021**, *13*, 567. https://doi.org/10.3390/cancers13030567

Received: 7 January 2021
Accepted: 28 January 2021
Published: 2 February 2021

Publisher's Note: MDPI stays neutral with regard to jurisdictional claims in published maps and institutional affiliations.

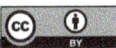

Copyright: © 2021 by the author. Licensee MDPI, Basel, Switzerland. This article is an open access article distributed under the terms and conditions of the Creative Commons Attribution (CC BY) license (https://creativecommons.org/licenses/by/4.0/).

Ultrasonography (US) was introduced in the thyroid field in the 1980s to guide the biopsy of palpable, scintigraphically cold nodules. Within a few years, US-guided fashion became the only modality to perform an optimal sampling of a thyroid lesion, and a significant decrease of unnecessary surgeries was recorded [1]. Subsequently, with the technological advancements of medical devices, the US examination of both thyroid and neck rapidly diffused and all thyroidologists, endocrinologists first, began to visit their patients with US alongside the physical examination and laboratory tests. US allows us to estimate the thyroid size, evaluate its echostructure and echogenicity, investigate visible and/or palpable thyroid nodules, and detect non-palpable ones. More importantly, the risk of malignancy of any thyroid lesion and the presence of neck lymph nodes metastases from thyroid cancer could be assessed [2]. Then, it seemed clear to all thyroidologists that US, due to its characteristics, had the potential to become the "extension" of their hands much more than the other imaging tools. At the turn of the 2000s, US examination was also integrated by color-flow Doppler analysis, elastosonography, and contrast-enhanced modality (CEUS) with the aim to detect thyroid carcinoma with higher accuracy [3–5]. Overall, since then, it came to light that US was essential to achieve an optimal standard of care of thyroid patients [6] and there was a terrific increase of studies reporting excellent reliability of US to diagnose thyroid cancer. Based on this literature, the US presentation of thyroid cancer is now well recognized and the presence of specific US features (i.e., strong hypoechogenicity, taller-than-wide shape, irregular or blurred margins, internal microcalcifications, apparent extrathyroidal extension) represent an important warning requiring biopsy. More recently, several attempts have been made to further improve the performance of US evaluation and some US-based risk stratification systems (RSSs) have been proposed by the most important international societies. These RSSs, often referred to as thyroid imaging reporting and data system (TIRADS), have been developed to establish a standard lexicon to describe the thyroid nodules, assign nodules to a malignancy risk class, and identify nodules requiring biopsy. The evidence-based studies indicate that the performance of RSSs is close to optimal [7,8]. However, some weaknesses might be present with their rigorous use and further improvements are needed. Particularly, the RSSs have been conceived starting from 20-year literature mainly focused on the US presentation of papillary carcinoma [9] and whether they are reliable to identify follicular and medullary thyroid cancers remains to be proven. Moreover, what will be the role of color-flow Doppler, elastosonography, and CEUS in the era of RSSs has to be defined.

Soon, thyroid US RSSs/TIRADSs will be used by all thyroidologists. Endocrinologists, surgeons, radiologists, nuclear medicine physicians, and cytopathologists focused on thyroid disease will have to be familiar with RSSs/TIRADSs terminology, as was the case when the cytological systems were introduced in clinical practice in 2000s. However, before using RSSs/TIRADSs in a multidisciplinary modality, we need further proofs and this special issue will try to address many of the current questions. Highly experienced thyroidologists focused on US are asked to contribute to this honorable aim.

Funding: This research received no external funding.

Conflicts of Interest: The author declares no conflict of interest.

References

1. Gharib, H.; Goellner, J.R.; Johnson, D.A. Fine-needle aspiration cytology of the thyroid. A 12-year experience with 11,000 biopsies. *Clin. Lab. Med.* **1993**, *13*, 699–709. [CrossRef]
2. Antonelli, A.; Miccoli, P.; Ferdeghini, M.; Di Coscio, G.; Alberti, B.; Iacconi, P.; Baldi, V.; Fallahi, P.; Baschieri, L. Role of neck ultrasonography in the follow-up of patients operated on for thyroid cancer. *Thyroid* **1995**, *5*, 25–28. [CrossRef]
3. Rago, T.; Vitti, P.; Chiovato, L.; Mazzeo, S.; De Liperi, A.; Miccoli, P.; Viacava, P.; Bogazzi, F.; Martino, E.; Pinchera, A. Role of conventional ultrasonography and color flow-doppler sonography in predicting malignancy in 'cold' thyroid nodules. *Eur. J. Endocrinol.* **1998**, *138*, 41–46. [CrossRef]
4. Rago, T.; Santini, F.; Scutari, M.; Pinchera, A.; Vitti, P. Elastography: New developments in ultrasound for predicting malignancy in thyroid nodules. *J. Clin. Endocrinol. Metab.* **2007**, *92*, 2917–2922. [CrossRef]
5. Trimboli, P.; Castellana, M.; Virili, C.; Havre, R.F.; Bini, F.; Marinozzi, F.; D'Ambrosio, F.; Giorgino, F.; Giovanella, L.; Prosch, H.; et al. Performance of contrast-enhanced ultrasound (CEUS) in assessing thyroid nodules: A systematic review and meta-analysis using histological standard of reference. *Radiol. Med.* **2020**, *125*, 406–415. [CrossRef]
6. Hegedüs, L. Clinical practice. The thyroid nodule. *N. Engl. J. Med.* **2004**, *351*, 1764–1771. [CrossRef]
7. Castellana, M.; Castellana, C.; Treglia, G.; Giorgino, F.; Giovanella, L.; Russ, G.; Trimboli, P. Performance of Five Ultrasound Risk Stratification Systems in Selecting Thyroid Nodules for FNA. *J. Clin. Endocrinol. Metab.* **2020**, *105*, dgz170. [CrossRef] [PubMed]
8. Castellana, M.; Grani, G.; Radzina, M.; Guerra, V.; Giovanella, L.; Deandrea, M.; Ngu, R.; Durante, C.; Trimboli, P. Performance of EU-TIRADS in malignancy risk stratification of thyroid nodules: A meta-analysis. *Eur. J. Endocrinol.* **2020**, *183*, 255–264. [CrossRef]
9. Trimboli, P.; Castellana, M.; Piccardo, A.; Romanelli, F.; Grani, G.; Giovanella, L.; Durante, C. The ultrasound risk stratification systems for thyroid nodule have been evaluated against papillary carcinoma. A meta-analysis. *Rev. Endocr. Metab. Disord.* **2020**. Available online: https://link.springer.com/article/10.1007%2Fs11154-020-09592-3 (accessed on 26 December 2020). [CrossRef]

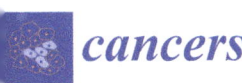

Review

Risk Stratification of Thyroid Nodules: From Ultrasound Features to TIRADS

Teresa Rago *[ID] and Paolo Vitti

Department of Clinical and Experimental Medicine, Endocrinology Section, University of Pisa, 56124 Pisa, Italy; paolo.vitti@med.unipi.it
* Correspondence: rago@endoc.med.unipi.it; Tel.: +39-050-997339

Simple Summary: Thyroid nodules are a frequent clinical issue. Their incidence has increased mainly due to the widespread use of neck ultrasound scans. Most thyroid nodules are asymptomatic, incidentally discovered, and benign at cytology. Thyroid ultrasound is the most sensitive diagnostic tool to evaluate patients with nodular thyroid disease. It is therefore important to use the ultrasound features to select nodules that require a fine-needle aspiration cytology.

Abstract: Thyroid nodules are common in iodine deficient areas, in females, and in patients undergoing neck irradiation. High-resolution ultrasonography (US) is important for detecting and evaluating thyroid nodules. US is used to determine the size and features of thyroid nodules, as well as the presence of neck lymph node metastasis. It also facilitates guided fine-needle aspiration (US-FNA). The most consistent US malignancy features of thyroid nodules are spiculated margins, microcalcifications, a taller-than-wide shape, and marked hypoechogenicity. Increased nodular vascularization is not identified as a predictor of malignancy. Thyroid elastosonography (USE) is also used to characterize thyroid nodules. In fact, a low elasticity of nodules at USE has been related to a higher risk of malignancy. According to their US features, thyroid nodules can be stratified into three categories: low-, intermediate-, and high-risk nodules. US-FNA is suggested for intermediate and high-risk nodules.

Keywords: thyroid nodule; thyroid cancer; ultrasonography; elastosonography; fine-needle aspiration

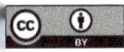

1. Introduction

Thyroid nodules are detected in 50–65% of healthy individuals, the majority being asymptomatic and discovered incidentally [1,2]. Most are benign and do not require treatment [1,2]—less than 5% being malignant. Thyroid nodules are more common in iodine deficiency areas, in females, and in patients undergoing neck irradiation. In rare cases, a thyroid nodule can cause compressive symptoms or hyperthyroidism, thus requiring treatment.

The risk factors associated with a higher probability of malignancy include a history of neck irradiation, a family history of medullary thyroid carcinoma or multiple endocrine neoplasia (MEN2), age < 20 years or >60 years, male sex, rapid growth, a firm and hard consistency, and the presence of suspicious cervical lymph nodes [3–8].

US is the most important diagnostic tool for detecting thyroid nodules [1,2,9,10]. In addition, US can be used to determine the size and features of palpable and nonpalpable nodules, to guide fine-needle aspiration (FNA), and to diagnose lymph node metastasis.

Although thyroid US has been considered as the cornerstone for the management of thyroid nodules, there is no clear consensus on nodule selection for US-guided FNA [11–14], on a standardized terminology for US features [15–20]. Due to their increased detection, thyroid nodules represent a clinical challenge [15–20]. Initial evaluation should include physical examination and investigation of risk factors, such as previous radiation exposure, family history of thyroid diseases, lump growth rate, and signs and symptoms of compression [1,2]. When there is a suspicion that a nodule is functioning (i.e., low TSH), thyroid scintigraphy is mandatory. US examination should always be recommended [1,2]. Several endocrine societies have developed various US-based guidelines and recommendations for managing thyroid nodules [16–22].

2. Real-Time US Findings of Thyroid Nodules

Size: Although the size of a thyroid nodule is not helpful in predicting malignancy, the size should be measured in all three dimensions and recorded for follow-up. Malignant nodules grow faster than benign nodules, but 90% of the latter grow by 15% during a 5-year follow-up period [23–25]. Cystic nodules show a slower growth than solid nodules [25]. Sudden growth of solid nodules may be a clinical manifestation of high-grade malignancy, such as anaplastic thyroid carcinoma or lymphoma [1,2].

There is no clear consensus on the definition of nodule growth. According to the American Thyroid Association (ATA) guidelines, a definition of growth is a 20% increase in the diameter of the nodule with a minimum 2 mm increase in 2 diameters [1]. Some authors prefer a 15% increase in lump volume as a definition of nodule growth [25,26]. However, inter-observer variability has been observed in small nodules, especially for a volume increase of less than 50%. Nodule growth is therefore defined as a 20% increase in diameter or a 50% increase in volume [1,27,28].

Aspect: Thyroid cancer is rare in cystic nodules, although 13–26% of thyroid cancers may have a cystic component [29,30]. Rarely, partially cystic nodules can be malignant [31]. In this case, papillary thyroid carcinoma may have an eccentric solid component with vascularization, or the presence of microcalcifications [29,31,32]. A lump is called spongiform when a microcystic appearance occupies more than 50% of the lump and is considered a sign of benignity with high specificity [33–35]. A nodule can be classified according to the ratio between the solid component and the cystic one as: solid ($\leq$10% of the cystic portion), predominantly solid (from >10% to $\leq$50% of the cystic portion), predominantly cystic (from >50% to $\leq$90% of the cystic portion), and cystic (>90% of the cystic portion) [33].

Shape: The shape of a nodule has gained diagnostic importance for the differentiation between benign and malignant nodules since the first observation by Kim et al. [36–38], who reported that a taller-than-wide shape had 93% specificity for diagnosing malignancy. In a larger multicenter study, a taller-than-wide shape was shown to be highly suggestive of malignancy with a specificity of 89% and a positive predictive value of 86% [33]. These results are explained by the growth pattern, because malignant nodules grow through the normal tissue plane in a centrifugal way, while benign nodules grow along the tissue plane in a parallel fashion [36–39]. In benign nodules, the shape can therefore be ovoid to round (the antero–posterior diameter is less or equal to its transverse diameter on a transverse plane).

Halo sign: Nodules may have a thin or thick halo. A halo or hypoechoic rim surrounding a nodule consists of a pseudocapsule due to fibrous connective tissue, compressed thyroid tissue, and chronic inflammatory process [40]. Although a completely uniform halo is suggestive of benignity with a specificity of 95% [41], more than half of benign nodules are devoid of a halo [30–40]. An uneven thick or incomplete halo due to a fibrotic pseudocapsular structure and inflammatory and necrotic process is observed in 10–12% of papillary thyroid carcinomas and is frequently associated with an irregular shape. On the other hand, 10–24% of papillary carcinomas have a complete or incomplete halo [29,30,41].

Margins: Previous studies have reported that both spiculated or microlobulated margins and poorly defined margins are suggestive of malignancy [36,42]. Nodule margins are ill-defined when they lack clear demarcation from the surrounding perinodular tissue for most of (>50%) their edge [33].

When the tumor infiltration of the margin is minimal, it manifests as an ill-defined margin. However, benign thyroid nodules are sometimes incompletely encapsulated and poorly marginated, and they can merge with normal tissue [43]. Therefore, an ill-defined margin is a nonspecific finding that can be observed in both benign and malignant nodules. Conversely, a spiculated margin is highly suggestive of malignancy with a specificity of

92% and a positive predictive value of 81% [33]. We thus suggest that the margin of a nodule is classified as follows: smooth, spiculated/microlobulated, or ill-defined.

Echogenicity: Marked hypoechogenicity is highly specific for malignancy with a specificity of 92–94% [33,36]. Although the thyroid parenchymal echogenicity is different in different individuals, it is used as a reference for nodule echogenicity. Neck strap muscles (the sternothyroid, sternocleidomastoid), characterized by very low echogenicity, are also used as a reference tissue [33,36]. The salivary glands may also be used as a standard of normal thyroid echogenicity in patients with hypoechogenicity. Nodule echogenicity is classified as follows: marked hypoechoic (nodule echogenicity is similar to that of the adjacent neck strap muscles), hypoechoic, isoechoic, or hyperechoic, compared with the echogenicity of the normal thyroid parenchyma.

Calcifications: A calcification is defined as an echogenic focus with or without back shadow. The absence of posterior shadow does not exclude calcification as some calcifications are too small to produce a posterior shadow. Punctate echogenic foci with reverberation artifacts are due to colloid materials and can be easily differentiated from calcifications on US. Some studies report that all types of calcifications seen on US increase the likelihood of malignancy. In particular, comet-tail artifacts can represent dense colloid, fibrin deposits and even microcalcifications. The presence of comet-tail artifacts in a cystic nodule is highly suggestive of benignity but may not rule out malignancy if present in a solid component. Moreover, the punctate echogenic foci do not necessarily represent the psammoma bodies that are observed in papillary thyroid carcinoma but may be dystrophic calcifications or microdeposit of dense colloid.

Calcifications can be observed in both benign and malignant nodules. We suggest classifying calcifications as follows: (i) microcalcifications—small dotted echogenic foci of 1 mm or less either with or without posterior shadow; (ii) macrocalcifications—dotted echogenic foci larger than 1 mm; (iii) coarse or peripheral and border calcifications.

At histology, microcalcifications correspond to psammoma bodies, which are round, laminar, crystalline, calcific deposits 10–100 µm, specific to papillary thyroid carcinoma. Microcalcifications are highly suggestive of malignancy with a specificity of 86–95% and a positive predictive value of 42–94% [33,36,42,44,45]. Large and irregular shaped dystrophic calcifications may be due to tissue necrosis and can be observed in benign and malignant nodules. The significance of peripheral, eggshell, or rim calcification is still debated in terms of differentiation between benign and malignant nodules. In longstanding hyperplastic nodules peripheral rim calcification may be present. However, the focal disruption of the eggshell structure associated with the presence on a thick and markedly hypoechoic halo can be predictive of malignancy [34,46–48].

3. Accessory Features

US in Lymph nodes: US examen of the cervical lymph nodes should be performed in all patients with thyroid nodules. The US appearance of a typical normal lymph node is hypoechogenicity, an oval shape and presence of the central hyperechoic streak corresponding to the hilum. On the other hand, a pathological lymph node can be cystic or solid, iso or hyperechoic, round or irregular in shape, and without the hilum [49]. The position of the described lymph nodes must be precisely located following Robbins' scheme [50]. In suspicious lymph nodes, an US-guided FNA should be performed for cytology and thyroglobulin or calcitonin measurement in the needle washout.

Extrathyroidal extension (EE): EE is characterized by protrusion into adjacent structures and/or rupture of the capsular margin of the thyroid neoplasm. In small tumors, the presence of EE is very important in deciding the type of surgery: lobectomy versus total thyroidectomy. The presence of minimal EE is not associate to a worse prognosis of the tumor. The US features that define EE are contact, degree of contact, and interruption of the capsule. Kwak reports that a greater than 25% contact between the thyroid nodule and the adjacent capsule is a useful US marker for predicting the presence of EE [51]. Capsular abutment has less specificity. On the other hand, the presence of more than 2 mm normal thyroid parenchyma between the nodule and a continuous capsule reduces the risk of microscopic extrathyroidal extension to less than 6% [51–54].

4. Color Doppler Flow Imaging (CDFI), Power Doppler US, and Superb Micro-Vascular Imaging (SMI)

US color Doppler or US power Doppler provide information on the vascularization of the nodules. Although vascularity is a nonspecific finding in thyroid cancer, it is found in 69–74% of cases [29]. Benign nodules are characterized by a perinodular flow which, however, can also be observed in 22% of carcinomas [29]. Intranodular vascularization is observed in carcinoma but has a low specificity, while chaotic vascularization is more specific, but with a very low sensitivity [35]. Some studies report that the resistance index, maximum systolic velocity, and vascularization pattern on a Doppler US do not differ between benign nodules and carcinomas [55–57]. Color and power Doppler only provide complementary information and are even less reliable for small nodules (<5 mm) due to the misinterpretation of perinodular vessels as an intranodular vascular signal. Therefore, several authors advise against the routine use of color and power Doppler US for thyroid nodules [1].

CDFI uses low-frequency, low-speed flow signals, while contrast-enhanced ultrasound (CEUS) detects low-frequency flow signals with a diameter of 10–30 µm and a flow rate of approximately 1 mm/s. CEUS is expensive and can cause an allergic reaction [58–61]. SMI is a recently introduced, non-invasive, inexpensive exam that highlights microflows and detects tissue signals, thus minimizing artifacts. There are few data in the literature on the usefulness of this investigation for the characterization of thyroid nodules [61].

In CEUS analysis, a high perfusion indicates an extensive microvasculature, whereas a low perfusion suggests a lower degree of microvasculature. Some reports have shown that malignant nodules had mainly hypo-enhancement [62–66], which can be due to fibrosis and neovascular damage by tumor cells, while benign nodules had hyper-enhancement or iso-enhancement, similar to normal tissue. Zang et al. reported a higher sensitivity and lower specificity of CEUS + SMI in 75 suspicious nodules, compared with CEUS or SMI alone [67].

5. US Elastosonography (USE)

USE determines the elasticity of tissue. Given that a carcinoma is harder than a normal thyroid parenchyma or a benign nodule, a high stiffness on USE has been suggested as a good predictor of malignancy [68–73]. Our group showed that low elasticity scores, indicative of a hard consistency, were associated with malignancy with a specificity of 100% and sensitivity of 97% [69]. The predictivity of the USE measurement was independent of the nodule size. In fact, a high sensitivity and specificity were found even in nodules with the largest diameter of 0.8–1 cm. In a large series of patients with indeterminate and non-diagnostic cytology, our group confirmed that high nodular stiffness is associated with malignancy. In this paper, we also simplified the classification of USE into 3 groups: score 1—nodules with uniform high elasticity, probably benign; score 3—nodules with uniform low elasticity, probably malignant; score 2—nodules with a non-homogeneous distribution of elasticity, suspicious. Since the vast majority of nodules with indeterminate and non-diagnostic cytology had a score of 1, they had a low probability of malignancy [74]. Our findings may limit the indications for surgical treatment to the subgroup of patients with the highest risk of cancer. We also showed that in 115 patients who underwent surgery for a suspicious cytology, or large nodules with suspicious US features and non-diagnostic cytology, low elasticity at USE was highly correlated with malignancy and also with the presence of fibrosis and expression of Gal-3 and FN-1 in the histological specimens [75]. A few pitfalls limit the diagnostic usefulness of USE, which is operator dependent. Moreover, cystic lesions, nodules with calcified shell and multinodular goiter with coalescent nodules are not suitable for USE evaluation.

6. US Risk Stratification Systems: The TIRADS

US-guided FNA is the main diagnostic tool for detecting malignancy in thyroid nodules. Its use should be restricted to thyroid nodules suspicious for malignancy. In fact, most scientific societies agree that US features should support the indications to perform US-guided FNA. Several classification systems have been proposed aimed at stratifying the risk of cancer in thyroid nodules [17–21].

However, apart from the well-recognized advantage, thyroid US also has drawbacks such as the poor reproducibility, due to the different equipment used, lack of a standardized US report and inter- and intra-operator variability. To address these main points, several US risk stratification systems (i.e., thyroid imaging reporting and data systems—TIRADS) have been developed to stratify the malignancy risk of a nodule and then suggest the need for US-guided FNA [76–82]. These systems are called TIRADS because they were modeled in line with the American Committee of Radiology BIRADS, which has been widely accepted in breast imaging.

The TIRADS classification is a point scale that categorizes the US of thyroid nodules from low to high suspicion, based on the number and combination of the predictors of malignancy [17]. Initially, Horvath et al. in 2009 [17] proposed a classification system, which assigned levels of malignancy risk to different patterns, involving 10 features. On the other hand, Park et al. devised an equation to predict the probability of malignancy based on 12 variables. Kwak proposed a simplified system in which nodules were stratified only on the basis of five US patterns [18].

So far, many professional societies have proposed US-based risk stratification systems. The Chinese-TIRADS was recently proposed from Chinese professional society and the revised 2021 Korean-TIRADS was very recently published [19,20]. The TIRADS classifications have been slightly modified over the years and different versions have been suggested by different guidelines, including EU-TIRADS provided by the European Thyroid Association [79], ACR-TIRADS by the American College of Radiology [22], and K-TIRADS by the Korean Society of Thyroid Radiology [20,21]. These different versions of TIRADS have been validated and have shown great diagnostic value in predicting thyroid malignancy. However, most of those studies were retrospective and the results heterogeneous, limiting their applicability in clinical practice. In a recent meta-analysis, Castellana et al. assessed the prevalence of malignancy in each EU-TIRADS, class 5 compared to classes 2, 3, and 4. The authors found that the prevalence of malignancy was 16% in class 2, 5.5% in 3, 20.6% in 4, and 83.3% in 5 [83,84]. These findings were very close to the estimates of the ETA experts. EU-TIRADS should therefore be considered as an accurate way of stratifying the risk of malignancy of thyroid nodules and performing US-guided FNA is not recommended in EU-TIRADS class 2 nodules. However, the risk of malignancy is greater in highly specialized centers than in primary care centers. This is linked to the fact that selected patients come to highly specialized centers. This explains why in EU-TIRADS there is an overestimation of the risk of malignancy.

A recent consensus of the Italian Thyroid Association, the Italian Society of Endocrinology, the Italian Society of Ultrasonography in Medicine and Biology, and the Ultrasound Chapter of the Italian Society of Medical Radiology considered that the main limitation of US is the poor reproducibility, due to the varying experience of the operators and the different performance and settings of the equipment. A simplified nodule risk stratification was therefore proposed, which is based on the predictive value of each US sign, classified and evaluated according to the strength of association with malignancy, but also to the estimated reproducibility between different operators [85]. The risk score was classified into four categories on the basis of the estimated specificity and reproducibility among different operators for each US feature (Table 1). The risk score is the sum of the single scores attributed to each US pattern.

Table 1. Stratification of the risk score based on the predictive value of each US feature associated with malignancy.

	US Features Associated with Malignancy		
	Low Specificity/High Reproducibility	Hypoechogenicity Thick Halo	Score Value 1
	High specificity/poor reproducibility	Microcalcifications irregular, disrupted, spiculated or lobulated margins, high stiffness at USE	Score Value 2
	High specificity/high reproducibility	Marked hypoechogenicity irregular shape, taller-than-wide	Score Value 3
	Very high specificity/high reproducibility/Accessory features	Extracapsular extension, suspicious lymph nodes	Score Value 4
Risk category	1. Low risk	Nodules with at least 2 US features associated with benignity * and no features associated with malignancy	
	2. Intermediate risk	Nodules with total risk score 1–3	
	3. High risk	Nodules with total risk score ≥4	

Modified by Rago et al. [85]. The risk score is the sum of the single scores attributed to each ultrasound feature. * Purely cystic nodules, mixed nodules with liquid content, spongiform nodules, oval shape, isoechoic/hyperechoic nodules with complete halo sign, isoechoic/hyperechoic nodules with complete halo sign and lamellar macrocalcifications, hyperechoic pseudonodular areas in thyroid autoimmune diseases.

7. Indication for FNA According to US Risk Stratification Systems

As noted above, the recommendation as to whether or not to perform US-guided FNA depends on US features associated with malignancy, size, and patient's history. US-FNA has a high sensitivity in small nodules with suspicious US features, while in large nodules, the sensitivity is reduced. Furthermore, considering that the prognosis of some tumors (such as follicular or Hurthle cell carcinoma) is related to the size of the nodule, it is important to recommend US-FNA in nodules > 2 cm in size, or in those that grow over time. Thus, most guidelines recommend FNA in solid nodules > 2 cm even when devoid of US signs suggestive of malignancy. A point of discussion is the size below which FNA is not indicated. In fact, the mortality and recurrence rate of thyroid cancer is directly proportional to the size of the nodules [1,2,19]. The ATA and ETA guidelines recommend US-guided FNA in sub-centimetric nodules only when suspicious features are present and in patients with a history of radiation exposure or familial thyroid cancer [1,2]. Thyroid carcinoma smaller than 5 mm compared with 6–10 mm diameter has a better survival and less recurrence at 5 years (<3% versus 14%) [1]. Recent studies thus recommend not performing US-guided FNA (Table 2) in nodules smaller than 5 mm, also due to the high rate of false positive US findings and the high rate of inadequate cytology [8].

In nodular goiter, US-guided FNA cannot be performed in all nodules. The risk of malignancy for patients with multiple thyroid nodules is not very different from the risk for patients with a single thyroid nodule [9,86]. According to the guidelines [1,2,78], in the presence of 2 or more nodules equal or greater than 1–1.5 cm, US-guided FNA is recommended for those with suspicious US features. If none of the nodules have suspicious US features, FNA of the largest nodule should be performed. All the guidelines agree that US-guided FNA should be advised in high and intermediate risk category nodules, and not the low-risk category.

In summary, the three main aims of using US risk stratification systems are the following: (i) to contribute to the optimal management strategy; (ii) to reduce the number of unnecessary investigations; (iii) to select those patients who should be operated on. The secondary objectives are to facilitate communication between professionals and patients, facilitate a cross-dialogue between clinicians and pathologists, and improve the inter-observer agreement of US reports.

Table 2. US risk stratification for malignancy and indication for US-FNA.

Risk Category	French [77] 2013		ATA [1] 2016		ACE/ACE-AME [2] 2016		Korean [20] 2021		ETA [79] 2018	
	M.R. (%)	FNA Size (cm)	M.R. (%)	FNA Size (cm)	M.R. (%)	FNA Size (cm)	M.R. (%)	FNA Size (cm)	M.R. (%)	FNA Size (cm)
High	100	≥ 1	70–90	>1	50–90	≥ 1	>60	>1–1.5	26–87	>10
Intermediate	69	≥ 1	10–20	≥ 1	5–15	>2	15–40	>2	6–17	>15
Low	6	≥ 1.5	5–10	≥ 1.5	1	≥ 2	3–10	≥ 1.5	2–4	>20
Very low	0.25	≥ 2	≥ 3	>2			<3			
Benign	0	NA	<1	NA				NA	0	NA
No Nodule										

M.R.—malignancy risk; N.A—not advised.

8. Conclusions

Today thyroid nodules are frequently detected by imaging techniques. Only a minority of these nodules will cause significant harm to health. Thyroid US is primarily responsible for this frequent detection, and is also the primary tool for stratifying the risk of cancer and the strength of US-guided FNA indication.

Funding: This research received no external funding.

Conflicts of Interest: The authors declare no conflict of interest.

Abbreviations

US	ultrasonography
FNA	fine-needle aspiration
US-FNA	ultrasound–guided fine-needle aspiration
USE	elastosonography
MEN-2	multiple endocrine neoplasia Type 2
TIRADS	thyroid imaging reporting and data systems
ATA	American Thyroid Association
ETA	European Thyroid Association
K-TIRADS	Korean Society of Thyroid Radiology
EE	extrathyroidal extension
AACE-AME	American Association of Clinical Endocrinologists, American College of Endocrinology, and Associazione Medici Endocrinologi Medical

References

1. Haugen, B.R.; Alexander, E.K.; Bible, K.C.; Doherty, G.M.; Mandel, S.J.; Nikiforov, Y.E.; Pacini, F.; Randolph, G.W.; Sawka, A.M.; Schlumberger, M.; et al. 2015 American Thyroid Association Management Guidelines for adult patients with thyroid nodules and differentiated thyroid cancer the American Thyroid Association Guidelines Task Force on thyroid nodules and differentiated thyroid cancer. *Thyroid* **2016**, *26*, 1–133. [CrossRef] [PubMed]
2. Gharib, H.; Papini, E.; Garber, J.R.; Duick, D.S.; Harrell, R.M.; Hegedus, L.; Paschke, R.; Valcavi, R.; Vitti, P. American Association of Clinical Endocrinologists, American College of Endocrinology, and Associazione Medici Endocrinologi Medical Guidelines for Clinical Practice for the Diagnosis and Management of Thyroid Nodules–2016 Update. *Endocr. Pract.* **2016**, *22*, 622–639. [CrossRef] [PubMed]
3. Tunbridge, W.M.G.; Evered, D.C.; Hall, R.; Appleton, D.; Brewis, M.; Clark, F.; Evans, J.G.; Young, E.; Bird, T.; Smith, P.A. The spectrum of thyroid disease in a community: The Whickham survey. *Clin. Endocrinol.* **1977**, *43*, 481–493. [CrossRef] [PubMed]
4. Tan, G.H.; Gharib, H. Thyroid incidentalomas: Management approaches to nonpalpable nodules discovered incidentally on thyroid imaging. *Ann. Intern. Med.* **1997**, *126*, 226–231. [CrossRef]
5. Aghini-Lombardi, F.; Antonangeli, L.; Martino, E.; Vitti, P.; Maccherini, D.; Leoli, F.; Rago, T.; Grasso, L.; Valeriano, R.; Balestrieri, A.; et al. The spectrum of thyroid disorders in an iodine-deficient community: The Pescopagano survey. *J. Clin. Endocrinol. Metab.* **1999**, *84*, 561–566. [CrossRef]
6. Cooper, D.S.; Doherty, G.M.; Haugen, B.R.; Kloos, R.T.; Lee, S.L.; Mandel, S.J.; Mazzaferri, E.L.; McIve, B.; Sherman, S.I.; Tuttle, R.M.; et al. Management Guidelines for Patients with Thyroid Nodules and Differentiated Thyroid Cancer. *Thyroid* **2006**, *16*, 109–142. [CrossRef]
7. Gharib, H.; Papini, E. Thyroid nodules: Clinical importance, assessment, and treatment. *Endocrinol. Metab. Clin. N. Am.* **2007**, *36*, 707–735. [CrossRef]
8. Rago, T.; Fiore, E.; Scutari, M.; Santini, F.; Di Coscio, G.; Romani, R.; Piaggi, P.; Ugolini, C.; Basolo, F.; Miccoli, P.; et al. Male sex, single nodularity, and young age are associated with the risk of finding a papillary thyroid cancer on fine-needle aspiration cytology in a large series of patients with nodular thyroid disease. *Eur. J. Endocrinol.* **2010**, *162*, 763–770. [CrossRef]
9. Mandel, S.J. Diagnostic use of ultrasonography in patients with nodular thyroid disease. *Endocr. Pract.* **2004**, *10*, 246–252. [CrossRef]
10. Rago, T.; Chiovato, L.; Aghini-Lombardi, F.; Grasso, L.; Pinchera, A.; Vitti, P. Non-palpable thyroid nodules in a borderline iodine-sufficient area: Detection by ultrasonography and follow-up. *J. Endocrinol. Investig.* **2001**, *24*, 770–776. [CrossRef]
11. Castro, M.R.; Gharib, H. Thyroid fine-needle aspiration biopsy: Progress, practice, and pitfalls. *Endocr. Pract.* **2003**, *9*, 128–136. [CrossRef] [PubMed]
12. Baskin, H.J. Chapter 5, Ultrasound of thyroid nodules. In *Thyroid Ultrasound and Ultrasound-Guided FNA Biopsy*; Baskin, H.J., Ed.; Springer: Boston, MA, USA, 2000; pp. 71–86.

13. Baloch, Z.W.; LiVolsi, V.A.; Asa, S.L.; Rosai, J.; Merino, M.J.; Randolph, G.; Vielh, P.; DeMay, R.M.; Sidawy, M.K.; Frable, W.J. Diagnostic terminology and morphologic criteria for cytologic diagnosis of thyroid lesions: A synopsis of the National Cancer Institute thyroid fine-needle aspiration state of the science conference. *Diagn. Cytopathol.* **2008**, *36*, 425–437. [CrossRef] [PubMed]
14. Nardi, F.; Basolo, F.; Crescenzi, A.; Fadda, G.; Frasoldati, A.; Orlandi, F.; Palombini, L.; Papini, E.; Zini, M.; Pontecorvi, A.; et al. Italian consensus for the classification and reporting of thyroid cytology. *J. Endocrinol. Investig.* **2014**, *37*, 593–599. [CrossRef]
15. Perros, P.; Boelaert, K.; Colley, S.; Evans, C.; Evans, R.M.; Gerrard Ba, G.; Gilbert, J.; Harrison, B.; Johnson, S.J.; Giles, T.E.; et al. British Thyroid Association. Guidelines for the management of thyroid cancer. *Clin. Endocrinol.* **2014**, *15*, 1–122. [CrossRef]
16. Frates, M.C.; Benson, C.B.; Doubilet, P.M.; Kunreuther, E.; Contreras, M.; Cibas, E.; Orcutt, J.; Moore, F.D., Jr.; Larsen, P.R.; Marqusee, E.; et al. Prevalence and distribution of carcinoma in patients with solitary and multiple thyroid nodules on sonography. *J. Clin. Endocrinol. Metab.* **2006**, *91*, 3411–3417. [CrossRef] [PubMed]
17. Hovarth, E.; Majlis, S.; Rossi, R.; Franco, C.; Niedmann, J.P.; Castro, A. An ultrasonogram reporting system for thyroid nodules stratifying cancer risk for clinical management. *J. Clin. Endocrinol. Metab.* **2009**, *90*, 1748–1751. [CrossRef]
18. Kwak, J.Y.; Han, K.H.; Yoon, J.H.; Moon, H.J.; Son, E.J.; Park, S.H.; Jung, H.K.; Choi, J.S.; Kim, B.M.; Kim, E.K. Thyroid imaging reporting and data system for US features of nodules: A step in establishing better stratification of cancer risk. *Radiology* **2011**, *260*, 892–899. [CrossRef]
19. Zhou, J.; Yin, L.; Wei, X.; Zhang, S.; Song, Y.; Luo, B.; Li, J.; Qian, L.; Cui, L.; Chen, W.; et al. 2020 Chinese guidelines for ultrasound malignancy risk stratification of thyroid nodules: The C-TIRADS. *Endocrine* **2020**, *70*, 256–279. [CrossRef]
20. Ha, E.J.; Chung, S.R.; Na, D.G.; Ahn, H.S.; Chung, J.; Lee, J.Y.; Park, J.S.; Yoo, R.E.; Baek, J.H.; Baek, S.M.; et al. 2021 Korean Thyroid Imaging Reporting and Data System and Imaging-Based Management of Thyroid Nodules: Korean Society of Thyroid Radiology Consensus Statement and Recommendations. *Korean J. Radiol.* **2021**, *22*, 2094–2123. [CrossRef]
21. Shin, J.H.; Baek, J.H.; Chung, J.; Ha, E.J.; Kim, J.H.; Lee, Y.H.; Lim, H.K.; Moon, W.J.; Na, D.G.; Park, J.S.; et al. Korean Society of Thyroid Radiology (KSThR) and Korean Society of Radiology, Ultrasonography diagnosis and imaging-based management of thyroid nodules: Revised Korean Society of Thyroid Radiology consensus statement and recommendations. *Korean J. Radiol.* **2016**, *17*, 370–395. [CrossRef]
22. Tessler, F.N.; Middleton, W.D.; Grant, E.G.; Hoang, J.K.; Berland, L.L.; Teefey, S.A.; Cronan, J.J.; Beland, M.D.; Desser, T.S.; Frates, M.C.; et al. ACR Thyroid Imaging, Reporting and Data System (TI-RADS): White paper of the ACR TI-RADS committee. *J. Am. Coll. Radiol.* **2017**, *14*, 587–595. [CrossRef]
23. Brander, A.E.; Viikinkoski, V.P.; Nickels, J.I.; Kivisaari, L.M. Importance of thyroid abnormalities detected at US screening: A 5-year follow-up. *Radiology* **2000**, *215*, 801–806. [CrossRef] [PubMed]
24. Kuma, K.; Matsuzuka, F.; Yokozawa, T.; Miyauchi, A.; Sugawara, M. Fate of untreated benign thyroid nodules: Results of long-term follow-up. *World J. Surg.* **1994**, *18*, 495–498. [CrossRef]
25. Durante, C.; Costante, G.; Lucisano, G.; Bruno, R.; Meringolo, D.; Paciaroni, A.; Puxeddu, E.; Torlontano, M.; Tumino, S.; Attard, M.; et al. The natural history of benign thyroid nodules. *JAMA* **2015**, *313*, 926–935. [CrossRef]
26. Alexander, E.K.; Hurwitz, S.; Heering, J.P.; Benson, C.B.; Frates, M.C.; Doubilet, P.M.; Cibas, E.S.; Larsen, P.R.; Marqusee, E. Natural history of benign solid and cystic thyroid nodules. *Ann. Intern. Med.* **2003**, *138*, 315–318. [CrossRef]
27. Papini, E.; Petrucci, L.; Guglielmi, R.; Panunzi, C.; Rinaldi, R.; Bacci, V.; Crescenzi, A.; Nardi, F.; Fabbrini, R.; Pacella, C.M. Long-term changes in nodular goiter: A 5-year prospective randomized trial of levothyroxine suppressive therapy for benign cold thyroid nodules. *J. Clin. Endocrinol. Metab.* **1998**, *83*, 780–783. [CrossRef] [PubMed]
28. Brauer, V.F.; Eder, P.; Miehle, K.; Wiesner, T.D.; Hasenclever, H.; Paschke, R. Interobserver variation for ultrasound determination of thyroid nodule volumes. *Thyroid* **2005**, *15*, 1169–1175. [CrossRef] [PubMed]
29. Chan, B.K.; Desser, T.S.; McDougall, I.R.; Weigel, R.J.; Jeffrey, R.B., Jr. Common and uncommon sonographic features of papillary thyroid carcinoma. *J. Ultrasound Med.* **2003**, *22*, 1083–1090. [CrossRef] [PubMed]
30. Watters, D.A.; Ahuja, A.T.; Evans, R.M.; Chick, W.; King, W.W.; Metreweli, C.; Li, A.K. Role of ultrasound in the management of thyroid nodules. *Am. J. Surg.* **1992**, *164*, 654–657. [CrossRef]
31. Lee, M.J.; Kim, E.K.; Kwak, J.Y.; Kim, M.J. Partially cystic thyroid nodules on ultrasound: Probability of malignancy and sonographic differentiation. *Thyroid* **2009**, *19*, 341–346. [CrossRef]
32. Hatabu, H.; Kasagi, K.; Yamamoto, K.; Iida, Y.; Misaki, T.; Hidaka, A.; Shibata, T.; Shoji, K.; Higuchi, K.; Yamabe, H.; et al. Cystic papillary carcinoma of the thyroid gland: A new sonographic sign. *Clin. Radiol.* **1991**, *43*, 121–124. [CrossRef]
33. Moon, W.J.; Jung, S.L.; Lee, J.H.; Na, D.G.; Baek, J.H.; Lee, Y.H.; Kim, J.; Kim, H.S.; Byun, J.S.; Lee, D.H. Benign and malignant thyroid nodules: US differentiation—multicenter retrospective study. *Radiology* **2008**, *247*, 762–770. [CrossRef] [PubMed]
34. Bonavita, J.A.; Mayo, J.; Babb, J.V.; Bennett, G.; Oweity, T.; Macari, M.; Yee, J. Pattern recognition of benign nodules at ultrasound of the thyroid: Which nodules can be left alone? *Am. J. Roentgenol.* **2009**, *193*, 207–213. [CrossRef] [PubMed]
35. Moon, W.J.; Kwag, H.J.; Na, D.G. Are there any specific ultrasound findings of nodular hyperplasia ("leave me alone" lesion) to differentiate it from follicular adenoma? *Acta Radiol.* **2009**, *50*, 383–388. [CrossRef]
36. Kim, E.K.; Park, C.S.; Chung, W.Y.; Oh, K.K.; Kim, D.I.; Lee, J.T.; Yoo, H.S. New sonographic criteria for recommending fine-needle aspiration biopsy of nonpalpable solid nodules of the thyroid. *Am. J. Roentgenol.* **2002**, *178*, 687–691. [CrossRef] [PubMed]
37. Cappelli, C.; Castellano, M.; Pirola, I.; Gandossi, E.; De Martino, E.; Cumetti, D.; Agosti, B.; Rosei, E.A. Thyroid nodule shape suggests malignancy. *Eur. J. Endocrinol.* **2006**, *155*, 27–31. [CrossRef]

38. Alexander, E.K.; Marqusee, E.; Orcutt, J.; Benson, C.B.; Frates, M.C.; Doubilet, P.M.; Cibas, E.S.; Atri, A. Thyroid nodule shape and prediction of malignancy. *Thyroid* **2004**, *14*, 953–958. [CrossRef]
39. Stavros, A.T.; Thickman, D.; Rapp, C.L.; Dennis, M.A.; Parker, S.H.; Sisney, G.A. Solid breast nodules: Use of sonography to distinguish between benign and malignant lesions. *Radiology* **1995**, *196*, 123–134. [CrossRef]
40. Propper, R.A.; Skolnick, M.L.; Weinstein, B.J.; Dekker, A. The non specificity of the thyroid halo sign. *J. Clin. Ultrasound* **1980**, *8*, 129–132. [CrossRef]
41. Lu, C.; Chang, T.C.; Hsiao, Y.L.; Kuo, M.S. Ultrasonographic findings of papillary thyroid carcinoma and their relation to pathologic changes. *J. Formos. Med. Assoc.* **1994**, *93*, 933–938.
42. Papini, E.; Guglielmi, R.; Bianchini, A.; Crescenzi, A.; Taccogna, S.; Nardi, F.; Panunzi, C.; Rinaldi, R.; Toscano, V.; Pacella, C.M. Risk of malignancy in nonpalpable thyroid nodules: Predictive value of ultrasound and color-Doppler features. *J. Clin. Endocrinol. Metab.* **2002**, *87*, 1941–1946. [CrossRef] [PubMed]
43. Reading, C.C.; Charboneau, J.W.; Hay, I.D.; Sebo, T.J. Sonography of thyroid nodules: A "classic pattern" diagnostic approach. *Ultrasound Q.* **2005**, *21*, 157–165. [CrossRef] [PubMed]
44. Khoo, M.L.; Asa, S.L.; Witterick, I.J.; Freeman, J.L. Thyroid calcification and its association with thyroid carcinoma. *Head Neck* **2002**, *24*, 651–655. [CrossRef] [PubMed]
45. Peccin, S.; de Castro, J.A.; Furlanetto, T.W.; Furtado, A.P.; Brasil, B.A.; Czepielewski, M.A. Ultrasonography: Is it useful in the diagnosis of cancer in thyroid nodules? *J. Endocrinol. Investig.* **2002**, *25*, 39–43. [CrossRef] [PubMed]
46. Kwak, M.S.; Baek, J.H.; Kim, Y.S.; Jeong, H.J. Patterns and significance of peripheral calcifications of thyroid tumors seen on ultrasound. *J. Korean Radiol. Soc.* **2005**, *53*, 401–405. [CrossRef]
47. Yoon, D.Y.; Lee, J.W.; Chang, S.K.; Choi, C.S.; Yun, E.J.; Seo, Y.L.; Kim, K.H.; Hwang, H.S. Peripheral calcification in thyroid nodules: Ultrasonographic features and prediction of malignancy. *J. Ultrasound Med.* **2007**, *26*, 1349–1355. [CrossRef] [PubMed]
48. Kim, B.M.; Kim, M.J.; Kim, E.K.; Kwak, J.Y.; Hong, S.W.; Son, E.J.; Kim, K.H. Sonographic differentiation of thyroid nodules with eggshell calcifications. *J. Ultrasound Med.* **2008**, *27*, 1425–1430. [CrossRef]
49. Leenhardt, L.; Erdogan, M.F.; Hegedus, L.; Mandel, S.J.; Paschke, R.; Rago, T.; Russ, G. European thyroid association guidelines for cervical ultrasound scan and ultrasound-guided techniques in the postoperative management of patients with thyroid cancer. *Eur. Thyroid J.* **2013**, *2*, 147–159. [CrossRef]
50. Robbins, K.T.; Shaha, A.R.; Medina, J.E.; Califano, J.A.; Wolf, G.T.; Ferlito, A.; Som, P.M.; Day, T.A. Consensus statement on the classification and terminology of neck dissection. *Arch. Otolaryngol. Head Neck Surg.* **2008**, *134*, 536–538. [CrossRef]
51. Kwak, J.Y.; Kim, E.K.; Youk, J.H.; Kim, M.J.; Son, E.J.; Choi, S.H.; Oh, K.K. Extrathyroid extension of well-differentiated papillary thyroid microcarcinoma on US. *Thyroid* **2008**, *18*, 609–614. [CrossRef]
52. Kim, S.J.; Ko, K.R.; Chung, K.W.; Lee, J.H. Predictive factors for extrathyroidal extension of papillary thyroid carcinoma based on preoperative sonography. *J. Ultrasound Med.* **2014**, *33*, 231–238. [CrossRef]
53. Moon, S.J.; Kim, D.W.; Kim, S.J.; Ha, T.K.; Park, H.K.; Jung, S.J. Ultrasound assessment of degrees of extrathyroidal extension in papillary thyroid microcarcinoma. *Endocr. Pract.* **2014**, *20*, 1037–1043. [CrossRef] [PubMed]
54. Ramundo, V.; Di Gioia, C.R.T.; Falcone, R.; Lamartina, L.; Biffoni, M.; Giacomelli, L.; Filetti, S.; Durante, C.; Grani, G. Diagnostic Performance of Neck Ultrasonography in the Preoperative Evaluation for Extrathyroidal Extension of Suspicious Thyroid Nodules. *World J. Surg.* **2020**, *44*, 2669–2674. [CrossRef] [PubMed]
55. Tamsel, S.; Demirpolat, G.; Erdogan, M.; Nart, D.; Karadeniz, M.; Uluer, H.; Ozgen, A.G. Power Doppler US patterns of vascularity and spectral Doppler US parameters in predicting malignancy in thyroid nodules. *Clin. Radiol.* **2007**, *62*, 245–251. [CrossRef] [PubMed]
56. Moon, H.J.; Kwak, J.Y.; Kim, M.J.; Son, E.J.; Kim, E.K. Can vascularity at power Doppler US help predict thyroid malignancy? *Radiology* **2010**, *255*, 260–269. [CrossRef] [PubMed]
57. Lee, S.K.; Rho, B.H.; Woo, S.K. Hürthle cell neoplasm: Correlation of gray-scale and power Doppler sonographic findings with gross pathology. *J. Clin. Ultrasound* **2010**, *38*, 169–176. [CrossRef]
58. Jiang, J.; Huang, L.; Zhang, H.; Ma, W.; Shang, X.; Zhou, Q.; Gao, Y.; Yu, S.; Qi, Y. Contrast-enhanced sonography of thyroid nodules. *J. Clin. Ultrasound* **2015**, *43*, 153–156. [CrossRef]
59. Ma, J.J.; Ding, H.; Xu, B.H.; Xu, C.; Song, L.J.; Huang, B.J.; Wang, W.P. Diagnostic performances of various gray-scale, color Doppler, and contrast-enhanced ultrasonography findings in predicting malignant thyroid nodules. *Thyroid* **2014**, *24*, 355–363. [CrossRef]
60. Trimboli, P.; Castellana, M.; Virili, C.; Havre, R.F.; Bini, F.; Marinozzi, F.; D'Ambrosio, F.; Giorgino, F.; Giovanella, L.; Prosch, H.; et al. Performance of contrast-enhanced ultrasound (CEUS) in assessing thyroid nodules: A systematic review and meta-analysis using histological standard of reference. *Radiol. Med.* **2020**, *125*, 406–415. [CrossRef]
61. Zhang, Y.; Zhou, P.; Tian, S.M.; Zhao, Y.F.; Li, J.L.; Li, L. Usefulness of combined use of contrast-enhanced ultrasound and TI-RADS classification for the differentiation of benign from malignant lesions of thyroid nodules. *Eur. Radiol.* **2017**, *27*, 1527–1536. [CrossRef]
62. Hong, Y.R.; Yan, C.X.; Mo, G.Q.; Luo, Z.Y.; Zhang, Y.; Wang, Y.; Huang, P.T. Conventional US, elastography, and contrast enhanced US features of papillary thyroid microcarcinoma predict central compartment lymph node metastases. *Sci. Rep.* **2015**, *5*, 7748. [CrossRef]

63. Phuttharak, W.; Somboonporn, C.; Hongdomnern, G. Diagnostic performance of gray-scale versus combined gray-scale with colour doppler ultrasonography in the diagnosis of malignancy in thyroid nodules. *Asian Pac. J. Cancer Prev.* **2009**, *10*, 759–764. [PubMed]
64. Forsberg, F.; Machado, P.; Segal, S.; Okamura, Y.; Guenette, G.; Rapp, C.; Lyshchik, A. Microvascular blood flow in the thyroid: Preliminary results with a novel imaging technique. In Proceedings of the 2014 IEEE International Ultrasonics Symposium, Chicago, IL, USA, 3–6 September 2014; pp. 2237–2240.
65. Cantisani, V.; Consorti, F.; Guerrisi, A.; Guerrisi, I.; Ricci, P.; Di Segni, M.; Mancuso, E.; Scardella, L.; Milazzo, F.; D'Ambrosio, F.; et al. Prospective comparative evaluation of quantitative-elastosonography (Q-elastography) and contrast-enhanced ultrasound for the evaluation of thyroid nodules: Preliminary experience. *Eur. J. Radiol.* **2013**, *82*, 1892–1898. [CrossRef] [PubMed]
66. Debnam, J.M.; Vu, T.; Sun, J.; Wei, W.; Krishnamurthy, S.; Zafereo, M.E.; Weitzman, S.P.; Garg, N.; Ahmed, S. Vascular flow on doppler sonography may not be a valid characteristic to distinguish colloid nodules from papillary thyroid carcinoma even when accounting for nodular size. *Gland Surg.* **2019**, *8*, 461–468. [CrossRef] [PubMed]
67. Zhang, L.; Gu, J.; Zhao, Y.; Zhu, M.; Wei, J.; Zhang, B. The role of multimodal ultrasonic flow imaging in Thyroid Imaging Reporting and Data System (TI-RADS) 4 nodules. *Gland Surg.* **2020**, *9*, 1469–1477. [CrossRef]
68. Lyshchik, A.; Higashi, T.; Asato, R.; Tanaka, S.; Ito, J.; Mai, J.; Pellot-Barakat, C.; Insana, M.F.; Brill, A.B.; Saga, T.; et al. Thyroid gland tumor diagnosis at US elastography. *Radiology* **2005**, *237*, 202–211. [CrossRef] [PubMed]
69. Rago, T.; Santini, F.; Scutari, M.; Pinchera, A.; Vitti, P. Elastography: New developments in ultrasound for predicting malignancy in thyroid nodules. *J. Clin. Endocrinol. Metab.* **2007**, *92*, 2917–2922. [CrossRef]
70. Rago, T.; Vitti, P. Role of thyroid ultrasound in the diagnostic evaluation of thyroid nodules. *Best Pract. Res. Clin. Endocrinol. Metab.* **2008**, *22*, 913–928. [CrossRef]
71. Hegedus, L. Can elastography stretch our understanding of thyroid histomorphology? *J. Clin. Endocrinol. Metab.* **2010**, *95*, 5213–5215. [CrossRef]
72. Trimboli, P.; Guglielmi, R.; Monti, S.; Misischi, I.; Graziano, F.; Nasrollah, N.; Amendola, S.; Morgante, S.N.; Deiana, M.G.; Valabrega, S.; et al. Ultrasound sensitivity for thyroid malignancy is increased by real-time elastography: A prospective multicenter study. *J. Clin. Endocrinol. Metab.* **2012**, *97*, 4524–4530. [CrossRef]
73. Magri, F.; Chytiris, S.; Capelli, V.; Gaiti, M.; Zerbini, F.; Carrara, R.; Malovini, A.; Rotondi, M.; Bellazzi, R.; Chiovato, L. Comparison of elastographic strain index and thyroid fine-needle aspiration cytology in 631 thyroid nodules. *J. Clin. Endocrinol. Metab.* **2013**, *12*, 4790–4797. [CrossRef] [PubMed]
74. Rago, T.; Scutari, M.; Santini, F.; Loiacono, V.; Piaggi, P.; Di Coscio, G.; Basolo, F.; Berti, P.; Pinchera, A.; Vitti, P. Real-time elastosonography: Useful tool for refining the presurgical diagnosis in thyroid nodules with indeterminate or nondiagnostic cytology. *J. Clin. Endocrinol. Metab.* **2010**, *95*, 5274–5280. [CrossRef] [PubMed]
75. Rago, T.; Scutari, M.; Loiacono, V.; Santini, F.; Tonacchera, M.; Torregrossa, L.; Giannini, R.; Borrelli, N.; Proietti, A.; Basolo, F.; et al. Low Elasticity of Thyroid Nodules on Ultrasound Elastography Is Correlated with Malignancy, Degree of Fibrosis, and High Expression of Galectin-3 and Fibronectin-1. *Thyroid* **2017**, *27*, 103–110. [CrossRef] [PubMed]
76. Park, J.Y.; Lee, H.J.; Jang, H.W.; Kim, H.K.; Yi, J.H.; Lee, W.; Kim, S.H. A proposal for a thyroid imaging reporting and data system for ultrasound features of thyroid carcinoma. *Thyroid* **2009**, *19*, 1257–1264. [CrossRef]
77. Russ, G.; Royer, B.; Bigorgne, C.; Rouxel, A.; Bienvenu-Perrard, M.; Leenhardt, L. Prospective evaluation of thyroid imaging reporting and data system on 4550 nodules with and without elastography. *Eur. J. Endocrinol.* **2013**, *168*, 649–655. [CrossRef]
78. Seo, H.; Na, D.G.; Kim, J.H.; Kim, K.W.; Yoon, J.W. Ultrasound based risk stratification for malignancy in thyroid nodules: A fourtier categorization system. *Eur. Radiol.* **2015**, *25*, 2153–2162. [CrossRef]
79. Russ, G.; Bonnema, S.J.; Erdogan, M.F.; Durante, C.; Ngu, R.; Leenhardt, L. European Thyroid Association Guidelines for Ultrasound Malignancy Risk Stratification of Thyroid Nodules in Adults: The EU-TIRADS. *Eur. Thyroid. J.* **2017**, *6*, 225–237. [CrossRef]
80. Maino, F.; Forleo, R.; Martinelli, M.; Fralassi, N.; Barbato, F.; Pilli, T.; Capezzone, M.; Brilli, L.; Ciuoli, C.; Cairano, G.; et al. Prospective validation of ATA and ETA sonographic pattern risk of thyroid nodules selected for FNAC. *J. Clin. Endocrinol. Metab.* **2018**, *103*, 2362–2368. [CrossRef]
81. Persichetti, A.; Di Stasio, E.; Guglielmi, R.; Bizzarri, G.; Taccogna, S.; Misischi, I.; Graziano, F.; Petrucci, L.; Bianchini, A.; Papini, E. Predictive value of malignancy of thyroid nodule ultrasound classification systems: A prospective study. *J. Clin. Endocrinol. Metab.* **2018**, *103*, 1359–1368. [CrossRef]
82. Richman, D.M.; Benson, C.B.; Doubilet, P.M.; Wassner, A.J.; Asch, E.; Cherella, C.E.; Smith, J.R.; Frates, M.C. Assessment of American College of Radiology Thyroid Imaging Reporting and Data System (TI-RADS) for Pediatric Thyroid Nodules. *Radiology* **2020**, *294*, 415–420. [CrossRef]
83. Castellana, M.; Castellana, C.; Treglia, G.; Giorgino, F.; Giovanella, L.; Russ, G.; Trimboli, P. Performance of five ultrasound risk stratification systems in selecting thyroid nodules for FNA. *J. Clin. Endocrinol. Metab.* **2020**, *105*, 1659–1669. [CrossRef] [PubMed]
84. Castellana, M.; Grani, G.; Radzina, M.; Guerra, V.; Giovanella, L.; Deandrea, M.; Ngu, R.; Durante, C.; Trimboli, P. Performance of EU-TIRADS in malignancy risk stratification of thyroid nodules: A meta-analysis. *Eur. J. Endocrinol.* **2020**, *183*, 255–264. [CrossRef] [PubMed]

85. Rago, T.; Cantisani, V.; Ianni, F.; Chiovato, L.; Garberoglio, R.; Durante, C.; Frasoldati, A.; Spiezia, S.; Farina, R.; Vallone, G.; et al. Thyroid ultrasonography reporting: Consensus of Italian Thyroid Association (AIT), Italian Society of Endocrinology (SIE), Italian Society of Ultrasonography in Medicine and Biology (SIUMB) and Ultrasound Chapter of Italian Society of Medical Radiology (SIRM). *J. Endocrinol. Investig.* **2018**, *41*, 1435–1443. [CrossRef]
86. Leenhardt, L.; Hejblum, G.; Franc, B.; Fediaevsky, L.D.; Delbot, T.; Le Guillouzic, D.; Ménégaux, F.; Guillausseau, C.; Hoang, C.; Turpin, G.; et al. Indications and limits of ultrasound-guided cytology in the management of nonpalpable thyroid nodules. *Clin. Endocrinol. Metab.* **1999**, *84*, 24–28. [CrossRef] [PubMed]

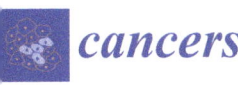

Article

Impact of the Hypoechogenicity Criteria on Thyroid Nodule Malignancy Risk Stratification Performance by Different TIRADS Systems

Nina Malika Popova [1,2,*], Maija Radzina [1,2,3,*], Peteris Prieditis [1,3], Mara Liepa [1,3], Madara Rauda [1] and Kaspars Stepanovs [1]

[1] Institute of Diagnostic Radiology, Pauls Stradins Clinical University Hospital, 1002 Riga, Latvia; peteris.prieditis@stradini.lv (P.P.); mara.liepa@rsu.lv (M.L.); madara.rauda@stradini.lv (M.R.); kstepanovs@gmail.com (K.S.)
[2] Faculty of Medicine, University of Latvia, 1004 Riga, Latvia
[3] Radiology Research Laboratory, Riga Stradins University, 1002 Riga, Latvia
* Correspondence: nina.popova@stradini.lv (N.M.P.); maija.radzina@rsu.lv (M.R.); Tel.: +371-26069563 (N.M.P.); +371-29623585 (M.R.)

Citation: Popova, N.M.; Radzina, M.; Prieditis, P.; Liepa, M.; Rauda, M.; Stepanovs, K. Impact of the Hypoechogenicity Criteria on Thyroid Nodule Malignancy Risk Stratification Performance by Different TIRADS Systems. Cancers 2021, 13, 5581. https://doi.org/10.3390/cancers13215581

Academic Editor: Stefan Delorme

Received: 31 August 2021
Accepted: 5 November 2021
Published: 8 November 2021

Publisher's Note: MDPI stays neutral with regard to jurisdictional claims in published maps and institutional affiliations.

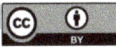

Copyright: © 2021 by the authors. Licensee MDPI, Basel, Switzerland. This article is an open access article distributed under the terms and conditions of the Creative Commons Attribution (CC BY) license (https://creativecommons.org/licenses/by/4.0/).

Simple Summary: This study is aimed at raising the question of the use of several TIRADS systems that stratify the risk of thyroid nodule malignancy. Approximately 5–20% of thyroid nodules are malignant, but most nodules are benign, and they are scored by FNA biopsy. One of the goals is to reduce the number of unnecessary FNA and the associated with-it possible complications for the patient and financial cost. Most TIRADS systems are based on the fact that one suspicious feature of a thyroid nodule classifies it as malignant, but there is a modified Kwak et al. system that is based on the count of malignant features. Therefore, this study is intended to estimate the specificity, sensitivity, and accuracy of the systems and, in the future, think about reducing the number of FNA biopsies. The result of this study can be important for all doctors who face thyroid changes, such as radiologists, ultrasonography specialists, and endocrinologists, those who must decide about the need for an FNA.

Abstract: Background: Various Thyroid Imaging and Reporting data systems (TIRADS) are used worldwide for risk stratification of thyroid nodules. Their sensitivity is high, while the specificity is suboptimal. The aim of the study was to compare several TIRADS systems and evaluate the effect of hypoechogenicity as a sign of risk of malignancy on the overall assessment of diagnostic accuracy. Methods: The prospective study includes 274 patients with 289 thyroid nodules to whom US and risk of malignancy were assessed according to four TIRADS systems—European (EU-TIRADS), Korean (K-TIRADS), TIRADS by American College of Radiology (ACR TIRADS), and modified Kwak et al. TIRADS (L-TIRADS) systems, in which mild hypoechogenicity is not included in malignancy risk suggestive signs. For all thyroid nodules, a fine needle aspiration (FNA) biopsy was performed and evaluated according to the Bethesda system. For all systems, diagnostic accuracy was calculated. Results: Assessing the echogenicity of the thyroid nodules: from 81 of isoechogenic nodules, 2 were malignant (2.1%), from 151 mild hypoechogenic, 18 (12%) were malignant, and from 48 marked hypoechogenic nodules, 16 (33%) were malignant. In 80 thyroid nodules, mild hypoechogenicity was the only sign of malignancy and none appeared malignant. Assessing various TIRADS systems on the same cohort, sensitivity, specificity, PPV, NPV, and accuracy, firstly for EU-TIRADS, they were 97.2%; 39.9%; 18.7%; 99.0%, and 73.3%, respectively; for K-TIRADS they were 97.2%; 46.6%; 20.6%; 99.2%, and 53.9%; for ACR-TIRADS they were 97.2%; 41.1%, 19.0%; 99.0%, and 48.0%, respectively; finally, for L-TIRADS they were 80.6%; 72.7%; 29.6%; 96.3%, and 73.3%. Conclusions: This comparative research has highlighted that applying different TIRADS systems can alter the number of necessary biopsies by re-categorization of the thyroid nodules. The main pattern that affected differences was inconsistent hypoechogenicity interpretation, giving the accuracy superiority to the systems that raise the malignancy risk with marked hypoechogenicity, at the same time with minor compensation for sensitivity.

Keywords: TIRADS; thyroid nodule; ultrasound; fine-needle aspiration biopsy

1. Introduction

The thyroid nodules are very common in the general population, and with the increase of imaging techniques, more thyroid nodules are accidentally detected [1]. Comparing the clinical examination with ultrasonographic examination, it was found that 46% of nodules (with a diameter >1 cm) detected with ultrasound (US) were not detected during the physical thyroid examination [2,3]. Therefore, nowadays the ultrasound (US) is the primary diagnostic method for patients with thyroid nodules. However, with the implementation of ultrasonography in the diagnosis of thyroid nodules, overdiagnosis and overtreatment occurs, which entails an increase in surgical operations and possible complications, as well as financial costs for the treatment of thyroid replacement therapy.

Nodular thyroid disease is relatively common. Most of the thyroid nodules are benign and asymptomatic, and their prevalence varies and accounts for about 85–93% in the population; in addition, 20% of them decrease in size over a lifetime [4]. About 80% of nodular thyroid diseases are caused by glandular hyperplasia, which occurs in up to 5% of the population. Its etiology includes iodine deficiency (endemic), hormonal diseases (congenital family forms) and poor iodine absorption because of certain medications [2]. Calcifications, which are often rough and perinodular, can occur during cyst degeneration. Pure cystic formation is rarely cancerous, but malignancy probability in the nodules with solid and cystic components reaches the prevalence of cancer in solid nodules [5].

Adenomas account for only 5% to 10% of all nodular thyroid diseases. In most cases, thyroid dysfunction is not observed, and less than 10% have hyperfunction, which can lead to thyrotoxicosis. Usually adenomas are solitary, but they can also develop as part of a multinodular formation [2].

Benign follicular adenoma is a true neoplasm characterized by compression of adjacent tissues and fibrous encapsulation. Cytologically, the features of follicular adenoma are usually indistinguishable from those of follicular carcinoma. Signs of follicular carcinoma are vascular and capsule infestations that can be detected during histology, so fine needle aspiration (FNA) is not considered as a reliable method to distinguish adenoma from carcinoma; therefore, tumors are usually removed surgically [6].

However, thyroid cancer is rare and accounts for less than 1% of all malignancies [4]. It accounts for 5% to 10% of all thyroid nodules and there are differentiated thyroid carcinomas, i.e., papillary, follicular, Hürthle cell carcinomas, as well as medullary and anaplastic thyroid carcinomas. Papillary thyroid carcinoma is the most common malignancy of the thyroid gland and accounts for about 80–85% of all thyroid cancers [7]. However, papillary carcinoma has an excellent prognosis with a 10-year survival rate of about 90% [8]. There are many histological subtypes of papillary carcinoma, but ultrasound features that are suggestive of this type of cancer are nodule hypoechogenicity, microlobulated or spiculated margins, microcalcifications in the structure, and taller-than-wide orientation [9].

Follicular carcinoma is the second most common thyroid cancer type and accounts for 10 to 15% of all thyroid cancer [10]. The challenge for the ultrasound specialist is to differentiate follicular carcinoma from follicular adenoma, but ultrasonographic features such as large, hypoechogenic nodule, lack of halo and absence of cystic component are more associated with follicular carcinoma than with adenoma [11].

Medullary thyroid carcinoma accounts for 3.5 to 10% of all thyroid cancers and is characterized by early lymphatic metastatic spread, aggressive invasion in adjacent tissues and organs, and has a poor prognosis. On the ultrasound examination, medullary carcinoma usually looks like papillary carcinoma and is perceived as a solid, hypoechogenic nodule, often with calcifications, which may look more visually coarser than in papillary carcinoma. Calcifications are observed in the primary tumor as well as in the metastatic lymph nodes [6].

Anaplastic thyroid carcinoma usually affects elderly people and is one of the deadliest solid thyroids tumors. It accounts for less than 2% of all thyroid cancers but has the worst prognosis, with 5-year mortality above 95%. The tumor manifests with a rapidly growing mass that extends beyond the gland and grows into adjacent structures. It does not tend to lymphogenic dissemination, but it aggressively grows in adjacent muscles and fat tissue. Sonographically, anaplastic cancer is usually hypoechogenic and often surrounds or grows into blood vessels and neck muscles. Often, these tumors cannot be properly evaluated by the ultrasound due to their large size. In this case, the extent of damage can be assessed more accurately by computed tomography or magnetic resonance imaging [6].

In this regard, the clinical challenge is to distinguish clinically significant malignant thyroid nodules and thus to identify patients who will require surgery for benign thyroid nodules and who will require long-term observation. That is why the main purpose of US thyroid nodule examination is to differentiate malignant nodules from benign [12–14].

In the past decade, several professional societies and research groups have implemented guidelines to provide a standardized assessment of ultrasonographic features of thyroid nodules, such as Thyroid Imaging Reporting and Data System (TIRADS), to assess the need for fine needle aspiration biopsy (FNA) [15].

Initially, in 2009, Horvath et al. introduced a thyroid malignancy risk stratification system—TIRADS [16], but it was difficult to implement, and as a result, several national thyroid associations introduced their own thyroid assessment models—American College of Radiology, European and Korean TIRADS systems.

Most variants of the TIRADS systems include mild hypoechogenic nodules in the potential risk group or TIRADS 4, however, several studies report that most thyroid nodules are mild hypoechogenic, both benign and malignant [17–20].

Several studies have been performed comparing thyroid malignancy risk assessment systems. The sensitivity of these systems is high enough, but specificity is quite low. Therefore, in this study we compare four TIRADS systems—Kwak et al., hereafter, referred to as L-TIRADS, European TIRADS (EU-TIRADS), Korean TIRADS (K-TIRADS) and American College of Radiology TIRADS (ACR-TIRADS) systems—including the sensitivity and specificity and evaluate the effect of hypoechogenicity as a sign of risk of malignancy on the overall assessment of diagnostic accuracy.

2. Materials and Methods

2.1. Study Design

This was a prospective multicentre study that was conducted in the period from 2019 to 2021. In total, 274 patients with 289 thyroid nodules underwent the conventional ultrasound (US) examination and all patients with clinical indication for fine needle aspiration biopsy (FNA) were included in the study. The study was approved by the institutional review boards and the responsible ethics committee.

2.2. Acquisition of Data

Without a regular clinical description of ultrasonographic examination, a standard protocol was additionally developed, with included patient data, suspicious ultrasound features of thyroid nodules, as well as all the necessary features for such systems as the TIRADS system used in Latvia (L-TIRADS), European (EU-TIRADS), Korean (K-TIRADS), and ACR TIRADS system. In addition, the protocol included such indicators as multinodular goiter, thyroiditis, suspicious lymph nodes in four groups of the neck—lateral and medial lymph node groups of right and left side.

2.3. US Examination

In the study, thyroid ultrasonography was performed with an ultrasonography device "Canon Aplio i800" with a linear probe i18LX5 (5–18 MHz), and with "Philips EPIQ 5G" with a linear probe eL 18-4. The ultrasound examination was performed by one of five certified radiologists with five and more years of experience. All ultrasound and biopsies, as well as documentation, were carried out by one radiologist. After ultrasound, the description documented the localization of the thyroid nodules, its size, contour, borders, shape, internal components, echogenicity, calcifications, vascularization, as well as the appearance of the thyroid parenchyma and lymph nodes of the neck.

2.4. Qualification of Thyroid Nodules by Modified Kwak et al. TIRADS, European TIRADS, Korean TIRADS, and ACR TIRADS Systems

Based on ultrasonographic features, each thyroid nodule was evaluated according to four TIRADS systems.

The modified Kwak et al. TIRADS system [21] that is used in Latvia (L-TIRADS) is based on the count of suspicious signs of ultrasound, which include marked hypoechogenicity, microcalcifications, taller than wide shape, irregular or microlobulated/ spiculated margins and metastatic lymph nodes. TIRADS 1—normal thyroid tissue without nodules. TIRADS 2 includes simple cysts, spongiform nodules, hyperechogenic nodules in patients with chronic autoimmune thyroiditis; multinodular hyperplastic goiter without separate bounded nodules; isolated macrocalcifications. TIRADS 3 includes partly cystic nodules; solid nodules with isoechogenic, hyperechogenic, moderately hypoechogenic structure, without any independent sign of malignancy (Figures 1 and 2). TIRADS 4A—one ultrasonographic sign of malignancy, 4B—two ultrasonographic signs of malignancy, 4C—three ultrasonographic signs of malignancy, and 5—four and more ultrasonographic signs of malignancy.

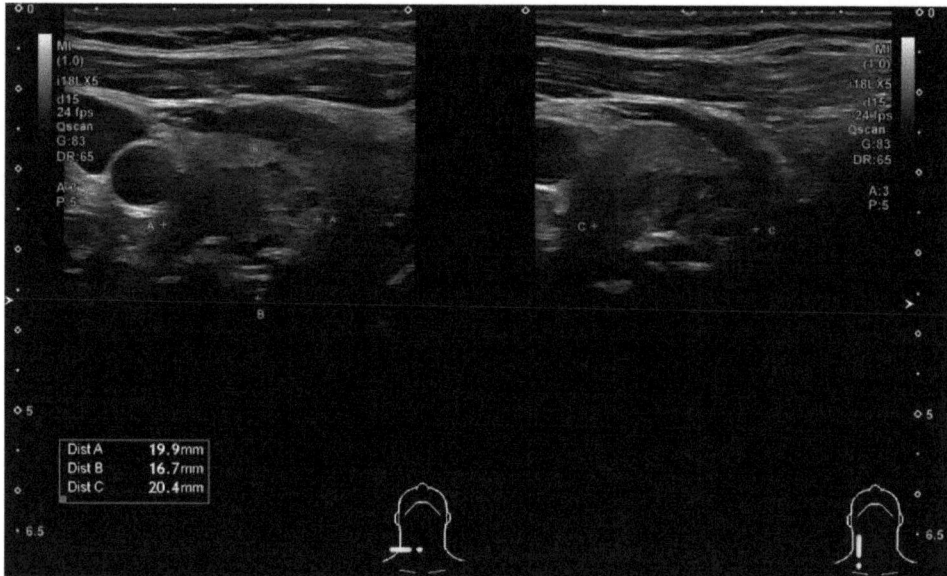

Figure 1. Hypoechogenic, ovoid, smooth, non-homogeneous solid thyroid nodule with cystic component and macrocalcification in its structure—categorized as TIRADS 3 by modified Kwak et al. (L-TIRADS), TIRADS 4 by European and Korean TIRADS, TIRADS 5 (5 points) by ACR TIRADS systems. FNA results—Bethesda 2 (benign).

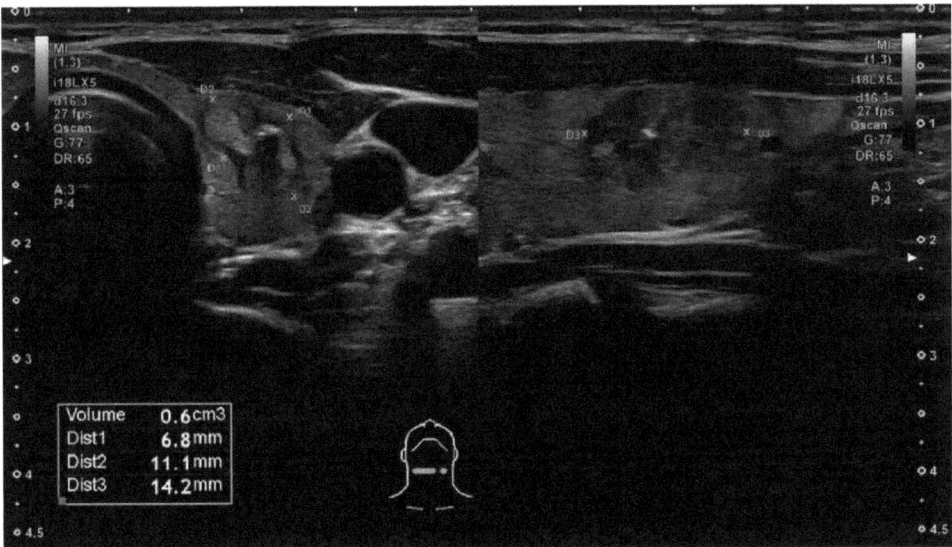

Figure 2. Hypoechogenic nodule, ovoid shape, smooth margins, non-homogeneous solid thyroid nodule with cystic component and macrocalcification in its structure—TIRADS 3 by modified Kwak et al. (L-TIRADS), TIRADS 4 by European and Korean TIRADS, TIRADS 5 by ACR TIRADS systems. FNA biopsy results—Bethesda 2.

According to the European TIRADS system [22] (EU-TIRADS), thyroid nodules were classified as EU-TIRADS 2 if it was a simple cyst or entirely spongiform nodule, EU-TIRADS 3—ovoid, smooth isoechogenic/ hyperechogenic nodule without high suspicion features, TIRADS 4—ovoid, smooth, mild hypoechogenic nodules without high suspicion features, and thyroid nodules were classified as TIRADS 5, if at least one of the following features of high suspicion were included—marked hypoechogenicity, irregular shape, and margins, microcalcifications, with the presence of solid component.

In accordance with the Korean TIRADS system [23] (K-TIRADS), thyroid nodules were classified as K-TIRADS 2 if it was a simple cyst, partially cystic nodule with comet tail artifact, or spongiform nodule. Partially cystic, iso/hyperechoic nodules without any suspicion features were classified as TIRADS 3, and with any suspicious US features such as microcalcification, non-parallel orientation, or spiculated/microlobulated margin such as TIRADS 4. Furthermore, as TIRADS 4 were classified thyroid nodules if they were solid, hypoechogenic without any suspicion US features. TIRADS 5 were classified as solid, hypoechogenic nodules with any suspicious US features—non-parallel orientation, spiculated/ microlobulated margin, and microcalcification in nodule structure.

American College of Radiology TIRADS (ACR TIRADS) [24] is based on points throughout the following categories: composition, echogenicity, shape, margin, and echogenic foci. Composition (select 1): cystic or almost completely cystic—0 points, spongiform—0 points, mixed cystic and solid—1 point, solid or almost completely solid—2 points. Echogenicity (select 1): anechogenic—0 points, hyperechogenic or isoechogenic—1 point, hypoechogenic—2 points, very hypoechogenic—3 points. Shape (select 1): wider-than-tall—0 points, taller-than-wide—3 points. Margin (select 1): smooth—0 points, ill-defined—0 points, lobulated or irregular—2 points, extrathyroidal extension—3 points. Echogenic foci (select all that apply): none or large comet-tail artifacts—0 points, macrocalcifications—1 point, peripheral (rim) calcifications—2 points, punctate echogenic foci—3 points. To determine ACR TIRADS level points from all categories need to be added—ACR-TIRADS 1—0 points, ACR-TIRADS 2—2 points, ACR-TIRADS 3—3 points, ACR-TIRADS 4—4 to 6 points, ACR-TIRADS 5—7 points and more.

2.5. Fine Needle Aspiration Biopsy (FNA)

The US-guided FNA biopsy was performed with a 23-gauge needle, three aspirations were performed according to the local standards, and the material was applied onto glass slides and sent for cytology evaluation [25,26]. Samples were analyzed by certified histopathologists with experience in thyroid pathologies, and thyroid nodule FNA materials were classified into Bethesda classification categories: I—non-diagnostic or unsatisfactory, II—benign, III—atypia of undetermined significance or follicular lesion of undetermined significance, IV—follicular neoplasm or suspicious of a follicular neoplasm, V—suspicious of malignancy, VI—malignant [27,28].

2.6. Statistical Analysis

IBM SPSS software, 22.0 version (IBM Corm., Armonk, NY, USA), MS Excel 2010 software were used to analyse statistical data and create graphs. Pearson correlation was used for correlation between Bethesda categories and all four TIRADS systems that were included in the study. Sensitivity (SEN), specificity (SPE), positive predictive value (PPV), negative predictive value (NPV), accuracy (ACC), 95% confidence interval (CI), area under curve (AUC) were calculated for each TIRADS system—L-TIRADS, EU-TIRADS, K-TIRADS, and ACR-TIRADS. Cronbach's Alpha was calculated for reliability between L-TIRADS and EU-TIRADS, L-TIRADS and K-TIRADS, L-TIRADS and ACR-TIRADS. The statistical significance level of this study was assumed to be p-value < 0.05.

3. Results

3.1. Characteristics of the Study Population

For a duration of 18 months, 289 thyroid nodule ultrasounds and fine-needle aspirations in 274 patients were analysed. Most patients were women (233; 85.1%), and only 41 (14.9%) men were included in this study. Using the binomial test, it was concluded that in our study the proportion of women and men (85.1%/14.9%) was statistically significantly different ($p < 0.001$). The age of the patients included ranged from 23 to 85 years, with a mean age of 55 years. The mean age was 55 years for women and 52 years for men. Most patients were in the age group from 60 to 69 years—69 patients (23 %).

3.2. Characteristics of the Thyroid Nodules

All 289 thyroid nodules included in the study underwent FNA biopsy, and the resulting cytological material was evaluated according to the Bethesda cytological classification, as shown in Figure 3. All 26 malignant nodules were surgically treated and proved to be papillary carcinomas.

In the study, 151 (52.6%) thyroid nodules were mild hypoechogenic compared to thyroid parenchyma, of which 133 (88.0%) were benign and 18 (12.0%) were malignant. A total of 48 thyroid nodules were marked hypoechogenic, compared to the neck muscles of which 32 (66.(6)%) were benign and 16 (33.(3)%) were malignant. From 81 (28.2%) isoechoic nodules 79 (97.5%) were benign, and only 2 (2.5%) were malignant, and all hyperechoic nodules (7; 2.4%) were benign (Figure 4). Using Spearman correlation, a negative, statistically significant, weak correlation between Bethesda classification and thyroid nodule echogenicity was found (rs = −0.187, $p = 0.002$).

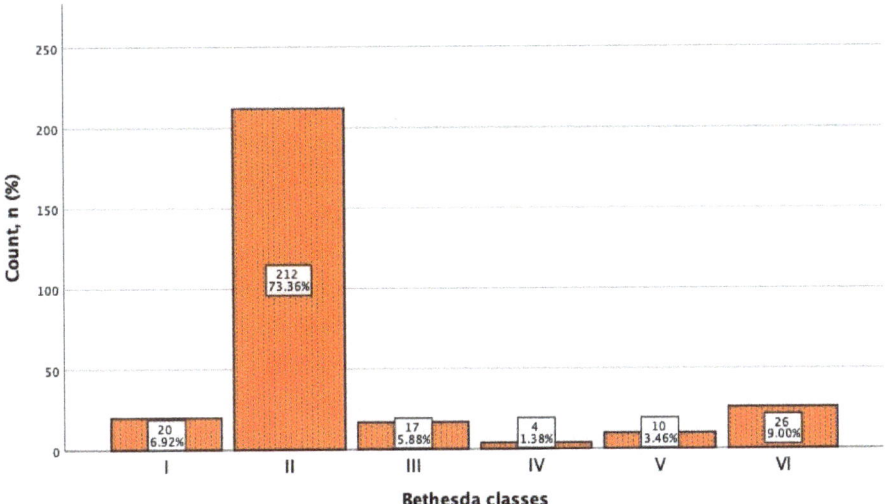

Figure 3. Incidence of cytological findings in thyroid nodules by Bethesda classes.

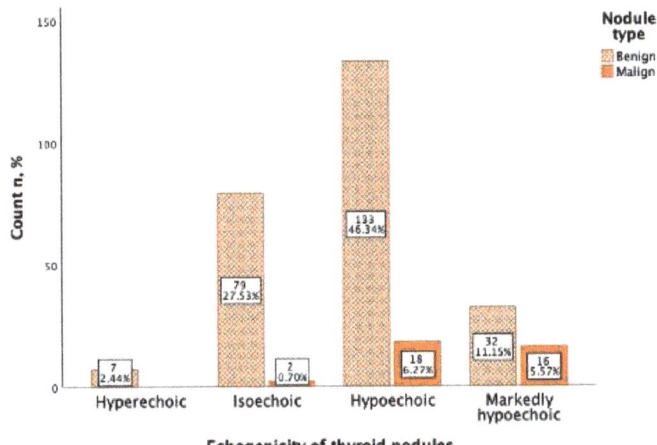

Figure 4. Thyroid nodule malignancy depending on nodule echogenicity. Benign nodules (orange) and malignant nodules (red) are displayed in four ultrasound echogenicity categories.

In the study of 231 thyroid nodules, the maximum diameter was noted, from which the majority (192; 83.1%) of thyroid nodules were more than 1 cm diameter (>1 cm), and 39 (16.9%) thyroid nodules were less than 1 cm diameter (<1 cm). From 192 thyroid nodules that were >1 cm diameter, 176 (91.6%) were benign, and 16 (8.4%) were malignant. Of the 39 thyroid nodules that were <1 cm diameter, 26 (66.(6)%) were benign, and 13 (33.(3)%) were malignant (Figure 5). Using Spearman correlation, it was found that there was a positive, statistically significant, weak correlation between the Bethesda classification and the thyroid maximum nodule diameter (rs = 0.283, p <0.001).

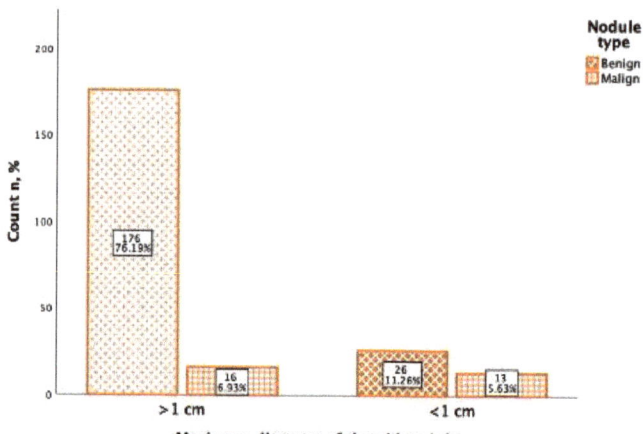

Figure 5. Thyroid nodule malignancy depending on the nodule maximal diameter. Benign nodules are marked with the oblique line pattern and malignant nodules with the check box pattern.

3.3. TIRADS Systems Data Analysis

A summary of thyroid nodules by cytological Bethesda category and L-TIRADS, EU-TIRADS, K-TIRADS, and ACR-TIRADS is shown in Tables 1–4. Most of the thyroid nodules were in the Bethesda category II or benign 212 (73.4%), although EU-TIRADS, K-TIRADS, ACR-TIRADS categorized them as TIRADS 3 category in 21.1 to 24.6% cases, the L-TIRADS system reached up to 46.4% cases, showing the superiority of the latter system because of mild hypoechogenicity interpretation as a benign sign.

Table 1. Summary of L-TIRADS categories by Bethesda classes.

		Bethesda Class					
		I	II	III	IV	V	VI
L-TIRADS, n (%)	2	-	2 (0.9)	-	-	-	-
	3	12 (4.2)	134 (46.4)	5 (1.7)	1 (0.3)	-	1 (0.3)
	4A	1 (0.3)	53 (18.3)	3 (1.0)	2 (0.7)	5 (1.7)	5 (1.7)
	4B	4 (1.4)	16 (5.5)	2 (0.7)	-	3 (1.0)	4 (1.4)
	4C	2 (0.7)	3 (1.0)	6 (2.1)	1 (0.3)	1 (0.3)	10 (3.5)
	5	1 (0.3)	4 (1.4)	1 (0.3)	-	1 (0.3)	6 (2.1)
Total, n (%)		20 (6.9)	212 (73.4)	17 (5.9)	4 (1.4)	10 (3.5)	26 (9.0)

Table 2. Summary of EU-TIRADS categories by Bethesda classes.

		Bethesda Class					
		I	II	III	IV	V	VI
EU-TIRADS, n (%)	2	-	4 (1.9)	-	-	-	-
	3	5 (1.7)	66 (22.8)	4 (1.4)	1 (0.3)	-	1 (0.3)
	4	7 (2.4)	73 (25.3)	2 (0.7)	-	-	-
	5	8 (2.8)	69 (23.9)	11 (3.8)	3 (1.0)	10 (3.5)	25 (8.7)
Total, n (%)		20 (6.9)	212 (73.4)	17 (5.7)	4 (1.4)	10 (3.5)	26 (9.0)

Table 3. Summary of K-TIRADS categories by Bethesda classes.

		Bethesda Class					
		I	II	III	IV	V	VI
K-TIRADS, n (%)	2	1 (0.3)	17 (5.9)	-	-	-	-
	3	6 (2.1)	71 (24.6)	3 (1.0)	1 (0.3)	-	1 (0.3)
	4	5 (1.7)	63 (21.8)	3 (1.0)	1 (0.3)	-	1 (0.3)
	5	8 (2.8)	61 (21.1)	11 (3.8)	2 (0.7)	10 (3.5)	24 (8.3)
Total, n (%)		20 (6.9)	212 (73.4)	17 (5.7)	4 (1.4)	10 (3.5)	26 (9.0)

Table 4. Summary of ACR-TIRADS categories by Bethesda classes.

		Bethesda Class					
		I	II	III	IV	V	VI
ACR-TIRADS, n (%)	1	1 (0.3)	2 (0.7)	-	-	-	-
	2	-	5 (1.7)	-	-	-	-
	3	6 (2.1)	61 (21.1)	3 (1.0)	1 (0.3)	-	1 (0.3)
	4	5 (1.7)	97 (33.6)	4 (1.4)	-	1 (0.3)	1 (0.3)
	5	8 (2.8)	47 (16.3)	10 (3.5)	3 (1.0)	9 (3.1)	24 (8.3)
Total, n (%)		20 (6.9)	212 (73.4)	17 (5.7)	4 (1.4)	10 (3.5)	26 (9.0)

Category I or non-diagnostic results were observed in 20 (6.9%) fine needle aspirations, category III of atypia of undetermined significance were in 17 (5.9%) cases.

IV category or suspicious of follicular neoplasm were in 4 (1.4%) cases, only the L-TIRADS system did not categorized these nodules as TIRADS 5, and the most accurate evaluation was performed by EU-TIRADS and ACR-TIRADS systems.

V category or suspicious of malignancy were in 10 (3.5%) cases, and malignant nodules or category VI were identified in 26 (9.0%) cases. Comparing EU-TIRADS, K-TIRADS, and ACR-TIRADS that showed similar rates of TIRADS 5 nodules in the Bethesda VI category (more than 8%), L-TIRADS categorized the Bethesda VI nodules in TIRADS category 4 A to C, resulting in the reduced sensitivity for TIRADS 5 (2.1%).

Using Pearson correlation, it was found that there was a positive, statistically significant, moderate correlation between Bethesda classification and L-TIRADS ($r = 0.509$, $p < 0.001$), as well as between Bethesda classification and EU-TIRADS ($r = 0.365$; $p < 0.001$), between Bethesda classification and K-TIRADS ($r = 0.365$; $p < 0.001$), and between Bethesda classification and ACR-TIRADS ($r = 0.384$; $p < 0.001$) systems there was also a positive, statistically significant, moderately strong correlation.

Table 5 compares the TIRADS systems and the number of benign and malignant thyroid nodules according to cytology (Bethesda 5 and 6), depending on the TIRADS category. L-TIRADS showed a markedly increased TIRADS 3 nodules category that was related to the interpretation of mild hypoechogenicity in these nodules in comparison to other systems. There was one malignant thyroid nodule in the TIRADS 3 category in all TIRADS systems. This nodule after check-up was an isoechogenic nodule without any suspicious ultrasound signs.

Table 6 reflects the comparison between TIRADS systems and percentual risk of malignancy of TIRADS categories. L-TIRADS showed lesser malignancy risk in the TIRADS 3 category and higher malignancy risk in TIRADS 5 category in comparison to other TIRADS systems 0.007% and 0.58%, respectively, suggestive of higher diagnostic accuracy in patient selection for FNA.

Table 5. Comparison between L-TIRADS, EU-TIRADS, K-TIRADS, and ACR-TIRADS categories.

Categories	Based on L-TIRADS	Based on EU-TIRADS	Based on K-TIRADS	Based on ARC-TIRADS
TIRADS 1 benign/malignant	-	-	-	2/0
TIRADS 2 benign/malignant	2/0	4/0	17/0	5/0
TIRADS 3 benign/malignant	140/1	71/1	75/1	65/1
TIRADS 4A * benign/malignant	58/10	75/0	67/1	101/2
TIRADS 4B benign/malignant	18/7	-	-	-
TIRADS 4C benign/malignant	10/7	-	-	-
TIRADS 5 benign/malignant	5/7	83/35	74/34	233/36

* 4A EU-TIRADS, K-TIRADS, and ACR-TIRADS considered as category 4. Excluded Bethesda I or non-informative material.

Table 6. Comparison between risk of malignancy (%) of L-TIRADS, EU-TIRADS, K-TIRADS, and ACR-TIRADS categories.

Categories	Based on L-TIRADS	Based on EU-TIRADS	Based on K-TIRADS	Based on ARC-TIRADS
Risk of malignancy of TIRADS categories (%)				
TIRADS1	-	-	-	0
TIRADS 2	0	0	0	0
TIRADS 3	0.007	0.013	0.013	0.015
TIRADS 4A *	0.147	0	0.014	0.019
TIRADS 4B	0.28			
TIRADS 4C	0.41			
TIRADS 5	0.58	0.29	0.31	0.13

* 4A EU-TIRADS, K-TIRADS, and ACR-TIRADS considered as category 4.

EU-TIRADS, K-TIRADS, and ACR-TIRADS had high sensitivity (SEN = 97.2%), however L-TIRADS showed higher specificity (SPE = 72.7%) and a better accuracy (ACC = 73.3, $p < 0.001$) than other systems—EU-TIRADS (ACC = 47.0, $p < 0.001$), K-TIRADS (ACC = 53.9, $p < 0.001$) and ACR-TIRADS (ACC = 48.0, $p < 0.001$). All TIRADS systems showed similar area under the ROC curve, but the L-TIRADS AUC value was better 0.766, followed by K-TIRADS with an AUC value 0.719 (Table 7, Figure 6).

Table 7. Pooled estimates of the sensitivity, specificity, PPV, NPV, accuracy, and area under curve (AUC).

TIRADS System	Included Values	SEN, %	SPE, %	PPV, %	NPV, %	ACC, %	95% CI	AUC	p-Value
L-TIRADS	TIRADS 4A-5	80.6	72.7	29.6	96.3	73.3	0.68–0.84	0.766	<0.0001
EU-TIRADS	TIRADS 4-5	97.2	39.9	18.7	99.0	47.0	0.61–0.76	0.686	<0.0001
K-TIRADS	TIRADS 4-5	97.2	46.6	20.6	99.2	53.9	0.65–0.79	0.719	<0.0001
ACR-TIRADS	TIRADS 4-5	97.2	41.1	19.0	99.0	48.0	0.61–0.76	0.692	<0.0001

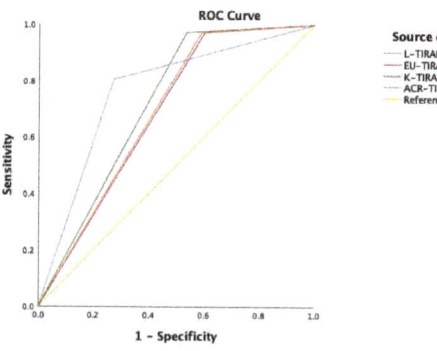

Figure 6. ROC curve analysis for TIRADS systems. L-TIRADS 4A-5 (blue line), EU-TIRADS 5 (red line), K-TIRADS 5 (green line), ACR-TIRADS 5 (orange line), reference line (yellow line).

In the comparison between L-TIRADS and EU-TIRADS, K-TIRADS, and ACR TI-RADS among the 126 thyroid nodules classified as TIRADS 5 by the EU-TIRADS, 23 were downgraded to 4C, 29 were downgraded to 4B, 57 were downgraded to 4A, 4 were downgraded to TIRADS 3, and 13 were categorized into the same TIRADS category. Among the 82 thyroid nodules classified as TIRADS 4 by the EU-TIRADS, 74 were downgraded to TIRADS 3 by L-TIRADS, and 8 were categorized into the same TIRADS category (Table 8).

Table 8. Comparison between the L-TIRADS and EU-TIRADS classifications.

L-TIRADS	EU-TIRADS				Total
	2	3	4	5	
2	1	1	0	0	2
3	3	74	74	4	155
4A	0	2	8	57	67
4B	0	0	0	29	29
4C	0	0	0	23	23
5	0	0	0	13	13
Total	4	77	82	126	289

A total of 113 thyroid nodules were classified as TIRADS 5 by the K-TIRADS, 23 were downgraded to 4C, 29 were downgraded to 4B, 48 were downgraded to 4A, 3 were downgraded to 3, and 13 were categorized into the same TIRADS category. Out of the 32 thyroid nodules classified as TIRADS 4 by the K-TIRADS, 56 were downgraded to TIRADS 3 by L-TIRADS, and 17 were categorized into the same TIRADS category (Table 9).

Table 9. Comparison between the L-TIRADS and K-TIRADS classifications.

L TIRADS	K-TIRADS				Total
	2	3	4	5	
2	1	1	0	0	2
3	15	81	56	3	155
4A	2	0	17	48	67
4B	0	0	0	29	29
4C	0	0	0	23	23
5	0	0	0	13	13
Total	18	82	73	113	289

In total, 103 thyroid nodules were classified as TIRADS 5 by the ACR-TIRADS, 23 were downgraded to 4C, 28 were downgraded to 4B, 34 were downgraded to 4A, 3 were downgraded to 3, and 12 were categorized into the same TIRADS category. In the group of the 108 thyroid nodules classified as TIRADS 4 by the ACR-TIRADS, 76 were downgraded to TIRADS 3 by L-TIRADS, 31 were categorized as TIRADS 4A, 1 was upgraded to TIRADS 4B, and 1 was upgraded to TIRADS 5 (Table 10).

Table 10. Comparison between the L-TIRADS and ACR-TIRADS classifications.

L TIRADS	ACR TIRADS					Total
	1	2	3	4	5	
2	1	0	1	0	0	2
3	2	5	69	76	3	155
4A	0	0	2	31	34	67
4B	0	0	0	1	28	29
4C	0	0	0	0	23	23
5	0	0	0	1	12	13
Total	3	5	71	108	103	287

The reliability between L-TIRADS and all three TIRADS systems with Cronbach's Alpha was comparable, between L-TIRADS and EU-TIRADS was 0.805, between L-TIRADS and K-TIRADS was 0.817, and between L-TIRADS and ACR-TIRADS was 0.794, respectively.

4. Discussion

This prospective comparative study includes ultrasound data from 289 thyroid nodules and fine-needle aspirations from 274 patients, with age ranging from 23 to 85 years (mean 55) and including predominantly women (85.1%), in accordance with the several studies that also noted a higher prevalence of thyroid nodules in women and noted that the incidence of thyroid nodules increases after the age of 50 [29,30]. A total of 26 nodules were proved to be malignant with papillary carcinoma.

Various TIRADS systems (ACR, EU-TIRADS, K-TIRADS, American Thyroid Association etc.) are used to define thyroid nodule risk of malignancy and to select patients for FNA. All systems are based on thyroid nodule malignancy features evaluation such as hypoechogenicity, microcalcifications, shape proportions (AP > LL), ill-defined and irregular margin. For these systems, diagnostic accuracy is similar, with high sensitivity and low specificity [31,32]. In our study, ACR TIRADS sensitivity, specificity, PPV, NPV and diagnostic accuracy were 97.2%; 41.1%, 19.0%; 99.0%, and 48.0%; for K-TIRADS—97.2%; 46.6%; 20.6%; 99.2%, and 53.9%; for EU-TIRADS —97.2%; 39.9%; 18.7%; 99.0%, and 73.3%, respectively, and these results are similar to other authors' research results [33–35].

Hypoechogenicity is one of the main but unspecific features of thyroid nodules on US [36]. The positive predictive value of this feature is weak (PPV and OR ranging from 3.57 to 6.63) [21,37]. In favor of making this pattern more selective, a lower echogenicity compared to muscle tissue termed "marked hypoechogenicity" has been introduced as a marker of increased risk of malignancy in solid nodules. It is reported that up to 55% of benign nodules appear hypoechoic compared to thyroid parenchyma, making nodules not marked as hypoechogenicity less specific, especially for sub-centimeter size [37]. The goal of the present study was to evaluate the diagnostic accuracy of the current TIRADS system. It was hypothesized that in accordance with the assumption of a higher malignancy in markedly hypoechogenic nodules, all remaining hypoechogenic lesions with equal or higher echogenicity compared to muscle tissue ("non-marked hypoechogenic nodules") would not be associated with an increased risk of malignancy and that their classification as grade 3 would significantly improve the predictive value of the TIRADS classification.

In the L-TIRADS system, which is the Kwak et al. modified version, mild hypoechogenicity is not included in the malignancy features. Mild hypoechogenic thyroid nodules, which do not have any other malignant features, are stratified as thyroid nodules with low risk of malignancy or TIRADS 3 category nodules, which results in higher specificity and diagnostic accuracy, 72.7% and 73.3%, respectively, and therefore showed different performance in comparison to the other systems with remaining high NPV 96.3% and a comprehensive decrease in sensitivity 80.6%. Based on the cytological response, among the nodules categorized as L-TIRADS 5, 58% were cytologically malignant (Bethesda 5 and 6), while from the nodules categorized as K-TIRADS, 5–31% were cytologically malignant, from nodules categorized as EU-TIRADS, 5–29% were cytologically malignant, and from thyroid nodules that were categorized as ACR-TIRADS 5, only 13% were cytologically malignant. Comparing EU-TIRADS, K-TIRADS, and ACR-TIRADS that showed similar rates of TIRADS 5 nodules in the Bethesda VI category (more than 8%), L-TIRADS categorized the Bethesda VI nodules in TIRADS category 4 A to C, resulting in the reduced sensitivity for TIRADS 5 to only 2.1%. This trade-off of the raised suspicion and lack of clear categorization of malignancy is compensated by the L-TIRADS system's high performance in the TIRADS 3 category with two-times higher true benign nodules (Bethesda 2).

The aim of TIRADS systems is to evaluate thyroid nodule risk of malignancy and to select patients for FNA. In these TIRADS systems, indications for FNA are based on thyroid nodule malignancy risk assessment or TIRADS category and size of the nodule [22,24,35].

Low TIRADS system specificity increases the number of FNA, which results in unnecessary manipulations, stress, and financial costs for the patients.

Analyzing echogenicity as malignancy risk evaluation criteria, it seems that only 12.0% of the mild hypoechogenic nodules were malignant, which means that this feature is not specific by itself, while among the marked hypoechogenic nodules, 66.6% were malignant, which means that every two out of three marked hypoechogenic nodules are malignant and this proves that this feature is specific for malignancy. The result of our study shows that mild hypoechogenicity cannot serve solely as a malignancy risk feature and may increase FNA rates unnecessarily. From 80 thyroid nodules, in which mild hypoechogenicity was the only possible malignancy sign, no cytological malignancy (Bethesda 5 and 6) by FNA was found. This approved the concept of mild hypoechogenicity with lower values to be considered as a sign of malignancy, as described in several TIRADS systems: ACR TI-RADS non-marked hypoechogenicity without other signs is classified as TIRADS 3 (mild suspicious), EU-TIRADS category 4 (intermediate risk) and K-TIRADS also as category 4 (intermediate suspicion) [22–24].

Regarding the size of the nodule—one of three nodules with a diameter less than 1 cm was malignant, but it should be noted that most of the small nodules firstly appear as relatively hypoechogenic and for these sub-centimeter nodules, FNA biopsy may be advised only if they have several signs of malignancy.

There were some limitations in our study, such as the examination of the thyroid gland was performed using two ultrasound machines, and in our study, there were several ultrasound specialists who performed examination and FNA, which could lead to different assessments and decisions about FNA of thyroid nodules. Furthermore, some of the patients had to be excluded from the study due to non-informative results of cytology, which may be due to imperfect ultrasound control during FNA, as well as changes in image quality. Lack of histology results in our cohort should be noted as a major limitation.

In conclusion, EU-TIRADS, K-TIRADS, and ACR-TIRADS showed high sensitivity, compared to L-TIRADS; however, the specificity and accuracy were higher for the L-TIRADS system. The main pattern that affected differences was inconsistent hypoechogenicity interpretation, giving accuracy superiority to the systems that raise the malignancy risk with marked hypoechogenicity and at the same time with minor compensation for sensitivity. This comparative research has highlighted that applying different TIRADS systems can alter the number of necessary biopsies by categorization of the mild hypoechogenic thyroid nodules as a low malignancy risk pattern.

Author Contributions: Conceptualization, N.M.P., M.R. (Maija Radzina) and P.P.; methodology, P.P. and M.R. (Madara Rauda); software N.M.P.; formal analysis, N.M.P., P.P. and M.R. (Madara Rauda); investigation, N.M.P., M.R. (Maija Radzina), P.P., M.L., M.R. (Madara Rauda) and K.S.; resources, N.M.P., M.R. (Maija Radzina), P.P., M.L., M.R. (Madara Rauda) and K.S.; data curation, N.M.P., P.P. and M.R. (Madara Rauda); writing—original draft preparation, N.M.P. and M.R.; writing—review and editing, visualization, N.M.P.; supervision, M.R. (Maija Radzina); project administration, M.R. (Madara Rauda). All authors have read and agreed to the published version of the manuscript.

Funding: This research has not received any external funding.

Institutional Review Board Statement: The study was conducted according to the guidelines of the Declaration of Helsinki and approved by the Research Ethics Commission of the Institute of Cardiology and Regenerative Medicine, University of Latvia, 10.2019-5. Patient data were fully anonymized before analysis.

Informed Consent Statement: Informed consent was obtained from all subjects involved in the study.

Data Availability Statement: Data are available from the corresponding author after appropriative review.

Conflicts of Interest: The authors declare no conflict of interest.

References

1. Basha, M.A.A.; Alnaggar, A.A.; Refaat, R.; El-Maghraby, A.M.; Refaat, M.M.; Elhamed, M.E.A.; Abdalla, A.A.E.-H.M.; Aly, S.A.; Hanafy, A.S.; Mohamed, A.E.M.; et al. The validity and reproducibility of the thyroid imaging reporting and data system (TI-RADS) in categorization of thyroid nodules: Multicentre prospective study. *Eur. J. Radiol.* **2019**, *117*, 184–192. [CrossRef] [PubMed]
2. Gharib, H.; Papini, E.; Paschke, R. Thyroid nodules: A review of current guidelines, practices, and prospects. *Eur. J. Endocrinol.* **2008**, *159*, 493–505. [CrossRef]
3. Gharib, H.; Papini, E.; Paschke, R.; Duick, D.S.; Valcavi, R.; Hegedüs, L.; Vitti, P.; Tseleni-Balafouta, S.; Baloch, Z.; Crescenzi, A.; et al. American Association of ClinicalEndocrinologists, Associazione Medici Endocrinologi, and European Thyroid Association Medical Guidelines for Clinical Practice for the Diagnosis and Management of Thyroid Nodules: Executive Summary of Recommendations. *Endocr. Pr.* **2010**, *16*, 468–475. [CrossRef] [PubMed]
4. Paschou, S.A.; Vryonidou, A.; Goulis, D.G. Thyroid nodules: A guide to assessment, treatment and follow-up. *Maturitas* **2017**, *96*, 1–9. [CrossRef] [PubMed]
5. Lee, M.-J.; Kim, E.-K.; Kwak, J.Y.; Kim, M.J. Partially Cystic Thyroid Nodules on Ultrasound: Probability of Malignancy and Sonographic Differentiation. *Thyroid* **2009**, *19*, 341–346. [CrossRef]
6. Solbiati, L.; Charboneau, J.W.; Cantisani, V.; Reading, C.; Mauri, G. The Thyroid Gland. In *Diagnostic Ultrasound*, 5th ed.; Elsevier: Philadelphia, PA, USA, 2018; pp. 691–731.
7. Limaiem, F.; Rehman, A.; Mazzoni, T. *Papillary Thyroid Carcinoma*; [Updated 16 September 2021]; StatPearls Publishing: Treasure Island, FL, USA, 2021.
8. Nixon, I.J.; Ganly, I.; Patel, S.G.; Palmer, F.L.; Whitcher, M.M.; Ghossein, R.; Tuttle, R.M.; Shaha, A.R.; Shah, J.P. Changing trends in well differentiated thyroid carcinoma over eight decades. *Int. J. Surg.* **2012**, *10*, 618–623. [CrossRef]
9. Shin, J.H. Ultrasonographic imaging of papillary thyroid carcinoma variants. *Ultrasonography* **2017**, *36*, 103–110. [CrossRef]
10. Parameswaran, R.; Hu, J.S.; En, N.M.; Tan, W.B.; Yuan, N.K. Patterns of metastasis in follicular thyroid carcinoma and the difference between early and delayed presentation. *Ann. R. Coll. Surg. Engl.* **2017**, *99*, 151–154. [CrossRef]
11. Sillery, J.C.; Reading, C.C.; Charboneau, J.W.; Henrichsen, T.L.; Hay, I.D.; Mandrekar, J.N. Thyroid Follicular Carcinoma: Sonographic Features of 50 Cases. *Am. J. Roentgenol.* **2010**, *194*, 44–54. [CrossRef]
12. Yang, R.; Zou, X.; Zeng, H.; Zhao, Y.; Ma, X. Comparison of Diagnostic Performance of Five Different Ultrasound TI-RADS Classification Guidelines for Thyroid Nodules. *Front. Oncol.* **2020**, *10*, 598225. [CrossRef]
13. American Thyroid Association Guidelines Taskforce on Thyroid; Cooper, D.S.; Doherty, G.; Haugen, B.R.; Kloos, R.T.; Lee, S.; Mandel, S.J.; Mazzaferri, E.L.; McIver, B.; Pacini, F.; et al. Revised American Thyroid Association Management Guidelines for Patients with Thyroid Nodules and Differentiated Thyroid Cancer. *Thyroid* **2009**, *19*, 1167–1214. [CrossRef] [PubMed]
14. Kim, E.-K.; Park, C.S.; Chung, W.Y.; Oh, K.K.; Kim, D.I.; Lee, J.T.; Yoo, H.S. New Sonographic Criteria for Recommending Fine-Needle Aspiration Biopsy of Nonpalpable Solid Nodules of the Thyroid. *Am. J. Roentgenol.* **2002**, *178*, 687–691. [CrossRef]
15. Baş, H.; Üstüner, E.; Kula, S.; Konca, C.; Demirer, S.; Elhan, A.H. Elastography and Doppler May Bring a New Perspective to TIRADS, Altering Conventional Ultrasonography Dominance. *Acad. Radiol.* **2021**, *13*, 1076. [CrossRef]
16. Horvath, E.; Majlis, S.; Rossi, R.; Franco, C.; Niedmann, J.P.; Castro, A.; Dominguez, M. An Ultrasonogram Reporting System for Thyroid Nodules Stratifying Cancer Risk for Clinical Management. *J. Clin. Endocrinol. Metab.* **2009**, *94*, 1748–1751. [CrossRef]
17. Lee, J.Y.; Na, D.G.; Yoon, S.J.; Gwon, H.Y.; Paik, W.; Kim, T.; Kim, J.Y. Ultrasound malignancy risk stratification of thyroid nodules based on the degree of hypoechogenicity and echotexture. *Eur. Radiol.* **2019**, *30*, 1653–1663. [CrossRef]
18. Bonavita, J.A.; Mayo, J.; Babb, J.; Bennett, G.; Oweity, T.; Macari, M.; Yee, J. Pattern Recognition of Benign Nodules at Ultrasound of the Thyroid: Which Nodules Can Be Left Alone? *Am. J. Roentgenol.* **2009**, *193*, 207–213. [CrossRef] [PubMed]
19. Wu, M.-H.; Chen, C.-N.; Chen, K.-Y.; Ho, M.-C.; Tai, H.-C.; Wang, Y.-H.; Chen, A.; Chang, K.-J. Quantitative analysis of echogenicity for patients with thyroid nodules. *Sci. Rep.* **2016**, *6*, 35632. [CrossRef] [PubMed]
20. Na, D.G.; Baek, J.H.; Sung, J.Y.; Kim, J.-H.; Kim, J.K.; Choi, Y.J.; Seo, H. Thyroid Imaging Reporting and Data System Risk Stratification of Thyroid Nodules: Categorization Based on Solidity and Echogenicity. *Thyroid* **2016**, *26*, 562–572. [CrossRef]
21. Kwak, J.Y.; Han, K.; Yoon, J.H.; Moon, H.J.; Son, E.J.; Park, S.H.; Jung, H.K.; Choi, J.S.; Kim, B.M.; Kim, E.-K. Thyroid Imaging Reporting and Data System for US Features of Nodules: A Step in Establishing Better Stratification of Cancer Risk. *Radiology* **2011**, *260*, 892–899. [CrossRef] [PubMed]
22. Russ, G.; Bonnema, S.J.; Erdogan, M.F.; Durante, C.; Ngu, R.; Leenhardt, L. European Thyroid Association Guidelines for Ultrasound Malignancy Risk Stratification of Thyroid Nodules in Adults: The EU-TIRADS. *Eur. Thyroid. J.* **2017**, *6*, 225–237. [CrossRef] [PubMed]
23. Shin, J.H.; Baek, J.H.; Chung, J.; Ha, E.J.; Kim, J.-H.; Lee, Y.H.; Lim, H.K.; Moon, W.-J.; Na, D.G.; Park, J.S.; et al. Ultrasonography Diagnosis and Imaging-Based Management of Thyroid Nodules: Revised Korean Society of Thyroid Radiology Consensus Statement and Recommendations. *Korean J. Radiol.* **2016**, *17*, 370–395. [CrossRef] [PubMed]
24. Tessler, F.N.; Middleton, W.D.; Grant, E.G.; Hoang, J.K.; Berland, L.L.; Teefey, S.A.; Cronan, J.J.; Beland, M.D.; Desser, T.S.; Frates, M.C.; et al. ACR Thyroid Imaging, Reporting and Data System (TI-RADS): White Paper of the ACR TI-RADS Committee. *J. Am. Coll. Radiol.* **2017**, *14*, 587–595. [CrossRef] [PubMed]
25. Abu-Yousef, M.; Larson, J.H.; Kuehn, D.; Wu, A.S.; Laroia, A. Safety of Ultrasound-Guided Fine Needle Aspiration Biopsy of Neck Lesions in Patients Taking Antithrombotic/Anticoagulant Medications. *Ultrasound Q.* **2011**, *27*, 157–159. [CrossRef]

26. Langer, J.E.; Baloch, Z.W.; McGrath, C.; Loevner, L.A.; Mandel, S.J. Thyroid Nodule Fine-Needle Aspiration. *Semin. Ultrasound, CT MRI* **2012**, *33*, 158–165. [CrossRef]
27. Cibas, E.S.; Ali, S.Z. The 2017 Bethesda System for Reporting Thyroid Cytopathology. *Thyroid* **2017**, *27*, 1341–1346. [CrossRef] [PubMed]
28. Cibas, E.S.; Ali, S.Z. The Bethesda System for Reporting Thyroid Cytopathology. *Am. J. Clin. Pathol.* **2009**, *132*, 658–665. [CrossRef] [PubMed]
29. Shen, Y.; Liu, M.; He, J.; Wu, S.; Chen, M.; Wan, Y.; Gao, L.; Cai, X.; Ding, J.; Fu, X. Comparison of Different Risk-Stratification Systems for the Diagnosis of Benign and Malignant Thyroid Nodules. *Front. Oncol.* **2019**, *9*, 378. [CrossRef]
30. Kwong, N.; Medici, M.; Angell, T.E.; Liu, X.; Marqusee, E.; Cibas, E.S.; Krane, J.F.; Barletta, J.A.; Kim, M.I.; Larsen, P.R.; et al. The Influence of Patient Age on Thyroid Nodule Formation, Multinodularity, and Thyroid Cancer Risk. *J. Clin. Endocrinol. Metab.* **2015**, *100*, 4434–4440. [CrossRef]
31. Kim, M.J.; Kim, E.-K.; Park, S.I.; Kim, B.M.; Kwak, J.Y.; Kim, S.J.; Youk, J.H. US-guided Fine-Needle Aspiration of Thyroid Nodules: Indications, Techniques, Results. *RadioGraphic* **2008**, *28*, 1869–1886. [CrossRef]
32. Ha, E.J.; Na, D.G.; Baek, J.H.; Sung, J.Y.; Kim, J.-H.; Kang, S.Y. US Fine-Needle Aspiration Biopsy for Thyroid Malignancy: Diagnostic Performance of Seven Society Guidelines Applied to 2000 Thyroid Nodules. *Radiology* **2018**, *287*, 893–900. [CrossRef]
33. Seifert, P.; Schenke, S.; Zimny, M.; Stahl, A.; Grunert, M.; Klemenz, B.; Freesmeyer, M.; Kreissl, M.C.; Herrmann, K.; Görges, R. Diagnostic Performance of Kwak, EU, ACR, and Korean TIRADS as Well as ATA Guidelines for the Ultrasound Risk Stratification of Non-Autonomously Functioning Thyroid Nodules in a Region with Long History of Iodine Deficiency: A German Multicenter Trial. *Cancers* **2021**, *13*, 4467. [CrossRef] [PubMed]
34. Koc, A.M.; Adıbelli, Z.H.; Erkul, Z.; Sahin, Y.; Dilek, I. Comparison of diagnostic accuracy of ACR-TIRADS, American Thyroid Association (ATA), and EU-TIRADS guidelines in detecting thyroid malignancy. *Eur. J. Radiol.* **2020**, *133*, 109390. [CrossRef] [PubMed]
35. Haugen, B.R.; Alexander, E.K.; Bible, K.C.; Doherty, G.M.; Mandel, S.J.; Nikiforov, Y.E.; Pacini, F.; Randolph, G.W.; Sawka, A.M.; Schlumberger, M.; et al. 2015 American Thyroid Association Management Guidelines for Adult Patients with Thyroid Nodules and Differentiated Thyroid Cancer: The American Thyroid Association Guidelines Task Force on Thyroid Nodules and Differentiated Thyroid Cancer. *Thyroid* **2016**, *26*, 1–133. [CrossRef] [PubMed]
36. Grani, G.; D'Alessandri, M.; Carbotta, G.; Nesca, A.; Del Sordo, M.; Alessandrini, S.; Coccaro, C.; Rendina, R.; Bianchini, M.; Prinzi, N.; et al. Grey-Scale Analysis Improves the Ultrasonographic Evaluation of Thyroid Nodules. *Medicine* **2015**, *94*, e1129. [CrossRef] [PubMed]
37. Choi, Y.J.; Kim, S.M.; Choi, S.I. Diagnostic Accuracy of Ultrasound Features in Thyroid Microcarcinomas. *Endocr. J.* **2008**, *55*, 931–938. [CrossRef] [PubMed]

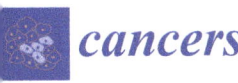

Review

Performance of Contrast-Enhanced Ultrasound in Thyroid Nodules: Review of Current State and Future Perspectives

Maija Radzina [1,2,3,*], Madara Ratniece [1], Davis Simanis Putrins [2,3], Laura Saule [1,3] and Vito Cantisani [4]

1. Radiology Research Laboratory, Riga Stradins University, LV-1007 Riga, Latvia; ratniece.madara@gmail.com (M.R.); laura.saule@rsu.lv (L.S.)
2. Medical Faculty, University of Latvia, LV-1004 Riga, Latvia; davisputrins@gmail.com
3. Diagnostic Radiology Institute, Paula Stradina Clinical University Hospital, LV-1002 Riga, Latvia
4. Department of Radiological, Anatomopathological and Oncological Sciences, Sapienza University of Rome, 00100 Rome, Italy; vito.cantisani@uniroma1.it
* Correspondence: maija.radzina@rsu.lv; Tel.: +371-29623585

Simple Summary: Ultrasound has been used as baseline imaging for thyroid nodules for decades; nevertheless, no single feature is sensitive or specific enough to exclude or confirm thyroid malignancy. Therefore, clinical practice and research still focus on less invasive diagnostic patterns to reduce unnecessary fine-needle aspiration biopsies or surgery. The main advantage of CEUS is the ability to assess the sequence and intensity of vascular perfusion and hemodynamics in the thyroid nodule, thus providing real-time characterization of nodule features, and considered a valuable new approach in the determination of benign vs. malignant nodules. In addition, contrast agents used in CEUS can help to guide treatment planning for minimally invasive procedures (e.g., ablation) and to provide accurate follow-up imaging to assess treatment efficacy in both benign and malignant nodules and associated lymph nodes. Examination protocol has almost reached standardization, although there are numerous controversies reported about the interpretation of qualitative and quantitative patterns that would require a systematic approach. This literature and current state review of CEUS in thyroid nodules address the existing concepts and highlights of the future perspectives.

Abstract: Ultrasound has been established as a baseline imaging technique for thyroid nodules. The main advantage of adding CEUS is the ability to assess the sequence and intensity of vascular perfusion and hemodynamics in the thyroid nodule, thus providing real-time characterization of nodule features, considered a valuable new approach in the determination of benign vs. malignant nodules. Original studies, reviews and six meta-analyses were included in this article. A total of 624 studies were retrieved, and 107 were included in the study. As recognized for thyroid nodule malignancy risk stratification by US, for acceptable accuracy in malignancy a combination of several CEUS parameters should be applied: hypo-enhancement, heterogeneous, peripheral irregular enhancement in combination with internal enhancement patterns, and slow wash-in and wash-out curve lower than in normal thyroid tissue. In contrast, homogeneous, intense enhancement with smooth rim enhancement and "fast-in and slow-out" are indicative of the benignity of the thyroid nodule. Even though overlapping features require standardization, with further research, CEUS may achieve reliable performance in detecting or excluding thyroid cancer. It can also play an operative role in guiding ablation procedures of benign and malignant thyroid nodules and metastatic lymph nodes, and providing accurate follow-up imaging to assess treatment efficacy.

Keywords: contrast-enhanced ultrasound (CEUS); thyroid nodules; thyroid cancer; papillary thyroid cancer; follicular thyroid cancer

Citation: Radzina, M.; Ratniece, M.; Putrins, D.S.; Saule, L.; Cantisani, V. Performance of Contrast-Enhanced Ultrasound in Thyroid Nodules: Review of Current State and Future Perspectives. *Cancers* **2021**, *13*, 5469. https://doi.org/10.3390/cancers13215469

Academic Editor: Stefan Delorme

Received: 31 August 2021
Accepted: 27 October 2021
Published: 30 October 2021

Publisher's Note: MDPI stays neutral with regard to jurisdictional claims in published maps and institutional affiliations.

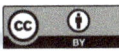

Copyright: © 2021 by the authors. Licensee MDPI, Basel, Switzerland. This article is an open access article distributed under the terms and conditions of the Creative Commons Attribution (CC BY) license (https://creativecommons.org/licenses/by/4.0/).

1. Introduction

Thyroid nodules are defined as discrete lesions within the thyroid gland that radiologically differ from the surrounding thyroid parenchyma [1]. With the increasingly widespread availability and use of diagnostic imaging modalities such as ultrasound (US), computed tomography (CT), magnetic resonance imaging (MRI) and positron emission tomography (PET), thyroid nodules have been more frequently identified [2]. The main goal of diagnostics in thyroid nodules is to exclude thyroid cancer by differentiating benign from malignant nodules [3,4]. The prevalence of thyroid nodules detected by ultrasound has been reported up to 50% in the general population [5], with a malignancy rate of 5–15% [1,6]. Despite the relatively high incidence, thyroid cancer mortality has remained rather stable over a longer period, with the ten-year relative survival rate reported to be greater than 90% [7]. The most common type of thyroid cancer is papillary carcinoma, accounting for 85% of all thyroid malignancies [8].

Due to the high incidence of thyroid nodules, a noninvasive and relatively easily accessible imaging modality is ultrasound, which has proven to be highly sensitive in the detection and characterization of different thyroid nodules [9], and is recommended as the first-line modality to be performed in all patients with suspected thyroid nodules [1,10]. Therefore this review will be dedicated to US. The US appearance of a nodule is crucial in the management of a patient, most importantly when deciding whether further investigation with fine-needle aspiration (FNAB) or routine follow-up is necessary [11]. By maximizing the detection of clinically relevant thyroid lesions and decreasing FNAB of benign nodules, the best patient outcomes and cost-effectiveness can be achieved due to reduced overdiagnosis and overtreatment [10].

To date, well known and guideline-approved malignancy US features have been defined, including solid composition, hypoechoic appearance, calcifications, ill-defined margins, "taller than wide" configuration, and a lack of "halo" [12]. However, no single feature is both sensitive and specific enough to exclude or confirm thyroid malignancy [10,13], for example calcifications can be seen in up to 40.2% of malignant and 22.2% of benign nodules as reported by Kim et al. [14]. In addition to the conventional B-mode imaging, color Doppler studies and methods for examining microvascular flow are also utilized in the evaluation of thyroid nodules, with marked hypervascularity being a commonly accepted indicator of potential malignancy in certain cases, although many guidelines recommend not to use vascularization to predict malignancy [15,16]. As such Doppler US is not recommended as a routine method for US malignancy risk stratification in the EU-TIRADS guidelines [11], and is also not considered to be a reliable indicator of malignancy in other guidelines, such as the ACR-TIRADS [17].

Ultrasound is used as the basis for several thyroid nodule risk stratification systems proposed by the American Thyroid Association (ATA), American College of Radiologists (ACR), European Thyroid Association (EU-TIRADS), and others, which are in place to increase the diagnostic confidence of thyroid nodule imaging. A widely used thyroid imaging reporting and data system (TI-RADS) has achieved good clinical value by improving the diagnostic accuracy and reducing unnecessary biopsies, and overall has affected the management of thyroid nodules [18]. However, TI-RADS staging largely depends on the operator, and several specific imaging features are not universally accepted in evaluation [10,19]. Furthermore, features of atypical benign and malignant nodules, especially TI-RADS 3 and 4 category, may overlap the routine US and even FNAB appears to prove half of all biopsied nodules as benign [20], and in up to one third of cases the results of cytology are inconclusive [2]. Therefore, problem-solving modalities of US have been introduced in the past two decades such as US elastography (strain elastography and shear-wave elastography [21,22] and contrast-enhanced ultrasound (CEUS), which have expanded the ability of conventional US.

The aim of this review was to analyze different aspects of CEUS in thyroid nodules, including technical considerations, qualitative and quantitative analysis of the following benign and malignant thyroid lesions: adenoma, goiter, thyroiditis, lymphoma, papillary, follicular, medullary and anaplastic thyroid cancer, while also providing an overview on its role in pre- and post-treatment nodule and specific lymph node local assessment.

2. Materials and Methods

In the present paper a comprehensive literature search of PubMed, Google Scholar and Scopus databases was conducted with MESH terms: "CEUS or Contrast-Enhanced Ultrasonography" and "thyroid nodule or thyroid cancer"; to investigate the role of CEUS in evaluation of efficacy of performed treatment on thyroid nodules and nodal involvement the MESH terms "CEUS or Contrast-Enhanced Ultrasonography" and "thyroid nodule or thyroid cancer" and "after treatment" were used. The search was updated from 2010 until June of 2021 and references of the retrieved articles were explored. Original studies, reviews and 6 meta-analyses were included in this article. A total of 624 studies were retrieved, and 107 were included in the study. To avoid bias, only studies with histological reference as the gold standard were included and all of the MESH terms should have been present in the titles or abstracts.

3. Results

3.1. The Technique of Contrast-Enhanced Ultrasound in Thyroid Imaging

The main advantage of CEUS is the ability to assess the sequence and intensity of vascular perfusion and hemodynamics in a thyroid nodule, therefore providing real-time characterization of nodule features after an intravenous bolus injection of a microbubble contrast agent (CA) [23]. Another advantage of CEUS is a lack of contrast media adverse effects or nephrotoxicity (1:10,000 vs. 1–12:100 of iodinated contrast agents) [24]. Adverse effects from CEUS microbubble contrast agents are shown to be sparse, which could be related to clearly intravascular distribution, and their overall safety is very reliable, especially when compared to the potential side effects of CT and MR and the use of their associated contrast agents [25,26].

In CEUS, both qualitative and quantitative evaluation is possible for thyroid nodules [27], and it has been shown by Trimboli et al. to have a good CEUS polled sensitivity of 85% across different studies and a specificity of 82%; in the recent meta-analysis, positive and negative predictive values were 83% and 85%, respectively [28].

A typical protocol for thyroid nodules CEUS examination includes low mechanical index (MI < 0.10) and the focus zone should be placed at the lower portion of the FOV [29] preferably including the entire nodule and surrounding thyroid tissue in the longitudinal plane. When the conventional B-mode image is properly adjusted and the CEUS mode activated, a microbubble contrast agent is injected as an intravenous bolus, generally with a dose of around 1.0–2.0 mL, followed by 5–10 mL of saline; however, specific amounts of CA and saline vary between operators and institutions [30–33]. A CEUS timer is started simultaneously with the injection of the contrast agent, and cine-clips of the scanning are stored digitally as raw data for 2–3 min before being processed, but the length of examination differs between sources and institutions, with most authors choosing a time period of at least 2 min [34,35]. Only one nodule can be evaluated for each injection of contrast agent.

First evaluation includes qualitative analysis—the presence of enhancement, washout and comparison to the normal thyroid parenchyma. After acquiring raw data, a more detailed post-processing of the nodule can be carried out using dedicated software, including quantitative analysis. The mainstay and basis of qualitative analysis include evaluation of contrast medium entry time in the nodule and peak enhancement, with contrast intensity being higher, lower or approximately identical to surrounding parenchyma (hyper-, hypo- or iso-enhancement, respectively), or absent enhancement [36]. The pattern is usually defined depending on the dynamics of contrast bubbles within the nodule: concentric in the case of centripetal enhancement (from the periphery) and centrifugal enhancement (towards the periphery). Non-concentric enhancement patterns include diffuse and eccentric enhancement when the contrast does not exhibit a particular directionality, and peripheral rim enhancement) [37–39]. Other qualitative indicators include contrast uptake homogeneity, with full enhancement, regardless of the enhancement degree, whereas heterogeneous nodules contain intra-nodular areas with various levels of enhancement; nodule borders (clearly differentiated from the surrounding parenchyma, or unclear); morphology (shape and regularity of form); and nodule size [40]. After contrast uptake, the contrast wash-out is observed: the timing of the beginning of washout and speed of this process relative to the surrounding parenchyma [41].

CEUS quantitative analysis is operator dependent: during the post-processing, the manually drawn region of interest (ROI) is placed within the nodule and surrounding parenchyma, subsequently generating variable color-coded curves, and most of the following quantitative parameters are automatically calculated and used for the analysis of the rise time, time to peak (time until peak intensity is reached), wash-in slope, peak intensity, mean transit time (intensity values are higher than the mean), and area under the time-intensity curve: all of these parameters can be used to characterize nodules and have been studied by multiple authors [29,37,42].

Despite the wide applications and interpretation possibilities provided by CEUS, no single feature is sensitive or specific enough for the determination of malignancy; moreover, there are no unified standards for quantitative and qualitative studies [27,28,43]. CEUS also suffers from various limitations that have contributed to the delay of its implementation in routine clinical practice: firstly technical, secondly interpretative, and finally economical. From the technical point of view, microbubble contrast agents last only 5–10 minutes, which shortens the time allowed for investigation, and some other tradeoffs have to be made regarding image quality in order to increase the lifespan of microbubbles, mainly lowering the MI, which simultaneously increases image noise [44–46]; in addition, the equipment requires specific software to perform US with low mechanical index, and together with extra contrast media costs they bring added expenses. CEUS is also a minimally-invasive diagnostic manipulation, although not more so than other methods of investigation which apply intravenous contrast media and are carried out routinely on a mass scale (e.g., computed tomography, magnetic resonance imaging) with significantly lower adverse reaction rates for CEUS, described above. Other authors also point out that CEUS depends on the experience and visual interpretation of the operator [47,48], especially in qualitative assessment. CEUS examination requires extended examination time, assistance of support medical personnel, post-procedural patient observation and, as it has not yet been approved for thyroid in the international guidelines, is not reimbursed in many countries. All of the above mentioned reasons may limit the wide use of CEUS and decrease its availability in certain cases.

3.2. CEUS of Thyroid Nodules: Benign vs. Malignant

Histologically normal thyroid parenchyma is rich in micro-vessels and therefore shows a rapid uniform enhancement after the administration of CA. Thyroid nodules, however, have a different vascularization pattern, therefore a different presentation on CEUS [49]. It has been reported that thyroid cancer cells secrete cytokines to stimulate angiogenesis, therefore increasing vascularization and causing distorted vessel distribution or arteriovenous fistula [50].

3.2.1. Qualitative Analysis of CEUS Enhancement Patterns

Enhancement patterns for CEUS within thyroid nodules are insufficient for the diagnosis of thyroid carcinoma, although several patterns have been described [39]. Some studies classify CEUS enhancement patterns as low-enhancing, iso-enhancing and high enhancement, with low enhancement most suggestive of malignancy and sensitivity, with specificity and accuracy of 82%, 85% and 84%, respectively [51–56]. In a study conducted by Zhang et al. [57] four contrast enhancement patterns were described as: homogenous, heterogeneous, ring-enhancement and no enhancement. In this study, there was a significant difference between benign and malignant nodules with a p value of <0.001. For benign nodules, ring enhancement was seen in 83% of cases, homogenous and heterogenous in 7.5%, and no enhancement in 1.9%. As for malignant nodules, 88.2% showed a heterogeneous enhancement, ring enhancement was observed in 5.9%, and homogenous enhancement also in 5.9% of the cases. Ring enhancement correlated with a benign disease, with a sensitivity and specificity of 83% and 94.1%, respectively. However, heterogeneous enhancement correlated with a malignant disease with sensitivity and specificity of 88.2% and 92.5%, respectively [57]. Most malignant nodules contain areas of fibrosis, calcification, or focal necrosis, which may cause heterogeneous enhancement.

In another similar study by Zhang et al. [39], 120 nodules were characterized using CEUS in which peripheral and internal enhancement patterns were determined. In contrast to previous statements, it was concluded that peripheral irregular ring enhancement pattern on CEUS detects malignancy and improves the diagnostic accuracy of CEUS in combination with internal enhancement patterns (sensitivity 97.6%, specificity 98.7%). Interestingly enough, the size of nodules with regular peripheral enhancing rings was significantly larger than with other types of peripheral rings [39], suggesting that the type of peripheral ring observed might be related to the size of the thyroid nodule.

In a 2016 study by Zhang et al. [9], 157 thyroid lesions were analyzed with CEUS. There was a statistically significant difference for the presence of peripheral ring enhancement and different enhancement patterns in benign and malignant thyroid nodules. Most malignant nodules (70.37%) were found to have a low enhancement, and the sensitivity, specificity and accuracy of this CEUS feature to diagnose thyroid cancer were 84.15%, 65.33% and 75.16%, respectively. The irregular peripheral ring pattern on CEUS had reached a sensitivity of 100%, specificity 94.12% and accuracy of 95% for diagnosing malignancy. In this study, the pattern of iso-enhancement with focal low-enhancing areas was also commonly associated with malignancy, with low-enhancing areas corresponding to interstitial fibrosis, but enhancing areas to malignant cells. Interestingly, the misdiagnosis rate with the conventional US was 57.33%, but only 34.67% for CEUS. This study also suggested the size of the lesion impacts the enhancement pattern on CEUS with small malignant lesions more often presenting as low enhancing, possibly due to an immature vascular network in microcarcinomas [9].

Pang et al. conducted a study in which regression analysis of CEUS for differentiating benign vs. malignant nodules showcased that the hypo-enhancement pattern was highly specific for malignancy [3]. The main reason that thyroid malignant tumors show a low blood supply is related to the complex neovascularization—once the growth outweighs neovascularization, necrosis and embolus formation within the tumor leads to hypo-enhancement on CEUS.

A different approach was taken in a study by Wu et al. where 229 lesions were analyzed with the conventional US and CEUS and divided into enhancement and non-enhancement groups as well as divided into two groups of different sizes, <10 mm and >10 mm. Five indicators were analyzed: arrival time, mode of entrance, echo intensity, homogeneity, and washout time. Within the subgroup of <10 mm there was a statistically significant difference between benign and malignant thyroid nodules for arrival time, mode of entrance and washout time; however, all five [30] indicators showed a statistically significant difference within the subgroup of >10 mm and the total group. The specificity for previously mentioned indicators ranged from 90–96% and diagnostic accuracy between 75–82%. As for the non-enhancement pattern, sensitivity and NPV were 95.5% and 95.8%, respectively [55].

In a recent study by Zhao et al. in 2018 the highest accuracy of 94.02%, sensitivity of 94.74% and specificity of 93.33% was achieved using TI-RADS in combination with CEUS for differentiation of malignant vs. benign nodules. The most prominent features of nodules pointing to malignancy on CEUS were low enhancement and rim-like enhancement [58]. In contrast, other authors reported rim-enhancement as a pattern for benign nodules [30].

Several studies suggest that using CEUS and TI-RADS together can help achieve the highest diagnostic accuracy [35]; for example, in a study by Zhang et al. the diagnostic accuracy of CEUS alone was 90%, for TI-RADS 90.3% and for the combination of both 96% [59]. Some studies report in addition that using conventional US, CEUS and real time elastography increases the sensitivity and specificity of all three methods, but elastography has often been reported as the most valuable tool [49,60,61]. In a study by Deng et al. the combination of US, CEUS and acoustic radiation force impulse (ARFI) markedly improved the diagnostic accuracy when compared to either combination of two modalities [62] and, as Sui et al. reported, the accuracy of CEUS alone was 85.32% vs. CEUS and strain elastography at 95.41% [63] and, according to the recent results [64], the SWE and TIRADS combination showed improved specificity compared with the TIRADS alone (0.917 vs. 0.896), suggesting that the combination method may be valuable in reducing unnecessary FNAB in certain patients. We have to keep in mind that several benign entities may show stiff patterns (e.g., Hashimoto and Riedel's thyroiditis) and malignancy may appear as soft lesions (e.g., follicular adenoma, carcinoma, Hurthle cell neoplasia) [65].

3.2.2. Quantitative Analysis of Thyroid Nodules in CEUS

Wang et al. conducted a study using CEUS on 135 patients with histologically proven thyroid nodules. Binary logistic regression indicated several features suggesting malignancy: slow wash-in, heterogeneous enhancement, ill-defined enhancement border and fast wash-out rate. The AUC in this study for TI-RADS, CEUS and the combination of both were 0.806, 0.934 and 0.950, respectively [66].

A similar study was carried out by Xu et al. in which 432 thyroid nodules were analyzed with CEUS and six suspicious features were pointed out as being specific in differentiating benign from malignant nodules: slow wash-in ($p = 0.001$), slow time to peak ($p = 0.002$), non-uniform enhancement ($p = 0.023$), irregular enhancement ($p = 0.002$), unclear enhancement boundary ($p = 0.012$) and no visible ring enhancement ($p = 0.004$) [34]. As in other studies, CEUS combined with TI-RADS showed better accuracy than any of the two alone, achieving a sensitivity of 85.66% and specificity of 83.33% [49,67].

In a study conducted by Jiang et al., the diagnostic value of CEUS for thyroid nodules with calcification was analyzed and the results for differentiating benign vs. malignant disease were as follows—for conventional US sensitivity and specificity 50% and 77%, for CEUS 90% and 92%, respectively. Moreover, quantitative analysis of CEUS in thyroid nodules was performed and revealed that time to enhancement and time to peak were greater in malignant nodules than benign, but the peak intensity or malignant nodules was significantly lower than in benign nodules [36].

Hu et al. carried out a study in which CEUS quantitative analysis was used for suspicious thyroid nodules. Benign thyroid nodules showed identically in slow-out and hypo-enhancement, but malignant nodules showed a slow-in, identical-out and more hypo-enhancing appearance compared to normal thyroid parenchyma [37,50].

For a comprehensive summary of existing research on qualitative and quantitative parameters in CEUS of thyroid nodules, see Table 1.

Table 1. Qualitative and quantitative CEUS parameter research summary.

Author	Year	Country	Nodules	Sensitivity	Specificity	AUC	Parameters
Zhang et al. [57]	2010	China	104	0.83	0.85	0.91	Qualitative
Nemec et al. [53]	2012	Austria	42	0.87	0.89	0.83	Quantitative
Cantisani et al. [54]	2013	Italy	53	0.78	0.83	0.87	Qualitative
Giusti et al. [49]	2013	Italy	73	0.86	0.91	0.94	Quantitative
Deng et al. [62]	2014	China	175	0.85	0.90	0.84	Qualitative
Jiang et al. [36]	2015	China	122	0.90	0.92	0.90	Quantitative
Wu et al. [55]	2016	China	229	0.95	0.95	0.77	Qualitative
Sui et al. [63]	2016	China	109	0.82	0.91	0.88	Qualitative
Zhang et al. [9]	2016	China	157	0.88	0.65	-	Qualitative
Zhang et al. [39]	2018	China	120	0.98	0.99	-	Qualitative
He et al. [30]	2018	China	88	0.79	0.95	-	Qualitative
Wang et al. [66]	2018	China	135	-	-	0.93	Qualitative/Quantitative
Zhao et al. [58]	2018	China	117	0.89	0.88	0.88	Qualitative
Xu et al. [68]	2019	China	432	0.86	0.83	0.87	Quantitative
Yang et al. [42]	2021	China	64	0.84	0.88	0.92	Quantitative
Yu et al. [69]	2014	Meta-analysis	597	0.85	0.87	0.91	-
Sun et al. [70]	2015	Meta-analysis	1154 nodules	0.88	0.90	0.94	-
Ma et al. [56]	2016	Meta-analysis	1127 patients	0.88	0.90	0.94	-
Zhang et al. [71]	2020	Meta-analysis	4827 nodules	0.87	0.83	0.93	-
Trimboli et al. [28]	2020	Meta-analysis	1515 nodules	0.85	0.82	-	-

3.3. Benign Thyroid Lesions

3.3.1. Thyroid Adenoma

Thyroid adenoma is a benign lesion with morphologically follicular or papillary architecture [72]. Adenomas may be hormonally active causing hyperthyroidism, also known as toxic adenomas, or appear inactive [72]. Cytologic features between follicular adenoma, carcinoma and follicular variants of papillary carcinoma overlap, suggestive of the difficult differential diagnosis [73], and pathological examination is required [74]. Jiang et al. conducted a study in which thyroid adenomas were analyzed by CEUS and mainly presented with a homogenous hyperenhancement; this is due to the fact that adenomas have a complete capsule with surrounding rich blood supply [36], as they mainly grow expansively, gradually pushing the arteries and veins towards the periphery of the tumor, with the continuous growth of new capillaries. Therefore, the contrast agent reaches the center of the nodule more slowly compared with the normal surrounding tissue and wash-out is equally slow, displaying a "fast-in and slow-out" imaging pattern (Figure 1). In a study by Schleder et al. CEUS was used in a preoperative setting to differentiate thyroid adenoma vs. carcinoma in a total of 101 patients. A statistically significant difference in microcirculation between adenoma and carcinoma was noted; adenoma was characterized by no wash-out or wash-out with a persisting edge in the late phase; in contrast, thyroid carcinomas showed a complete wash-out in the late phase with CEUS sensitivity, specificity, PPV and NPV of 81%, 92%, 97% and 63%, respectively [75].

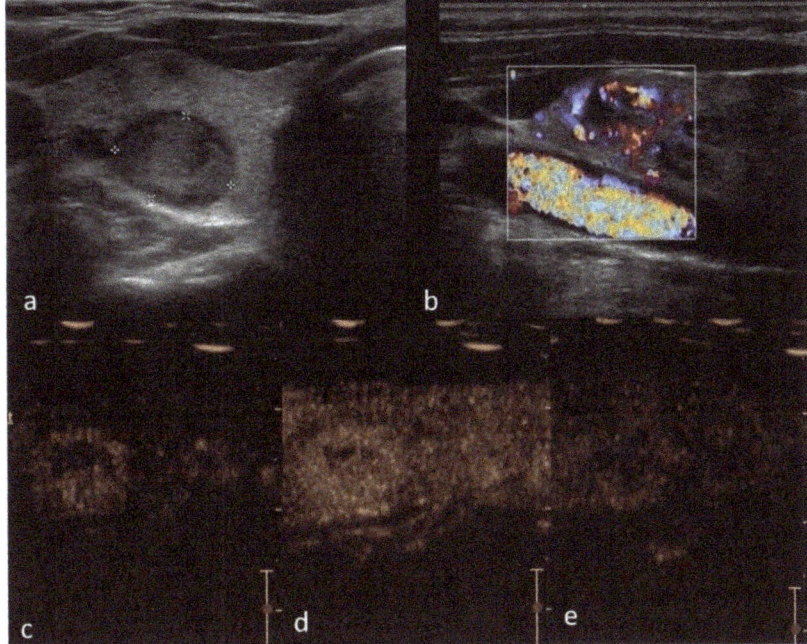

Figure 1. Right lobe hypoechoic lesion with halo sign, TIRADS 3, Bethesda 2, Follicular hyperplasia (**a**)—B mode hypo-echogenicity of the structure; (**b**) color Doppler shows hypervascularity in peripheral part of the lesion; (**c**) contrast enhancement is predominantly peripheral with smooth ring enhancement, with areas of rapid and intense vascularization in periphery and slow in the center (**d**) and suggestive slow wash-out (**e**) in comparison to the adjacent parenchyma.

3.3.2. Nodular Goiter

Multinodular goiter is characterized by an increased volume in the thyroid gland ranging from uni-nodular to multinodular and cystic enlargement of the gland [76], volume exceeding 19 mL for women and 25 mL for men as reported in a study by Teng et al. [77].

A study by Jiang et al. analyzed 62 cases of nodular goiter with CEUS and revealed predominantly homogeneous iso-enhancement due to lack of fibrous capsules and no difference in vascularization between the nodule and surrounding thyroid parenchyma, therefore the internal perfusion is similar in nodular goiters and normal thyroid. However, six cases showed inhomogeneous hypo-enhancement that could be attributed to the development pattern of nodular goiter where at the late hyperplasia stage necrosis, liquefaction and hemorrhage occur [36].

Furthermore, nodular goiter has been described as having regular high enhancing rings similar to thyroid adenoma aiding the differentiation between benign and malignant disease by using CEUS [9,75].

In a study conducted by He et al. 35 nodular goiters and 15 nodular goiters with hyperplasia were analyzed and various enhancement patterns were observed, most commonly wash-in and wash-out, similarly to thyroid parenchyma. Interestingly enough, six cases of nodular goiter in this study were misdiagnosed as malignancy due to an inhomogeneous low enhancement pattern [30].

3.3.3. Thyroiditis and Lymphoma

Hashimoto's thyroiditis is a rather common endocrine disorder and is the leading cause of hypothyroidism in iodine-sufficient parts of the world [78]. The inflammation in the thyroid gland contributes to a 40–80 times greater risk for developing primary thyroid lymphoma in comparison with patients without thyroiditis [79]. On ultrasound, Hashimoto's thyroiditis background with a heterogeneously decreased thyroid echogenicity and hypervascularity may cause overlap between benign and malignant findings [71].

In 2015 a study on the value of CEUS was analyzed in diagnosing thyroid nodules coexisting with Hashimoto's thyroiditis. Sixty-two nodules in a study of 48 patients were evaluated—peak intensity and enhancement pattern showed statistically significant differences between malignant and benign thyroid nodules and heterogeneous enhancement was highly suggestive of malignancy in patients with co-existing autoimmune thyroiditis with sensitivity and specificity of 97.6% and 85.7%, respectively [80].

Moreover, it is also suggested to add CEUS in subacute thyroiditis where lesions are hypoechoic with irregular margins, suggestive of malignancy, and additionally elastography data confirm suspicious stiff areas, while CEUS shows peripheral or iso-enhancement and would lead to follow-up and conservative treatment instead of surgery.

Another similar study by Yang et al. investigated the diagnostic performance of CEUS in differentiating primary thyroid lymphoma (PTL) and nodular Hashimoto's thyroiditis (NHL) in patients with a known background of autoimmune thyroiditis. Sixty-four thyroid nodules were analyzed out of which 31 were primary thyroid lymphoma and 33 were nodular autoimmune thyroiditis. All 64 lesions presented as hypoechoic solid nodules on conventional US, but PTL was more often associated with mixed vascularity and NHT with peripheral vascularity on Doppler US. As for CEUS, most PTL lesions presented as hypo-enhanced, with the centripetal heterogeneous pattern. There were statistically significant differences between peak intensity and AUC for PTL and NHT. The diagnostic accuracy of CEUS for diagnosing PTL in patients with autoimmune thyroiditis was around 70.3–75%. The best results were accomplished if the combination of quantitative parameters, PI, TTP and AUC ratios, were used and, if combined with CEUS imaging features, showed an AUROC of 0.92 (95% CI, 0.82–0.97) [42].

In a study conducted by Wei et al. primary thyroid lymphoma was studied in 20 patients with the conventional US and 10 patients with CEUS. The conventional B mode ultrasound appearances of PTL were classified and were as follows: all cases were of hypoechoic appearance, 12 were the diffuse mass type, six of multiple nodular type and two cases of mixed type. As for CEUS, 8 out of 10 cases showed a diffuse homogenous enhancement and two cases were a diffuse heterogeneous enhancement which was linked to necrosis within the tumor. By performing quantitative analysis on CEUS parameters, TTP of the primary tumor or affected lymph nodes was longer than that of the ipsilateral common carotid artery ($p = 0.004$) [81].

3.4. Thyroid Cancer in CEUS

There are several known subtypes of thyroid cancer, the most commonly described pattern of malignancy being a low enhancement on CEUS—particularly due to lack of blood supply and insufficient neovascularization, as well as interstitial fibrosis, especially in the central parts [41,82]. Qualitative patterns on CEUS suggesting malignancy include incomplete ring enhancement, heterogeneous enhancement and wash-out in the late phases; furthermore, such parameters suggestive of malignancy in the quantitative analysis include polyphasic washout curves, early arrival time and shorter TTP [54] (see Figure 2).

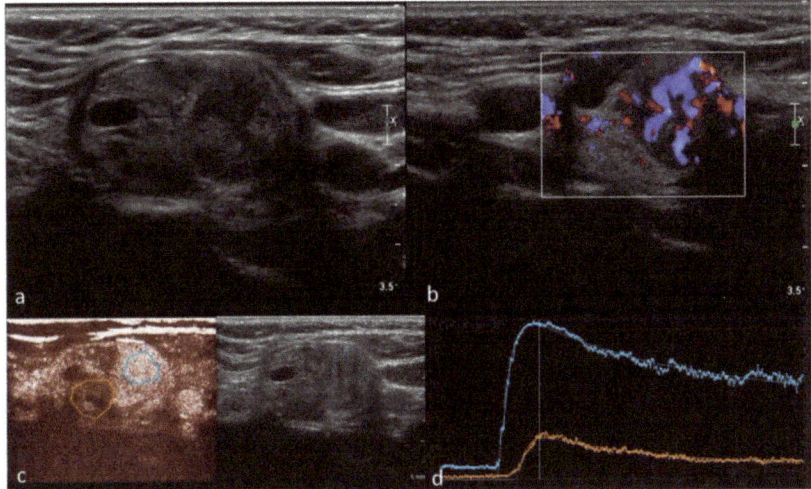

Figure 2. Right lobe heterogeneous lesion, TIRADS 4, Bethesda 5, Papillary cancer (**a**)—B mode hypo-echogenicity of the structure with cystic components; (**b**) Color Doppler shows hypervascularity in one part of the lesion, (**c**) contrast enhancement is heterogeneous with areas of low vascularization suggestive of malignancy and (**d**) confirming quantitative difference within the malignant tumor parts (yellow—necrotic areas, blue—intense enhancement and slow wash-out curve).

Hornung et al. quantitatively analyzed 22 malignant thyroid nodules with CEUS, out of which 14 were papillary, seven follicular and one medullary carcinoma. On CEUS 19 out of 22 tumors presented with a significant early arterial irregular vascularization starting at the periphery, in all 22 cases wash-out in the late arterial phase was present. AUC representing the amount of CA reaching different regions of the nodule was higher at the edge than in the center of the tumor. Interestingly, irregular peripheral vascularization by Power Doppler was only detected in 8 out of 22 patients [50]. Usually, in the literature, studies are dedicated to papillary carcinoma or are mixed studies with few other subtypes included.

3.4.1. Papillary Thyroid Carcinoma (PTC)

Papillary carcinoma is the most common histological type of thyroid cancer accounting for approximately 85% and is often diagnosed in women between the third and fifth decades of life. The prognosis is excellent with a survival rate of approximately 90% at 20 years [8,83].

Papillary carcinomas morphologically are usually 2–3 cm in size on average, usually white and with an invasive appearance, characterized by a central core of fibrovascular tissue surrounded by cells with crowded oval nuclei [84].

In a study by Jiang et al. 49 papillary carcinomas were analyzed with CEUS; 44 had microcalcifications, of which 42 had inhomogeneous hypo-enhancement on CEUS [36]. A similar study by Ma et al. examined papillary carcinomas and found that a low enhancement pattern on CEUS is the most common finding for this type of tumor [52]. The reason for decreased blood supply in papillary carcinomas may be due to calcified psammoma bodies that affect tumor angiogenesis [14].

In 2015 a study was conducted by Li et al. where the performance of CEUS in diagnosing papillary thyroid microcarcinomas (<1cm in diameter) was studied. The correct diagnostic rate of CEUS was 85%, sensitivity 88% and specificity 80% for diagnosing microcarcinomas in 73 patients, but t0he use of CEUS had no clear advantages for diagnosing thyroid microcarcinomas as there were no statistically significant differences between malignant and benign nodules [61]. Furthermore, an interesting study by Gao et al. also suggests that blood-rich enhancement on CEUS is associated with a non-excellent response after thyroidectomy in a study on 306 patients with PTC [85].

A quantitative CEUS analysis of 62 patients with PTC was performed by Zhou et al., where the correlation between CEUS features and histologically determined micro-vessel density (MVD) was studied. The main peak intensity of PTC was lower than that of the surrounding thyroid parenchyma; moreover, a positive correlation was observed between peak intensity and MVD in PTC suggesting that quantitative analysis of CEUS could help determine PTC [86].

The correct staging of thyroid cancer through the identification of metastatic lymph nodes is essential for proper clinical and surgical management, for treatment planning and prognostic evaluation. Jia Zhan showed that homogeneity, cystic change or calcification, and above all intensity at peak time, were the three strongest independent predictors for malignancy in lymph nodes on CEUS [87]. In addition, benign nodes show a centrifugal progression of enhancement, while a prominent centripetal enhancement is more often observed in metastatic nodes.

3.4.2. Follicular Thyroid Carcinoma (FTC)

Follicular carcinoma is the second most common thyroid malignancy classically accounting for 10–15% of all thyroid malignancies, though a decrease in incidence has been reported recently [88]. This cancer is more often diagnosed in women between the fifth and sixth decades of life. Cumulative incidence of all-cause deaths for FTC was 24% and 45% at 10 and 20 years, respectively, as showcased by Su et al. [89].

In the case of FTC surgical biopsy or excision is usually required to make the diagnosis, though over 80% of all follicular neoplasms prove to be benign [90]. It has been reported that for the detection of FTC with the predominantly internal flow, Color Doppler Ultrasound (CDUS) can be useful [91], a meta-analysis revealing that sensitivity and specificity and specificity for CDUS in predicting malignant follicular thyroid neoplasms is 85% and 86%, respectively [91,92]. Lesions showing iso-enhancement with a focal low-enhancement region should be considered malignant if the inflammatory cause has been excluded [9].

He at al. conducted a study in which only one case of FTC was analyzed with CEUS showing a fast wash-in and slow wash-out with homogenous intense enhancement without ring enhancement, similar to that of a follicular adenoma; moreover, on CDUS this lesion was rich in blood flow. This study reports that CEUS, however, cannot accurately distinguish between FTC and follicular adenoma as the only pathological diagnostic criteria for FTC was tumor invasion of the margin or blood vessels [30]. Further research on CEUS sensitivity and specificity for diagnosing FTC is required.

3.4.3. Medullary Thyroid Carcinoma (MTC)

Medullary thyroid carcinomas (MTC) are rare tumors accounting for approximately 5% of all thyroid malignancies. MTC arises from parafollicular C cells of the thyroid [93] which secrete calcitonin and carcinoembryonic antigen. These are also sensitive markers in the process of MTC diagnosis, follow up and prognosis, but rare cases of calcitonin-negative MTC have been reported [94] requiring a more complex approach, possibly including CEUS. MTC can be associated with Multiple Endocrine Neoplasia type 2 (MEN2). It has to be noted that the prognosis of MTC is markedly worse than that of papillary or follicular thyroid cancer with 10-year survival being around 74% as reported by a recent study of 140 patients with MTC [95].

In a study by Zhang et al. the value of peripheral enhancement pattern for diagnosing thyroid cancer was assessed, including two cases of medullary thyroid carcinoma. One of the cases showed an irregular no-enhancement pattern that is more typical of malignant lesions, but the other carcinoma showed a regular high-enhancing ring that characterizes mostly benign lesions. The latter carcinoma was large (>5cm), heterogenous and showed a well-defined margin and rich blood flow on the conventional US, mimicking a benign lesion, which contributed to a misdiagnosis; however, such cases are sparsely reported [39].

3.4.4. Anaplastic Thyroid Cancer (ATC)

Anaplastic thyroid cancer is a rare type of thyroid tumor accounting for approximately 2–5% of all thyroid malignancies and is associated with a high mortality rate [94]. The estimated incidence is around 1–2 cases per million in a year and the peak incidence is between the sixth and seventh decades of life [96]. Histological variants of ATC include giant-cell, spindle-cell and squamoid-cell tumors. Up to 20–30% of cases morphologically show areas of necrosis and hemorrhage [96].

Only one case of ATC scanned with the conventional B mode ultrasound, CD and CEUS has been reported in the literature by Proiti et al. The diagnosis was confirmed by FNAB. On the conventional US the lesion showed a heterogeneous hypoechoic structure with irregular margins and was solitary with a maximum diameter of 3 cm. With CD no significant internal vascularity was noted, but some peripheral vessels were present. As for CEUS, a bolus of 4.8 mL of CA was used, the lesion showed an overall markedly reduced vascularity. Quantitative analysis of CEUS parameters was performed, average TTP index was 2 and average peak index was 3.4 [96]. Guisti et al. reported that a peak index of less than 1 and TTP index greater than 1 are characteristic of malignancy [49]. Additional research is required for further determination of diagnostic patterns for ATC.

For an accuracy comparison of CEUS in benign and malignant thyroid nodules, see Table 2.

Table 2. CEUS performance in benign and malignant thyroid lesions.

Thyroid Lesion	CEUS Characteristics	Sensitivity	Specificity	PPV	NPV
Benign Thyroid Lesions					
Thyroid Adenoma [74]	homogenous hyperenhancement, "fast-in and slow-out" no wash-out or wash-out with persisting edge in the late phase	0.81	0.92	0.97	0.63
Malignant thyroid lesions					
Primary thyroid lymphoma [41]	hypo-enhanced, with centripetal heterogeneous pattern, lower PI, AUC, TTP than thyroid parenchyma	0.84	0.88	0.87	0.85
Papillary thyroid carcinoma [35,60]	inhomogeneous hypo-enhancement lower PI than parenchyma	0.88–0.90	0.8–0.92	0.8	0.93
Pooled					
Benign and malignant [27,97]	histology as reference	0.85–0.88	0.82–0.90	0.83	0.85

PI—peak intensity, TTP—time to peak, AUC—area under the time–intensity curve.

3.5. CEUS before and after Local Treatment

Thermal ablation has been frequently applied in recent years to reduce the invasiveness of treatment in benign thyroid nodules, recurrent thyroid cancer, and metastatic cervical lymph nodes. For solid and mixed structure nodules, the most commonly used are the following—laser (LA) and radiofrequency ablation (RFA) [98,99], microwave ablation [100,101], and, lately, high-frequency ultrasound (HIFU) [102,103]. Percutaneous ethanol injection efficacy is reported based on a proportion of solid and cystic components and is effective in the treatment of predominantly cystic nodules (>90%) [104]. The primary outcome of image-guided thermal ablations was associated with a volume reduction ratio (VRR) at 6, 12, 24, and 36 months of 60%, 66%, 62%, and 53% [28].

CEUS helps to clarify boundaries between viable and nonviable tissue before and after treatment (Figure 3). This could be helpful in obtaining a more precise and reproducible measurement of the ablated area right after the ablation procedure and in the follow-up imaging—early term (3 months) and intermediate-term (6 and 12 months) are suggested intervals for follow-up with long term monitoring up to 1–2 years, to assess regrowth and to address the misinterpretation of post-treatment appearances (hypo-echogenicity), mimicking malignancy in cases of limited history data [105].

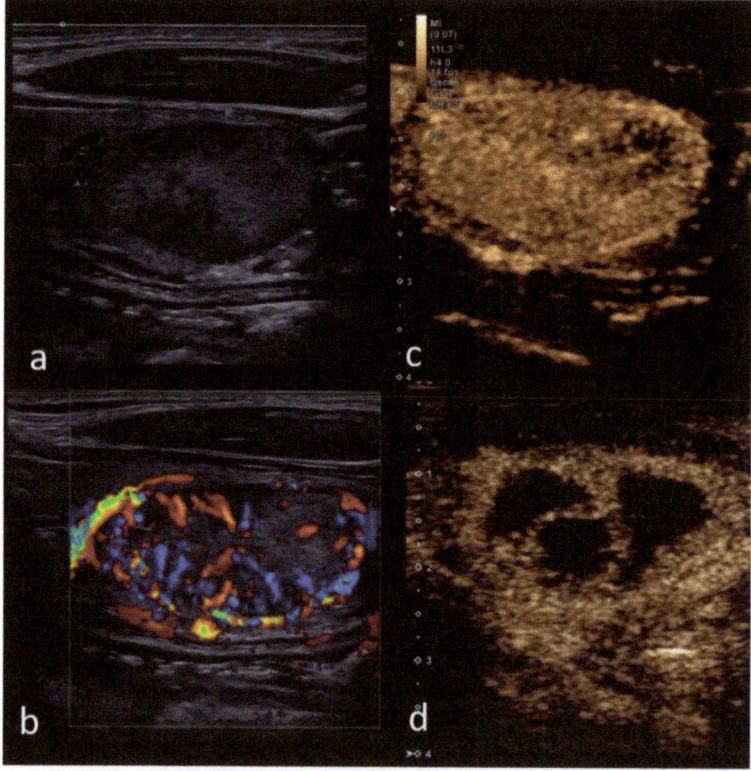

Figure 3. Right lobe heterogeneous lesion, TIRADS 3, Bethesda 2, Follicular adenoma, (**a**) B mode mildly heterogeneous structure with cystic components; (**b**) Color Doppler shows hypervascularity in periphery of the lesion, (**c**) contrast enhancement is predominantly hyper-vascular and homogeneous with minor parts of lower vascularization prior to the ablation treatment; (**d**) 6 months after radiofrequency ablation volume reduction by 52% has been reached, and avascular necrotic areas (black areas) are well delineated within nodule for further treatment planning.

A recent systematic review reported that regrowth may be a distinct process from nodule shrinkage; furthermore, it may depend on the nodule behaviour and technical issues such as operator experience, the lack of treatment of the nodule's margins related to the feeding artery or draining vein, and the size and the position of the nodule which influence the quality of an RFA treatment. Due to the above mentioned difficulties in performing RFA, CEUS rather than non-enhanced ultrasound may be of particular use in determining local treatment outcome in cases with thyroid nodules proximal to critical structures, as well as large thyroid nodules [106–108].

Contrast-enhanced ultrasound can improve ultrasound diagnostic accuracy for cervical lymph nodes staging after papillary thyroid carcinoma diagnosis. It can be useful for characterizing focal US alterations in patients with suspicions of nodal metastatic involvement, where perfusion defects are a sign of metastatic involvement: poor or absent vascularization can be identified in widespread metastatic infiltration, corresponding to areas of necrosis.

4. Discussion

An increase in thyroid nodule prevalence has been recorded in the last few years. High-resolution ultrasonography is the most important modality for the evaluation of a thyroid nodule. The latest guidelines have proposed criteria for risk stratification that categorizes the thyroid nodules and risk of malignancy in TIRADS systems. However, the differential diagnosis for nodules with intermediate and low suspicion is still difficult. Conventional ultrasound features such as hypo-echogenicity, irregular margins, a taller-than-wide shape, a solid internal component and microcalcification are predictive of non-follicular thyroid carcinoma. CEUS enhancement provides additional significant patterns for differentiating benign and malignant nodules with intermediate and low suspicion (5–20% malignancy risk). This risk can increase to 38.5% if the nodule shows heterogeneous enhancement [109]. With nodular goiter and subacute thyroiditis, a visible peripheral enhancement may be observed, as they are hyperplastic or atrophic in architecture. While some cases may present with low enhancement or no enhancement in subacute thyroiditis, the majority of benign nodules, including adenoma show a tendency of "fast in and slow out" enhancement, which poses a risk for misdiagnosis. There are also various meta-analyses [56,69,70], systematic reviews and original articles [35] showing controversial statements about ring enhancement as predictor of malignancy or feature of the benign nodule, leaving the community with the question as to whether CEUS in clinical practice can be associated with any additional benefit. Nevertheless, four meta-analyses [28,56,69,70] showed that both the sensitivity and specificity of CEUS were more than 85% and 82%, while PPV and NPV were 83% and 85%, respectively. Although CEUS exhibits high sensitivity and specificity, there remains a missed diagnosis rate of 12.5% and a misdiagnosis rate of 13.67% [110]. The present review showed that no isolated CEUS feature is capable of predicting thyroid malignancy with acceptable diagnostic accuracy. We have to underline that only a few papers reported on specific CEUS features of certain subtypes of the tumors such as follicular, medullary and anaplastic cancers. However, as recognized for thyroid nodule malignancy risk stratification by the US, for acceptable accuracy in malignancy a combination of several CEUS parameters should be applied: hypo-enhancement, heterogeneous, peripheral irregular enhancement in combination with internal enhancement patterns and slow wash-in and wash-out curve lower than in normal thyroid tissue. In contrast, homogeneous, intense enhancement with smooth rim enhancement, intense wash-in and slow wash-out are indicative of benignity of the thyroid nodule. In cases of indeterminate lesions by conventional US and in cases of diagnostic inconsistencies between CEUS and SWE, combined scores and further fine-needle aspiration biopsy is recommended to improve diagnostic accuracy. Furthermore, many recent studies suggest that artificial intelligence algorithms increase the accuracy of diagnosing benign versus malignant thyroid nodules, especially in the TI-RADS 4 and 5 categories, and help reduce the rate of unnecessary FNAB from 62% to 35% [111–113]. In 2020, Xu et al. published a meta-analysis which included 19 papers with 4781 thyroid nodules, analyzing the performance of Computer Aided Diagnosis (CAD) systems performance in differentiation of malignant thyroid nodules: the deep learning-based system showed a sensitivity of 87% and a specificity of 85%. The authors concluded that CAD systems could help, but that experienced radiologists may be superior to CAD systems, especially for real-time diagnosis [68], highlighting yet another tool that could aid differential diagnosis in the near future.

5. Conclusions

In conclusion, with current further research, CEUS appears to achieve reliable performance in detecting or excluding thyroid cancer. It can also play an operative role in guiding ablation procedures on benign and malignant thyroid nodules and metastatic lymph nodes and has a promising role in the detection of extra-nodular extension in malignancy and in the evaluation of treatment response. However, there is a need for a prospective multicenter study, with a tailored approach by TIRADS categories and histology reference, to define indication and standardized qualitative techniques and parameters in order to confirm the usefulness of CEUS.

Author Contributions: Conceptualization, M.R. (Maija Radzina); methodology, M.R. (Maija Radzina); writing—original draft preparation, M.R. (Madara Ratniece), D.S.P., M.R. (Maija Radzina) and V.C.; writing—review and editing, L.S.; visualization, M.R. (Maija Radzina); supervision, M.R. (Maija Radzina). All authors have read and agreed to the published version of the manuscript.

Funding: This research received no external funding.

Conflicts of Interest: Maija Radzina has received the speaker honoraria from Bracco and Canon, other co-authors have nothing to disclose.

References

1. Haugen, B.R.; Alexander, E.K.; Bible, K.C.; Doherty, G.M.; Mandel, S.J.; Nikiforov, Y.E.; Pacini, F.; Randolph, G.W.; Sawka, A.M.; Schlumberger, M.; et al. 2015 American Thyroid Association Management Guidelines for Adult Patients with Thyroid Nodules and Differentiated Thyroid Cancer: The American Thyroid Association Guidelines Task Force on Thyroid Nodules and Differentiated Thyroid Cancer. *Thyroid* **2016**, *26*, 1–133. [CrossRef] [PubMed]
2. Durante, C.; Grani, G.; Lamartina, L.; Filetti, S.; Mandel, S.J.; Cooper, D.S. The Diagnosis and Management of Thyroid Nodules: A Review. *JAMA* **2018**, *319*, 914–924. [CrossRef] [PubMed]
3. Pang, T.; Huang, L.; Deng, Y.; Wang, T.; Chen, S.; Gong, X.; Liu, W. Logistic Regression Analysis of Conventional Ultrasonography, Strain Elastosonography, and Contrast-Enhanced Ultrasound Characteristics for the Differentiation of Benign and Malignant Thyroid Nodules. *PLoS ONE* **2017**, *12*, e0188987. [CrossRef]
4. Chng, C.; Kurzawinski, T.R.; Beale, T. Value of Sonographic Features in Predicting Malignancy in Thyroid Nodules Diagnosed as Follicular Neoplasm on Cytology. *Clin. Endocrinol.* **2015**, *83*, 711–716. [CrossRef] [PubMed]
5. Jiang, H.; Tian, Y.; Yan, W.; Kong, Y.; Wang, H.; Wang, A.; Dou, J.; Liang, P.; Mu, Y. The Prevalence of Thyroid Nodules and an Analysis of Related Lifestyle Factors in Beijing Communities. *Int. J. Environ. Res. Public Health* **2016**, *13*, 442. [CrossRef]
6. Bomeli, S.R.; LeBeau, S.O.; Ferris, R.L. Evaluation of a Thyroid Nodule. *Otolaryngol. Clin. N. Am.* **2010**, *43*, 229–238. [CrossRef] [PubMed]
7. Vigneri, R.; Malandrino, P.; Vigneri, P. The Changing Epidemiology of Thyroid Cancer. *Curr. Opin. Oncol.* **2015**, *27*, 1–7. [CrossRef] [PubMed]
8. Kuhn, E.; Teller, L.; Piana, S.; Rosai, J.; Merino, M.J. Different Clonal Origin of Bilateral Papillary Thyroid Carcinoma, with a Review of the Literature. *Endocr. Pathol.* **2012**, *23*, 101–107. [CrossRef]
9. Zhang, Y.; Luo, Y.; Zhang, M.; Li, J.; Li, J.; Tang, J. Diagnostic Accuracy of Contrast-Enhanced Ultrasound Enhancement Patterns for Thyroid Nodules. *Med. Sci. Monit.* **2016**, *22*, 4755–4764. [CrossRef]
10. Melany, M.; Chen, S. Thyroid Cancer Ultrasound Imaging and Fine-Needle Aspiration Biopsy. *Endocrinol. Metab. Clin.* **2017**, *46*, 691–711. [CrossRef] [PubMed]
11. Russ, G.; Bonnema, S.J.; Erdogan, M.F.; Durante, C.; Ngu, R.; Leenhardt, L. European Thyroid Association Guidelines for Ultrasound Malignancy Risk Stratification of Thyroid Nodules in Adults: The EU-TIRADS. *Eur. Thyroid J.* **2017**, *6*, 225–237. [CrossRef] [PubMed]
12. Shin, J.H.; Baek, J.H.; Chung, J.; Ha, E.J.; Kim, J.; Lee, Y.H.; Lim, H.K.; Moon, W.-J.; Na, D.G.; Park, J.S.; et al. Ultrasonography Diagnosis and Imaging-Based Management of Thyroid Nodules: Revised Korean Society of Thyroid Radiology Consensus Statement and Recommendations. *Korean J. Radiol.* **2016**, *17*, 370–395. [CrossRef]

3. Ozel, A.; Erturk, S.M.; Ercan, A.; Yılmaz, B.; Basak, T.; Cantisani, V.; Basak, M.; Karpat, Z. The Diagnostic Efficiency of Ultrasound in Characterization for Thyroid Nodules: How Many Criteria Are Required to Predict Malignancy? *Med. Ultrason.* **2012**, *14*, 24–28.
4. Kim, B.K.; Choi, Y.S.; Kwon, H.J.; Lee, J.S.; Heo, J.J.; Han, Y.J.; Park, Y.-H.; Kim, J.H. Relationship between Patterns of Calcification in Thyroid Nodules and Histopathologic Findings. *Endocr. J.* **2013**, *60*, 155–160. [CrossRef] [PubMed]
5. Sultan, L.R.; Xiong, H.; Zafar, H.M.; Schultz, S.M.; Langer, J.E.; Sehgal, C.M. Vascularity Assessment of Thyroid Nodules by Quantitative Color Doppler Ultrasound. *Ultrasound Med. Biol.* **2015**, *41*, 1287–1293. [CrossRef]
6. Lu, R.; Meng, Y.; Zhang, Y.; Zhao, W.; Wang, X.; Jin, M.; Guo, R. Superb Microvascular Imaging (SMI) Compared with Conventional Ultrasound for Evaluating Thyroid Nodules. *BMC Med. Imaging* **2017**, *17*, 65. [CrossRef] [PubMed]
7. Tessler, F.N.; Middleton, W.D.; Grant, E.G.; Hoang, J.K.; Berland, L.L.; Teefey, S.A.; Cronan, J.J.; Beland, M.D.; Desser, T.S.; Frates, M.C.; et al. ACR Thyroid Imaging, Reporting and Data System (TI-RADS): White Paper of the ACR TI-RADS Committee. *J. Am. Coll. Radiol.* **2017**, *14*, 587–595. [CrossRef]
8. Kwak, J.Y.; Han, K.H.; Yoon, J.H.; Moon, H.J.; Son, E.J.; Park, S.H.; Jung, H.K.; Choi, J.S.; Kim, B.M.; Kim, E.-K. Thyroid Imaging Reporting and Data System for US Features of Nodules: A Step in Establishing Better Stratification of Cancer Risk. *Radiology* **2011**, *260*, 892–899. [CrossRef]
9. Grani, G.; Lamartina, L.; Ascoli, V.; Bosco, D.; Biffoni, M.; Giacomelli, L.; Maranghi, M.; Falcone, R.; Ramundo, V.; Cantisani, V.; et al. Reducing the Number of Unnecessary Thyroid Biopsies while Improving Diagnostic Accuracy: Toward the "Right" TIRADS. *J. Clin. Endocrinol. Metab.* **2019**, *104*, 95–102. [CrossRef]
10. Bongiovanni, M.; Spitale, A.; Faquin, W.C.; Mazzucchelli, L.; Baloch, Z.W. The Bethesda System for Reporting Thyroid Cytopathology: A Meta-Analysis. *Acta Cytol.* **2012**, *56*, 333–339. [CrossRef]
11. Cantisani, V.; David, E.; Grazhdani, H.; Rubini, A.; Radzina, M.; Dietrich, C.; Durante, C.; Lamartina, L.; Grani, G.; Valeria, A.; et al. Prospective Evaluation of Semiquantitative Strain Ratio and Quantitative 2D Ultrasound Shear Wave Elastography (SWE) in Association with TIRADS Classification for Thyroid Nodule Characterization. *Ultraschall Der Medizin Eur. J. Ultrasound* **2019**, *40*, 495–503. [CrossRef] [PubMed]
12. Săftoiu, A.; Gilja, O.; Sidhu, P.; Dietrich, C.; Cantisani, V.; Amy, D.; Bachmann-Nielsen, M.; Bob, F.; Bojunga, J.; Brock, M.; et al. The EFSUMB Guidelines and Recommendations for the Clinical Practice of Elastography in Non-Hepatic Applications: Update 2018. *Ultraschall Der Medizin Eur. J. Ultrasound* **2019**, *40*, 425–453. [CrossRef]
13. Greis, C. Quantitative Evaluation of Microvascular Blood Flow by Contrast-Enhanced Ultrasound (CEUS). *Clin. Hemorheol. Microcirc.* **2011**, *49*, 137–149. [CrossRef]
14. Chang, E.H. An Introduction to Contrast-Enhanced Ultrasound for Nephrologists. *Nephron* **2018**, *138*, 176–185. [CrossRef]
15. Hu, C.; Feng, Y.; Huang, P.; Jin, J. Adverse Reactions after the Use of SonoVue Contrast Agent: Characteristics and Nursing Care Experience. *Medicine* **2019**, *98*, e17745. [CrossRef] [PubMed]
16. Yusuf, G.T.; Sellars, M.E.; Deganello, A.; Cosgrove, D.O.; Sidhu, P.S. Retrospective Analysis of the Safety and Cost Implications of Pediatric Contrast-Enhanced Ultrasound at a Single Center. *Am. J. Roentgenol.* **2017**, *208*, 446–452. [CrossRef] [PubMed]
17. Sidhu, P.; Cantisani, V.; Dietrich, C.; Gilja, O.; Saftoiu, A.; Bartels, E.; Bertolotto, M.; Calliada, F.; Clevert, D.-A.; Cosgrove, D.; et al. The EFSUMB Guidelines and Recommendations for the Clinical Practice of Contrast-Enhanced Ultrasound (CEUS) in Non-Hepatic Applications: Update 2017 (Short Version). *Ultraschall Der Medizin Eur. J. Ultrasound* **2018**, *39*, 154–180. [CrossRef]
18. Trimboli, P.; Castellana, M.; Virili, C.; Havre, R.F.; Bini, F.; Marinozzi, F.; D'Ambrosio, F.; Giorgino, F.; Giovanella, L.; Prosch, H.; et al. Performance of Contrast-Enhanced Ultrasound (CEUS) in Assessing Thyroid Nodules: A Systematic Review and Meta-Analysis Using Histological Standard of Reference. *Radiol. Med.* **2020**, *125*, 406–415. [CrossRef]
19. Zhan, J.; Ding, H. Application of Contrast-Enhanced Ultrasound for Evaluation of Thyroid Nodules. *Ultrasonography* **2018**, *37*, 288–297. [CrossRef]
20. He, Y.; Wang, X.Y.; Hu, Q.; Chen, X.X.; Ling, B.; Wei, H.M. Value of Contrast-Enhanced Ultrasound and Acoustic Radiation Force Impulse Imaging for the Differential Diagnosis of Benign and Malignant Thyroid Nodules. *Front. Pharm.* **2018**, *9*, 1363. [CrossRef]
21. Jiao, Z.; Luo, Y.; Song, Q.; Yan, L.; Zhu, Y.; Xie, F. Roles of Contrast-Enhanced Ultrasonography in Identifying Volume Change of Benign Thyroid Nodule and Optical Time of Secondary Radiofrequency Ablation. *BMC Med. Imaging* **2020**, *20*, 79. [CrossRef] [PubMed]
22. Hong, Y.-R.; Yan, C.-X.; Mo, G.-Q.; Luo, Z.-Y.; Zhang, Y.; Wang, Y.; Huang, P.-T. Conventional US, Elastography and Contrast Enhanced US Features of Papillary Thyroid Microcarcinoma Predict Central Compartment Lymph Node Metastases. *Sci. Rep.* **2015**, *5*, 7748. [CrossRef] [PubMed]
23. Piskunowicz, M.; Back, S.J.; Darge, K.; Humphries, P.D.; Jüngert, J.; Ključevšek, D.; Lorenz, N.; Mentzel, H.-J.; Squires, J.H.; Huang, D.Y. Contrast-Enhanced Ultrasound of the Small Organs in Children. *Pediatr. Radiol.* **2021**, 1–16. [CrossRef]
24. Wang, Y.; Dong, T.; Nie, F.; Wang, G.; Liu, T.; Niu, Q. Contrast-Enhanced Ultrasound in the Differential Diagnosis and Risk Stratification of ACR TI-RADS Category 4 and 5 Thyroid Nodules with Non-Hypovascular. *Front. Oncol.* **2021**, *11*, 662273. [CrossRef]
25. Xu, Y.; Qi, X.; Zhao, X.; Ren, W.; Ding, W. Clinical Diagnostic Value of Contrast-Enhanced Ultrasound and TI-RADS Classification for Benign and Malignant Thyroid Tumors: One Comparative Cohort Study. *Medicine* **2019**, *98*, e14051. [CrossRef] [PubMed]
26. Jiang, J.; Shang, X.; Wang, H.; Xu, Y.-B.; Gao, Y.; Zhou, Q. Diagnostic Value of Contrast-Enhanced Ultrasound in Thyroid Nodules with Calcification. *Kaohsiung J. Med. Sci.* **2015**, *31*, 138–144. [CrossRef]

37. Hu, Y.; Li, P.; Jiang, S.; Li, F. Quantitative Analysis of Suspicious Thyroid Nodules by Contrast-Enhanced Ultrasonography. *Int. J. Clin. Exp. Med.* **2015**, *8*, 11786–11793.
38. Yuan, Z.; Quan, J.; Yunxiao, Z.; Jian, C.; Zhu, H. Contrast-Enhanced Ultrasound in the Diagnosis of Solitary Thyroid Nodules. *J. Cancer Res. Ther.* **2015**, *11*, 41–45. [CrossRef] [PubMed]
39. Zhang, Y.; Zhang, M.; Luo, Y.; Li, J.; Wang, Z.; Tang, J. The Value of Peripheral Enhancement Pattern for Diagnosing Thyroid Cancer Using Contrast-Enhanced Ultrasound. *Int. J. Endocrinol.* **2018**, *2018*, 1–7. [CrossRef] [PubMed]
40. Li, X.; Gao, F.; Li, F.; Han, X.; Shao, S.; Yao, M.; Li, C.; Zheng, J.; Wu, R.; Du, L. Qualitative Analysis of Contrast-Enhanced Ultrasound in the Diagnosis of Small, TR3–5 Benign and Malignant Thyroid Nodules Measuring ≤1 cm. *Br. J. Radiol.* **2020**, *93*, 20190923. [CrossRef]
41. Chen, H.Y.; Liu, W.Y.; Zhu, H.; Jiang, D.W.; Wang, D.H.; Chen, Y.; Li, W.; Pan, G. Diagnostic Value of Contrast-Enhanced Ultrasound in Papillary Thyroid Microcarcinoma. *Exp. Ther. Med.* **2016**, *11*, 1555–1562. [CrossRef] [PubMed]
42. Yang, L.; Zhao, H.; He, Y.; Zhu, X.; Yue, C.; Luo, Y.; Ma, B. Contrast-Enhanced Ultrasound in the Differential Diagnosis of Primary Thyroid Lymphoma and Nodular Hashimoto's Thyroiditis in a Background of Heterogeneous Parenchyma. *Front. Oncol.* **2021**, *10*, 2861. [CrossRef] [PubMed]
43. Cantisani, V.; Bertolotto, M.; Weskott, H.P.; Romanini, L.; Grazhdani, H.; Passamonti, M.; Drudi, F.M.; Malpassini, F.; Isidori, A.; Meloni, F.M.; et al. Growing Indications for CEUS: The Kidney, Testis, Lymph Nodes, Thyroid, Prostate, and Small Bowel. *Eur. J. Radiol.* **2015**, *84*, 1675–1684. [CrossRef] [PubMed]
44. Paefgen, V.; Doleschel, D.; Kiessling, F. Evolution of Contrast Agents for Ultrasound Imaging and Ultrasound-Mediated Drug Delivery. *Front. Pharmacol.* **2015**, *6*, 197. [CrossRef] [PubMed]
45. Dietrich, C.; Averkiou, M.; Nielsen, M.; Barr, R.; Burns, P.; Calliada, F.; Cantisani, V.; Choi, B.; Chammas, M.; Clevert, D.-A.; et al. How to Perform Contrast-Enhanced Ultrasound (CEUS). *Ultrasound Int. Open* **2018**, *4*, E2–E15. [CrossRef] [PubMed]
46. Baun, J. Contrast-Enhanced Ultrasound: A Technology Primer. *J. Diagn. Med. Sonogr.* **2017**, *33*, 446–452. [CrossRef]
47. Sano, F.; Uemura, H. The Utility and Limitations of Contrast-Enhanced Ultrasound for the Diagnosis and Treatment of Prostate Cancer. *Sensors* **2015**, *15*, 4947–4957. [CrossRef] [PubMed]
48. Necas, M.; Keating, J.; Abbott, G.; Curtis, N.; Ryke, R.; Hill, G. How to set-up and perform contrast-enhanced ultrasound. *Australas. J. Ultrasound Med.* **2019**, *22*, 86–95. [CrossRef]
49. Giusti, M.; Orlandi, D.; Melle, G.; Massa, B.; Silvestri, E.; Minuto, F.; Turtulici, G. Is There a Real Diagnostic Impact of Elastosonography and Contrast-Enhanced Ultrasonography in the Management of Thyroid Nodules? *J. Zhejiang Univ. Sci. B* **2013**, *14*, 195–206. [CrossRef] [PubMed]
50. Hornung, M.; Jung, E.M.; Georgieva, M.; Schlitt, H.J.; Stroszczynski, C.; Agha, A. Detection of Microvascularization of Thyroid Carcinomas Using Linear High Resolution Contrast-Enhanced Ultrasonography (CEUS). *Clin. Hemorheol. Microcirc.* **2012**, *52*, 197–203. [CrossRef]
51. Jiang, J.; Shang, X.; Zhang, H.; Ma, W.; Xu, Y.; Zhou, Q.; Gao, Y.; Yu, S.; Qi, Y. Correlation Between Maximum Intensity and Microvessel Density for Differentiation of Malignant from Benign Thyroid Nodules on Contrast-Enhanced Sonography. *J. Ultrasound Med.* **2014**, *33*, 1257–1263. [CrossRef] [PubMed]
52. Ma, B.; Jin, Y.; Suntdar, P.S.; Zhao, H.; Jiang, Y.; Zhou, J. Contrast-Enhanced Ultrasonography Findings for Papillary Thyroid Carcinoma and Its Pathological Bases. *Sichuan Da Xue Xue Bao Yi Xue Ban* **2014**, *45*, 997–1000. [PubMed]
53. Nemec, U.; Nemec, S.F.; Novotny, C.; Weber, M.; Czerny, C.; Krestan, C.R. Quantitative Evaluation of Contrast-Enhanced Ultrasound after Intravenous Administration of a Microbubble Contrast Agent for Differentiation of Benign and Malignant Thyroid Nodules: Assessment of Diagnostic Accuracy. *Eur. Radiol.* **2012**, *22*, 1357–1365. [CrossRef] [PubMed]
54. Cantisani, V.; Consorti, F.; Guerrisi, A.; Guerrisi, I.; Ricci, P.; Segni, M.D.; Mancuso, E.; Scardella, L.; Milazzo, F.; D'Ambrosio, F.; et al. Prospective Comparative Evaluation of Quantitative-Elastosonography (Q-Elastography) and Contrast-Enhanced Ultrasound for the Evaluation of Thyroid Nodules: Preliminary Experience. *Eur. J. Radiol.* **2013**, *82*, 1892–1898. [CrossRef] [PubMed]
55. Wu, Q.; Wang, Y.; Li, Y.; Hu, B.; He, Z.-Y. Diagnostic Value of Contrast-Enhanced Ultrasound in Solid Thyroid Nodules with and without Enhancement. *Endocrine* **2016**, *53*, 480–488. [CrossRef] [PubMed]
56. Ma, X.; Zhang, B.; Ling, W.; Liu, R.; Jia, H.; Zhu, F.; Wang, M.; Liu, H.; Huang, J.; Liu, L. Contrast-enhanced Sonography for the Identification of Benign and Malignant Thyroid Nodules: Systematic Review and Meta-analysis. *J. Clin. Ultrasound* **2016**, *44*, 199–209. [CrossRef] [PubMed]
57. Zhang, B.; Jiang, Y.-X.; Liu, J.-B.; Yang, M.; Dai, Q.; Zhu, Q.-L.; Gao, P. Utility of Contrast-Enhanced Ultrasound for Evaluation of Thyroid Nodules. *Thyroid* **2010**, *20*, 51–57. [CrossRef] [PubMed]
58. Zhao, H.; Liu, X.; Lei, B.; Cheng, P.; Li, J.; Wu, Y.; Ma, Z.; Wei, F.; Su, H. Diagnostic Performance of Thyroid Imaging Reporting and Data System (TI-RADS) Alone and in Combination with Contrast-Enhanced Ultrasonography for the Characterization of Thyroid Nodules. *Clin. Hemorheol. Microcirc.* **2019**, *72*, 95–106. [CrossRef] [PubMed]
59. Zhang, Y.; Zhou, P.; Tian, S.-M.; Zhao, Y.-F.; Li, J.-L.; Li, L. Usefulness of Combined Use of Contrast-Enhanced Ultrasound and TI-RADS Classification for the Differentiation of Benign from Malignant Lesions of Thyroid Nodules. *Eur. Radiol.* **2017**, *27*, 1527–1536. [CrossRef] [PubMed]

60. Zhou, X.; Zhou, P.; Hu, Z.; Tian, S.M.; Zhao, Y.; Liu, W.; Jin, Q. Diagnostic Efficiency of Quantitative Contrast-Enhanced Ultrasound Indicators for Discriminating Benign from Malignant Solid Thyroid Nodules. *J. Ultrasound Med.* **2018**, *37*, 425–437. [CrossRef]
61. Li, F.; Zhang, J.; Wang, Y.; Liu, L. Clinical Value of Elasticity Imaging and Contrast-Enhanced Ultrasound in the Diagnosis of Papillary Thyroid Microcarcinoma. *Oncol. Lett.* **2015**, *10*, 1371–1377. [CrossRef]
62. Deng, J.; Zhou, P.; Tian, S.; Zhang, L.; Li, J.; Qian, Y. Comparison of Diagnostic Efficacy of Contrast-Enhanced Ultrasound, Acoustic Radiation Force Impulse Imaging, and Their Combined Use in Differentiating Focal Solid Thyroid Nodules. *PLoS ONE* **2014**, *9*, e90674. [CrossRef]
63. Sui, X.; Liu, H.-J.; Jia, H.-L.; Fang, Q.-M. Contrast-Enhanced Ultrasound and Real-Time Elastography in the Differential Diagnosis of Malignant and Benign Thyroid Nodules. *Exp. Ther. Med.* **2016**, *12*, 783–791. [CrossRef]
64. Hang, J.; Li, F.; Qiao, X.; Ye, X.; Li, A.; Du, L. Combination of Maximum Shear Wave Elasticity Modulus and TIRADS Improves the Diagnostic Specificity in Characterizing Thyroid Nodules: A Retrospective Study. *Int. J. Endocrinol.* **2018**, *2018*, 1–8. [CrossRef] [PubMed]
65. Cosgrove, D.; Barr, R.; Bojunga, J.; Cantisani, V.; Chammas, M.C.; Dighe, M.; Vinayak, S.; Xu, J.-M.; Dietrich, C.F. WFUMB Guidelines and Recommendations on the Clinical Use of Ultrasound Elastography: Part 4—Thyroid. *Ultrasound Med. Biol.* **2017**, *43*, 4–26. [CrossRef] [PubMed]
66. Wang, Y.; Nie, F.; Liu, T.; Yang, D.; Li, Q.; Li, J.; Song, A. Revised Value of Contrast-Enhanced Ultrasound for Solid Hypo-Echoic Thyroid Nodules Graded with the Thyroid Imaging Reporting and Data System. *Ultrasound Med. Biol.* **2018**, *44*, 930–940. [CrossRef] [PubMed]
67. Liu, Y.; Wu, H.; Zhou, Q.; Gou, J.; Xu, J.; Liu, Y.; Chen, Q. Diagnostic Value of Conventional Ultrasonography Combined with Contrast-Enhanced Ultrasonography in Thyroid Imaging Reporting and Data System (TI-RADS) 3 and 4 Thyroid Micronodules. *Med. Sci. Monit. Int. Med. J. Exp. Clin. Res.* **2016**, *22*, 3086–3094. [CrossRef] [PubMed]
68. Xu, L.; Gao, J.; Wang, Q.; Yin, J.; Yu, P.; Bai, B.; Pei, R.; Chen, D.; Yang, G.; Wang, S.; et al. Computer-Aided Diagnosis Systems in Diagnosing Malignant Thyroid Nodules on Ultrasonography: A Systematic Review and Meta-Analysis. *Eur. Thyroid J.* **2020**, *9*, 186–193. [CrossRef] [PubMed]
69. Yu, D.; Han, Y.; Chen, T. Contrast-Enhanced Ultrasound for Differentiation of Benign and Malignant Thyroid Lesions. *Otolaryngol. Head Neck Surg.* **2014**, *151*, 909–915. [CrossRef]
70. Sun, B.; Lang, L.; Zhu, X.; Jiang, F.; Hong, Y.; He, L. Accuracy of Contrast-Enhanced Ultrasound in the Identification of Thyroid Nodules: A Meta-Analysis. *Int. J. Clin. Exp. Med.* **2015**, *8*, 12882–12889. [PubMed]
71. Zhang, J.; Zhang, X.; Meng, Y.; Chen, Y. Contrast-Enhanced Ultrasound for the Differential Diagnosis of Thyroid Nodules: An Updated Meta-Analysis with Comprehensive Heterogeneity Analysis. *PLoS ONE* **2020**, *15*, e0231775. [CrossRef]
72. Mulita, F.; Anjum, F. *Thyroid Adenoma*; StatPearls 4AD: Treasure Island, FL, USA, 2021.
73. Yoon, J.H.; Kim, E.-K.; Youk, J.H.; Moon, H.J.; Kwak, J.Y. Better Understanding in the Differentiation of Thyroid Follicular Adenoma, Follicular Carcinoma, and Follicular Variant of Papillary Carcinoma: A Retrospective Study. *Int. J. Endocrinol.* **2014**, *2014*, 1–9. [CrossRef] [PubMed]
74. Duggal, R.; Rajwanshi, A.; Gupta, N.; Vasishta, R.K. Interobserver Variability amongst Cytopathologists and Histopathologists in the Diagnosis of Neoplastic Follicular Patterned Lesions of Thyroid. *Diagn. Cytopathol.* **2011**, *39*, 235–241. [CrossRef] [PubMed]
75. Schleder, S.; Janke, M.; Agha, A.; Schacherer, D.; Hornung, M.; Schlitt, H.J.; Stroszczynski, C.; Schreyer, A.G.; Jung, E.M. Preoperative Differentiation of Thyroid Adenomas and Thyroid Carcinomas Using High Resolution Contrast-Enhanced Ultrasound (CEUS). *Clin. Hemorheol. Microcirc.* **2015**, *61*, 13–22. [CrossRef] [PubMed]
76. Hegedüs, L. Thyroid ultrasound. *Endocrin. Metab. Clin.* **2001**, *30*, 339–360. [CrossRef]
77. Teng, W.; Shan, Z.; Teng, X.; Guan, H.; Li, Y.; Teng, D.; Jin, Y.; Yu, X.; Fan, C.; Chong, W.; et al. Effect of Iodine Intake on Thyroid Diseases in China. *N. Engl. J. Med.* **2006**, *354*, 2783–2793. [CrossRef]
78. Ragusa, F.; Fallahi, P.; Elia, G.; Gonnella, D.; Paparo, S.R.; Giusti, C.; Churilov, L.P.; Ferrari, S.M.; Antonelli, A. Hashimotos' Thyroiditis: Epidemiology, Pathogenesis, Clinic and Therapy. *Best Pract. Res. Clin. Endocrinol.* **2019**, *33*, 101367. [CrossRef]
79. Walsh, S.; Lowery, A.J.; Evoy, D.; McDermott, E.W.; Prichard, R.S. Thyroid Lymphoma: Recent Advances in Diagnosis and Optimal Management Strategies. *Oncologist* **2013**, *18*, 994–1003. [CrossRef]
80. Zhao, R.; Zhang, B.; Yang, X.; Jiang, Y.; Lai, X.; Zhu, S.; Zhang, X. Diagnostic Value of Contrast-Enhanced Ultrasound of Thyroid Nodules Coexisting with Hashimoto's Thyroiditis. *Zhongguo Yi Xue Ke Xue Yuan Xue Bao Acta Acad. Med. Sin.* **2015**, *37*, 66–70. [CrossRef]
81. Wei, X.; Li, Y.; Zhang, S.; Li, X.; Gao, M. Evaluation of Primary Thyroid Lymphoma by Ultrasonography Combined with Contrast-Enhanced Ultrasonography: A Pilot Study. *Indian J. Cancer* **2015**, *52*, 546–550. [CrossRef]
82. Moon, H.J.; Kwak, J.Y.; Kim, M.J.; Son, E.J.; Kim, E.-K. Can Vascularity at Power Doppler US Help Predict Thyroid Malignancy? *Radiology* **2010**, *255*, 260–269. [CrossRef] [PubMed]
83. Ito, Y.; Miyauchi, A.; Kihara, M.; Fukushima, M.; Higashiyama, T.; Miya, A. Overall Survival of Papillary Thyroid Carcinoma Patients: A Single-Institution Long-Term Follow-Up of 5897 Patients. *World J. Surg.* **2018**, *42*, 615–622. [CrossRef]
84. LiVolsi, V.A. Papillary Thyroid Carcinoma: An Update. *Mod. Pathol.* **2011**, *24* (Suppl. S2), S1–S9. [CrossRef] [PubMed]

85. Gao, L.; Xi, X.; Gao, Q.; Tang, J.; Yang, X.; Zhu, S.; Zhao, R.; Lai, X.; Zhang, X.; Zhang, B.; et al. Blood-Rich Enhancement in Ultrasonography Predicts Worse Prognosis in Patients with Papillary Thyroid Cancer. *Front. Oncol.* **2021**, *10*, 546378. [CrossRef] [PubMed]
86. Zhou, Q.; Jiang, J.; Shang, X.; Zhang, H.-L.; Ma, W.-Q.; Xu, Y.-B.; Wang, H.; Li, M. Correlation of Contrast-Enhanced Ultrasonographic Features with Microvessel Density in Papillary Thyroid Carcinomas. *Asian Pac. J. Cancer Prev.* **2014**, *15*, 7449–7452. [CrossRef]
87. Zhan, J.; Diao, X.-H.; Chen, Y.; Wang, W.-P.; Ding, H. Homogeneity Parameter in Contrast-Enhanced Ultrasound Imaging Improves the Classification of Abnormal Cervical Lymph Node after Thyroidectomy in Patients with Papillary Thyroid Carcinoma. *Biomed. Res. Int.* **2019**, *2019*, 1–8. [CrossRef]
88. Crea, C.D.; Raffaelli, M.; Sessa, L.; Ronti, S.; Fadda, G.; Bellantone, C.; Lombardi, C.P. Actual Incidence and Clinical Behaviour of Follicular Thyroid Carcinoma: An Institutional Experience. *Sci. World J.* **2014**, *2014*, 952095. [CrossRef]
89. Su, D.-H.; Chang, T.-C.; Chang, S.-H. Prognostic Factors on Outcomes of Follicular Thyroid Cancer. *J. Formos. Med. Assoc.* **2019**, *118*, 1144–1153. [CrossRef]
90. Sharma, C. Diagnostic Accuracy of Fine Needle Aspiration Cytology of Thyroid and Evaluation of Discordant Cases. *J. Egypt Natl. Cancer Inst.* **2015**, *27*, 147–153. [CrossRef]
91. Yang, G.C.H.; Fried, K.O. Most Thyroid Cancers Detected by Sonography Lack Intranodular Vascularity on Color Doppler Imaging: Review of the Literature and Sonographic-Pathologic Correlations for 698 Thyroid Neoplasms. *J. Ultrasound Med.* **2017**, *36*, 89–94. [CrossRef]
92. Iared, W.; Shigueoka, D.C.; Cristófoli, J.C.; Andriolo, R.; Atallah, A.N.; Ajzen, S.A.; Valente, O. Use of Color Doppler Ultrasonography for the Prediction of Malignancy in Follicular Thyroid Neoplasms. *J. Ultrasound Med.* **2010**, *29*, 419–425. [CrossRef]
93. Somnay, Y.; Schneider, D.; Mazeh, H. Thyroid: Medullary Carcinoma. *Atlas Genet. Cytogenet. Oncol. Haematol.* **2013**, *17*, 291–296. [CrossRef] [PubMed]
94. Gambardella, C.; Offi, C.; Patrone, R.; Clarizia, G.; Mauriello, C.; Tartaglia, E.; Capua, F.D.; Martino, S.D.; Romano, R.M.; Fiore, L.; et al. Calcitonin Negative Medullary Thyroid Carcinoma: A Challenging Diagnosis or a Medical Dilemma? *BMC Endocr. Disord.* **2019**, *19* (Suppl. S1), 45. [CrossRef] [PubMed]
95. Simões-Pereira, J.; Bugalho, M.J.; Limbert, E.; Leite, V. Retrospective Analysis of 140 Cases of Medullary Thyroid Carcinoma Followed-up in a Single Institution. *Oncol. Lett.* **2016**, *11*, 3870–3874. [CrossRef]
96. Proiti, M.; Andreano, A.; Schiaffino, S.; Turtulici, G.; Laeseke, P.; Meloni, M. Contrast-Enhanced Ultrasound of Anaplastic Thyroid Cancer: A Case Report and Review of the Literature. *Ultrasound Int. Open* **2015**, *1*, E27–E29. [CrossRef] [PubMed]
97. Nagaiah, G.; Hossain, A.; Mooney, C.J.; Parmentier, J.; Remick, S.C. Anaplastic Thyroid Cancer: A Review of Epidemiology, Pathogenesis, and Treatment. *J. Oncol.* **2011**, *2011*, 542358. [CrossRef] [PubMed]
98. Bernardi, S.; Giudici, F.; Cesareo, R.; Antonelli, G.; Cavallaro, M.; Deandrea, M.; Giusti, M.; Mormile, A.; Negro, R.; Palermo, A.; et al. Five-Year Results of Radiofrequency and Laser Ablation of Benign Thyroid Nodules: A Multicenter Study from the Italian Minimally Invasive Treatments of the Thyroid Group. *Thyroid* **2020**, *30*, 1759–1770. [CrossRef]
99. Mauri, G.; Gennaro, N.; Lee, M.K.; Baek, J.H. Laser and Radiofrequency Ablations for Benign and Malignant Thyroid Tumors. *Int. J. Hyperther.* **2019**, *36*, 13–20. [CrossRef]
100. Teng, D.-K.; Li, W.-H.; Du, J.-R.; Wang, H.; Yang, D.-Y.; Wu, X.-L. Effects of Microwave Ablation on Papillary Thyroid Microcarcinoma: A Five-Year Follow-up Report. *Thyroid* **2020**, *30*, 1752–1758. [CrossRef]
101. Yan, J.; Qiu, T.; Lu, J.; Wu, Y.; Yang, Y. Microwave Ablation Induces a Lower Systemic Stress Response in Patients than Open Surgery for Treatment of Benign Thyroid Nodules. *Int. J. Hyperther.* **2018**, *34*, 1–5. [CrossRef]
102. Trimboli, P.; Pelloni, F.; Bini, F.; Marinozzi, F.; Giovanella, L. High-Intensity Focused Ultrasound (HIFU) for Benign Thyroid Nodules: 2-Year Follow-up Results. *Endocrine* **2019**, *65*, 312–317. [CrossRef]
103. Monpeyssen, H.; Hamou, A.B.; Hegedus, L.; Ghanassia, E.; Juttet, P.; Persichetti, A.; Bizzarri, G.; Bianchini, A.; Guglielmi, R.; Raggiunti, B.; et al. High-Intensity Focused Ultrasound (HIFU) Therapy for Benign Thyroid Nodules: A 3-Year Retrospective Multicenter Follow-up Study. *Int. J. Hyperther.* **2020**, *37*, 1301–1309. [CrossRef]
104. Kim, Y.J.; Baek, J.H.; Ha, E.J.; Lim, H.K.; Lee, J.H.; Sung, J.Y.; Kim, J.K.; Kim, T.Y.; Kim, W.B.; Shong, Y.K. Cystic versus Predominantly Cystic Thyroid Nodules: Efficacy of Ethanol Ablation and Analysis of Related Factors. *Eur. Radiol.* **2012**, *22*, 1573–1578. [CrossRef] [PubMed]
105. Papini, E.; Monpeyssen, H.; Frasoldati, A.; Hegedüs, L. 2020 European Thyroid Association Clinical Practice Guideline for the Use of Image-Guided Ablation in Benign Thyroid Nodules. *Eur. Thyroid J.* **2020**, *9*, 172–185. [CrossRef] [PubMed]
106. Schiaffino, S.; Serpi, F.; Rossi, D.; Ferrara, V.; Buonomenna, C.; Alì, M.; Monfardini, L.; Sconfienza, L.M.; Mauri, G. Reproducibility of Ablated Volume Measurement Is Higher with Contrast-Enhanced Ultrasound than with B-Mode Ultrasound after Benign Thyroid Nodule Radiofrequency Ablation—A Preliminary Study. *J. Clin. Med.* **2020**, *9*, 1504. [CrossRef] [PubMed]
107. Yan, L.; Luo, Y.; Xiao, J.; Lin, L. Non-Enhanced Ultrasound Is Not a Satisfactory Modality for Measuring Necrotic Ablated Volume after Radiofrequency Ablation of Benign Thyroid Nodules: A Comparison with Contrast-Enhanced Ultrasound. *Eur. Radiol.* **2021**, *31*, 3226–3236. [CrossRef]
108. Bernardi, S.; Palermo, A.; Grasso, R.F.; Fabris, B.; Stacul, F.; Cesareo, R. Current Status and Challenges of US-Guided Radiofrequency Ablation of Thyroid Nodules in the Long Term: A Systematic Review. *Cancers* **2021**, *13*, 2746. [CrossRef]

9. Xi, X.; Gao, L.; Wu, Q.; Fang, S.; Xu, J.; Liu, R.; Yang, X.; Zhu, S.; Zhao, R.; Lai, X.; et al. Differentiation of Thyroid Nodules Difficult to Diagnose with Contrast-Enhanced Ultrasonography and Real-Time Elastography. *Front. Oncol.* **2020**, *10*, 112. [CrossRef]
10. Chen, M.; Zhang, K.-Q.; Xu, Y.-F.; Zhang, S.-M.; Cao, Y.; Sun, W.-Q. Shear Wave Elastography and Contrast-Enhanced Ultrasonography in the Diagnosis of Thyroid Malignant Nodules. *Mol. Clin. Oncol.* **2016**, *5*, 724–730. [CrossRef]
11. Peng, S.; Liu, Y.; Lv, W.; Liu, L.; Zhou, Q.; Yang, H.; Ren, J.; Liu, G.; Wang, X.; Zhang, X.; et al. Deep Learning-Based Artificial Intelligence Model to Assist Thyroid Nodule Diagnosis and Management: A Multicentre Diagnostic Study. *Lancet Digit. Health* **2021**, *3*, e250–e259. [CrossRef]
12. Buda, M.; Wildman-Tobriner, B.; Hoang, J.K.; Thayer, D.; Tessler, F.N.; Middleton, W.D.; Mazurowski, M.A. Management of Thyroid Nodules Seen on US Images: Deep Learning May Match Performance of Radiologists. *Radiology* **2019**, *292*, 181343. [CrossRef] [PubMed]
13. Wu, G.-G.; Lv, W.-Z.; Yin, R.; Xu, J.-W.; Yan, Y.-J.; Chen, R.-X.; Wang, J.-Y.; Zhang, B.; Cui, X.-W.; Dietrich, C.F. Deep Learning Based on ACR TI-RADS Can Improve the Differential Diagnosis of Thyroid Nodules. *Front. Oncol.* **2021**, *11*, 575166. [CrossRef]

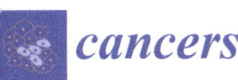

Article

Exploring the Performance of Ultrasound Risk Stratification Systems in Thyroid Nodules of Pediatric Patients

Lorenzo Scappaticcio [1,*], Maria Ida Maiorino [1], Sergio Iorio [1], Giovanni Docimo [2], Miriam Longo [1], Anna Grandone [3], Caterina Luongo [3], Immacolata Cozzolino [4], Arnoldo Piccardo [5], Pierpaolo Trimboli [6], Emanuele Miraglia Del Giudice [3], Katherine Esposito [7] and Giuseppe Bellastella [1]

[1] Division of Endocrinology and Metabolic Diseases, University of Campania "L. Vanvitelli", 80138 Naples, Italy; mariaida.maiorino@unicampania.it (M.I.M.); sergio.iorio@unicampania.it (S.I.); miriam.longo@unicampania.it (M.L.); giuseppe.bellastella@unicampania.it (G.B.)
[2] Division of Thyroid Surgery, University of Campania "L. Vanvitelli", 80138 Naples, Italy; giovanni.docimo@unicampania.it
[3] Department of Woman, Child, General and Specialized Surgery, University of Campania "L. Vanvitelli", 80138 Naples, Italy; anna.grandone@unicampania.it (A.G.); caterina.luongo@unicampania.it (C.L.); emanuele.miragliadelgiudice@unicampania.it (E.M.D.G.)
[4] Pathology Unit, Department of Mental and Physical Health and Preventive Medicine, University of Campania "L. Vanvitelli", 80138 Naples, Italy; immacolata.cozzolino@unicampania.it
[5] Department of Nuclear Medicine, E.O. Ospedali Galliera, 16128 Genoa, Italy; arnoldo.piccardo@galliera.it
[6] Clinic for Endocrinology and Diabetology, Regional Hospital of Lugano, Ente Ospedaliero Cantonale, 6900 Lugano, Switzerland; pierpaolo.trimboli@eoc.ch
[7] Department of Medical and Advanced Surgical Sciences, University of Campania "L. Vanvitelli", 80138 Naples, Italy; katherine.esposito@unicampania.it
* Correspondence: lorenzo.scappaticcio@unicampania.it; Tel.: +39-3293154461

Citation: Scappaticcio, L.; Maiorino, M.I.; Iorio, S.; Docimo, G.; Longo, M.; Grandone, A.; Luongo, C.; Cozzolino, I.; Piccardo, A.; Trimboli, P.; et al. Exploring the Performance of Ultrasound Risk Stratification Systems in Thyroid Nodules of Pediatric Patients. *Cancers* **2021**, *13*, 5304. https://doi.org/10.3390/cancers13215304

Academic Editors: Kennichi Kakudo, Barbara Jarzab and Amedeo Columbano

Received: 28 August 2021
Accepted: 20 October 2021
Published: 22 October 2021

Publisher's Note: MDPI stays neutral with regard to jurisdictional claims in published maps and institutional affiliations.

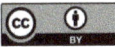

Copyright: © 2021 by the authors. Licensee MDPI, Basel, Switzerland. This article is an open access article distributed under the terms and conditions of the Creative Commons Attribution (CC BY) license (https://creativecommons.org/licenses/by/4.0/).

Simple Summary: Although pediatric thyroid nodules are uncommon, they need high clinical expertise and alert since they carry a greater risk of malignancy compared with those presenting in adults. Since there are no specific ultrasound (US)-based risk stratification systems (RSSs) for pediatric thyroid nodules, the application of adult-based RSSs in the pediatric population could represent a step forward in the care of children and adolescents with thyroid nodules. We compared the diagnostic performance of the main US-based RSSs *i.e., the American College of Radiology (ACR), European (EU), Korean (K) Thyroid Imaging Reporting and Data Systems (TI-RADSs) and ATA US RSS criteria) for detecting malignant thyroid lesions in pediatric patients. For ACR TI-RADS and EU-TIRADS, we found a sensitivity of 41.7%, and, for K-TIRADS and ATA US RSS, we found a sensitivity of 50%. The four US-based RSSs (i.e., ACR-TIRADS, EU-TIRADS, K-TIRADS, and ATA US RSS) have suboptimal performance in managing pediatric patients with thyroid nodules, with one-half of cancers without indication for FNA according to their recommendations. All thyroidologists, as well as the panelists of next TIRADSs, should be aware of these findings.

Abstract: Neck ultrasound (nUS) is the cornerstone of clinical management of thyroid nodules in pediatric patients, as well as adults. The current study was carried out to explore and compare the diagnostic performance of the main US-based risk stratification systems (RSSs) (i.e., the American College of Radiology (ACR), European (EU), Korean (K) TI-RADSs and ATA US RSS criteria) for detecting malignant thyroid lesions in pediatric patients. We conducted a retrospective analysis of consecutive children and adolescents who received a diagnosis of thyroid nodule. We included subjects with age <19 years having thyroid nodules with benign cytology/histology or final histological diagnosis. We excluded subjects with (a) a previous malignancy, (b) a history of radiation exposure, (c) cancer genetic susceptibility syndromes, (d) lymph nodes suspicious for metastases of thyroid cancer at nUS, (e) a family history of thyroid cancer, or (f) cytologically indeterminate nodules without histology and nodules with inadequate cytology. We included 41 nodules in 36 patients with median age 15 years (11–17 years). Of the 41 thyroid nodules, 29 (70.7%) were benign and 12 (29.3%) were malignant. For both ACR TI-RADS and EU-TIRADS, we found a sensitivity of 41.7%. Instead, for both K-TIRADS and ATA US RSS, we found a sensitivity of 50%. The missed malignancy rate for ACR-TIRADS and EU-TIRADS was 58.3%, while that for K-TIRADS and ATA US RSS was 50%. The unnecessary FNA prevalence for ACR TI-RADS and EU-TIRADS was 58.3%, while that for K-TIRADS and ATA US RSS was 76%. Our findings suggest that the four US-based RSSs (i.e., ACR-TIRADS, EU-TIRADS, K-TIRADS, and ATA US RSS) have suboptimal performance in managing pediatric patients with thyroid nodules, with one-half of cancers without indication for FNA according to their recommendations.

Keywords: pediatric thyroid nodules; neck ultrasound

1. Introduction

Compared with those of adults, pediatric thyroid nodules have molecular and pathological peculiarities that promoted the development of unique pediatric guidelines [1–3]. The prevalence of ultrasound-detected thyroid nodules varies from 0.5% [4] to 1.6% [5] in the child population. Although pediatric thyroid nodules are uncommon, they need high clinical expertise and alert since they carry a greater risk of malignancy compared with those presenting in adults (22–26% versus 5–10%) [1,6,7]. Moreover, children with thyroid cancer are more likely than adults to have cervical lymph node metastases, extrathyroidal extension, and pulmonary metastases at the time of diagnosis, as well as persistence/recurrence of disease [1].

Neck ultrasound (nUS) is the cornerstone of the clinical management of thyroid nodule in pediatric patients, as well as adults [8–12]. According to the American Thyroid Association (ATA) guidelines [1], sonographic evaluation of thyroid nodules in children should be modeled on 2009 ATA guidelines for adults [13]. However, when exploring thyroid nodules at nUS in childhood, some peculiar aspects should be kept in mind: first, the fact that the size is a rather questionable parameter in children because thyroid volume changes with age; second, increased intranodular vascularity is apparently more common in malignant nodules; third, a diffusely infiltrative form of papillary thyroid cancer (PTC) is relatively frequent; fourth, the clinical context is of paramount importance when interpreting sonographic features [1,14,15].

US-based risk stratification systems (RSSs), often referred to as Thyroid Imaging Reporting and Data Systems (TIRADSs), have been developed to establish a standard lexicon to describe thyroid nodules, to associate nodules with a malignancy risk class, and to detect malignant nodules requiring fine-needle aspiration (FNA) [16]. RSSs mainly apply to PTC [17], since they have a lower performance in the detection of follicular thyroid carcinoma [18], medullary thyroid carcinoma [19,20], anaplastic thyroid carcinoma [21], and autonomously functioning thyroid nodules [22]. Moreover, RSSs have been extensively validated in the adult population [23], but not in children [24] and older adults [25]. Yet, the clinical context of patients is not considered in RSSs, and whether a patient's age can modify their reliability is a matter of debate [25].

Since single thyroid US features are not highly accurate predictors of benign or malignant etiology of thyroid nodules in children, and specific RSSs for pediatric thyroid nodules are lacking, the application of adult-based RSSs in the pediatric population could represent a step forward in the care of children and adolescents with thyroid nodules [6,8]. Specifically, exploring the reliability of RSSs in the management of pediatric nodules could serve to create standardized diagnostic algorithms for childhood aimed at increasing our ability to detect thyroid cancer early.

To our knowledge, few studies [11,24] evaluated the diagnostic performance of RSSs in malignancy risk stratification of pediatric thyroid nodules with discordant results, and further studies on this topic are mandatory [24].

Therefore, the current study was carried out to explore and compare the diagnostic performance of the main RSSs (i.e., the American College of Radiology (ACR) [26], European (EU) [27], Korean (K) [28] TI-RADSs and ATA US RSS criteria [29]) for detecting malignant thyroid lesions in pediatric patients, in terms of risk stratification and reliability in the indication for FNA.

2. Materials and Methods

2.1. Study Design and Patients

In the current study, the Standards for Reporting Diagnostic Accuracy (STARD) statement was followed [30]. Specifically, we conducted a retrospective analysis of consecutive children and adolescents who received a diagnosis of thyroid nodule at a single referral center (i.e., Division of Endocrinology and Metabolic Diseases, University of Campania "L. Vanvitelli"—Naples, Italy) from January 2017 to March 2021. We gathered information (i.e., demographic, laboratory, imaging, and pathological details) from medical records included in the hospital database of pediatric patients referred to our multidisciplinary team since they developed clinical manifestations suspicious for hypothyroidism or thyrotoxicosis or were investigated for palpable thyroid nodules.

Subjects fulfilling the following criteria were enrolled in the current study: (a) age <19 years; (b) thyroid nodule(s) with benign cytology/histology or final histological diagnosis (i.e., benignity or malignancy); (c) complete data (i.e., hormonal and antibodies profile including serum calcitonin; at least two clear B-Mode US images for each nodule).

Patients were excluded if they had (a) a previous malignancy, (b) a history of radiation exposure, (c) cancer genetic susceptibility syndromes, (d) lymph nodes suspicious for metastases of thyroid cancer at nUS, (e) a family history of thyroid cancer (i.e., at least one relative), or (f) cytologically indeterminate nodules without histology and nodules showing inadequate cytology.

The Ethics Committee of the University Hospital "L. Vanvitelli" (Naples, Italy) approved the study, and written consent was obtained from all the participants.

2.2. Thyroid Ultrasonography

Thyroid ultrasonography was performed by the same experienced operator (S.I.) using an ultrasound device (MyLab^{TM}Six, Esaote) with a 7–14 MHz wide-band linear transducer. The color gain was adjusted so that artefacts were prevented. The examination of ultrasonographic features of thyroid nodules, along with thyroid vascularity and volume, were systematically conducted for patients presenting for thyroid assessment to our division.

In the current study, US images were reviewed, and ACR-TIRADS, EU-TIRADS, K-TIRADS, and ATA US RSS criteria were applied to each nodule for categorization separately by two experienced thyroidologists (L.S., G.B.) who were unaware of the nodule's cytopathology and histopathology, as well as of laboratory and imaging results. In the case of discordant US categorization, a consensus with the help of a third reviewer (P.T.) (also unaware of pathology or any other patient data) was reached.

2.3. Thyroid Nodule Pathology

In the Division of Anatomic Pathology of our institution, all FNAs were reported according to the revised Italian Consensus for the Classification and Reporting of Thyroid Cytology [31] and the final pathology (i.e., histology of the thyroid nodule after surgery) according to the World Health Organization (WHO) book on endocrine tumor classification [32]. For our pediatric thyroid nodules, benignity at cytological or histological exam and malignancy at histopathology were reference standard for the calculation of the diagnostic performance of US RSSs. Indication to perform FNA of thyroid nodules was made by the clinician (i.e., endocrinologist or pediatrician) according to US features, laboratory, other imaging (i.e., scintigraphy, if necessary), individual risk of malignancy, and patient/family preference. Indeterminate nodules at cytology often underwent surgery, or they were followed up on the basis of in-house molecular testing results, US features, and patient/family preference.

2.4. Statistical Analysis

Continuous variables were described as median and interquartile range (IQR). Categorical variables were presented as number (percentage). The diagnostic performance of the main RSSs was expressed through predictivity tests (i.e., sensitivity, specificity, positive (PPV) and negative (NPV) predictive value, and accuracy, with specific 95% confidence intervals), which were calculated according to Galen and Gambino [33], and the unnecessary FNA prevalence, defined as the number of benign nodules among the FNA-required nodules. Specifically, we employed assessments of malignant versus benign nodules in order to be able to report the estimates of accuracy on a lesion basis.

The interobserver agreement was evaluated by Cohen's kappa statistic, where the kappa value (k) denotes the strength of agreement and is interpreted as follows: 0–0.2, poor; 0.2–0.4, fair; 0.4–0.6, moderate; 0.6–0.8, good; 0.8–1.0 very good. Statistical significance was defined as a p-value < 0.05. Statistical analysis was performed by MedCalc software version 9 (Mariakerke, Belgium).

3. Results

There were 81 thyroid nodules in 71 patients undergoing both nUS and FNA in the initial database. After applying our exclusion criteria, in our study, we finally included 41 nodules in 36 patients (Figure 1). Twenty-six patients were female (72.2%), and ten patients were male (27.8%). Median age was 15 years (11–17 years), with the final cohort including 12 prepubertal and 24 postpubertal patients. The nUS indication was the following: autoimmune chronic thyroiditis (±hypothyroidism) in 17 patients (47.2%); excluding thyroid disease in nine patients (25.0%); palpable thyroid nodules (±goiter) in six patients (16.7%); Graves' hyperthyroidism in four patients (11.1%). Among the 36 patients, 28 (77.8%) had a solitary thyroid nodule, and eight patients (22.2%) had multiple thyroid nodules. The median nodule's maximal dimension was 13 mm (10–16 mm). Of the 41 thyroid nodules, 29 (70.7%) were benign (of which six (20.7%) underwent surgery) and 12 (29.3%) were malignant. Serum calcitonin was negative in all cases.

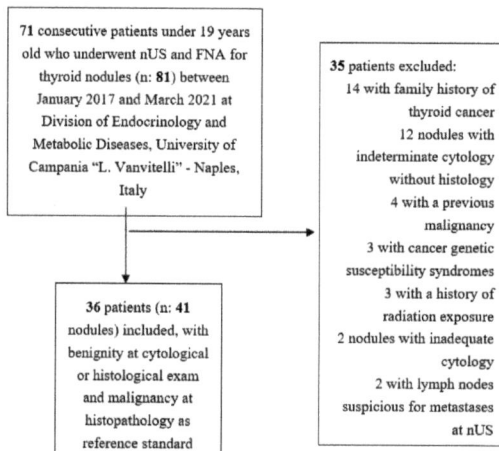

Figure 1. Flowchart of patient selection. nUS, neck ultrasound; FNA, fine-needle aspiration.

Most cancers were papillary carcinoma (10 (83.3%) of 12, nine conventional variants, including one multifocal and one follicular variant), followed by follicular carcinoma (two (16.7%) of 12). Median maximal dimension of malignant thyroid nodules was 10 mm (7–13). The characteristics of our patients are shown in Table 1.

Table 1. Main characteristics of our patients (n = 36).

Characteristics	
Age at diagnosis, years (IQR)	15 (11–17)
Females/males (n)	26/10
Reasons to perform nUS	
• autoimmune chronic thyroiditis, n (%)	17 (47.2)
• no thyroid disease, n (%)	9 (25)
• palpable thyroid nodules, n (%)	6 (16.7)
• Graves' hyperthyroidism, n (%)	4 (11.1)
Nodules	
• maximal dimension, mm (IQR)	13 (10–16)
• solitary, n (%)	28 (77.8)
• multiple, n (%)	8 (22.2)
Benign nodules/malignant nodules, n (%)	29/12 (70.7/29.3)
• benign with surgery Malignant nodules,	6/29 (20.7)
• maximal dimension, mm (IQR)	10 (7–13)
• PTC, n (%)	10 (83.3)
• FTC, n (%)	2 (16.7)

IQR, interquartile range; nUS, neck ultrasound; mm, millimeter; PTC, papillary thyroid cancer; FTC, follicular thyroid cancer.

The distribution of thyroid nodules according to the ACR-TIRADS, EU-TIRADS, K-TIRADS, and ATA US RSS risk levels is summarized in Table 2. The highest number of nodules (16 of 41 nodules) fell into the intermediate-risk category (i.e., TR4, EU-TIRADS 4, K-TIRADS 4, intermediate suspicion). A 100% cancer prevalence was observed in the high-risk class (i.e., TR5, EU-TIRADS 5, K-TIRADS 5, high suspicion). While 6/12 (50%) of cancers were assessed by the highest-risk category (i.e., TR5, EU-TIRADS 5, K-TIRADS 5, high suspicion), the remaining half were classified as at low or intermediate risk in all US RSSs.

Table 3 shows the recommended management of nodules in this cohort based on the ACR-TIRADS, EU-TIRADS, K-TIRADS, and ATA US RSS criteria. Among 29 benign nodules, according to ACR TI-RADS and EU-TIRADS criteria, seven (24.1%) would have undergone FNA, while 22 (75.9%) would have been followed up without FNA. Instead, among 29 benign nodules, according to K-TIRADS and ATA US RSS criteria, 19 (65.5%) would have undergone FNA, while 10 (34.5%) would have been followed up without FNA. According to the ACR TI-RADS and EU-TIRADS criteria, five (41.7%) of the 12 malignant nodules would have undergone FNA, and seven (58.3%) would have been assigned follow-up without FNA. According to the K-TIRADS and ATA US RSS criteria, six (50%) of the 12 malignant nodules would have undergone FNA, and six (50%) would have been assigned follow-up without FNA. The unnecessary FNA prevalence for ACR TI-RADS and EU-TIRADS was 58.3%, while that for K-TIRADS and ATA US RSS was 76%.

Table 4 resumes the reliability of the four RRSs in correctly indicating FNA. Specifically, for ACR TI-RADS and EU-TIRADS, we found the following results: sensitivity 41.7%, specificity 75.9%, PPV 41.7%, NPV 75.9%, and accuracy 65.9%. Instead, for K-TIRADS and ATA US RSS, we found the following results: sensitivity 50%, specificity 34.5%, PPV 24%, NPV 62.5%, and accuracy 39%. The interobserver agreement in classifying nodules according to ACR-TIRADS, EU-TIRADS, K-TIRADS, and ATA US RSS was good with k-values of 0.7, 0.61, 0.66, and 0.62, respectively ($p \leq 0.002$ in all cases).

Table 2. Distribution of 41 thyroid nodules according to the ACR-TIRADS, EU-TIRADS, K-TIRADS, and ATA US RSS risk levels in 36 patients in our cohort.

ACR-TIRADS	Benign Nodules (n)	Malignant Nodules (n)	Total Nodules (n)	Cancer Prevalence (%)
• TR1	4	0	4	0
• TR2	4	1	5	20
• TR3	7	3	10	30
• TR4	14	2	16	12.5
• TR5	0	6	6	100
EU-TIRADS				
• 2	7	1	8	12.5
• 3	8	3	11	27.3
• 4	14	2	16	12.5
• 5	0	6	6	100
K-TIRADS				
• 2	7	1	8	12.5
• 3	8	3	11	27.3
• 4	14	2	16	12.5
• 5	0	6	6	100
ATA US RSS				
• benign	0	0	0	0
• very low suspicion	5	0	5	0
• low suspicion	10	4	14	28.6
• intermediate suspicion	14	2	16	12.5
• high suspicion	0	6	6	100

TIRADS, Thyroid Imaging Reporting and Data System; US RSS, ultrasound-based risk stratification system; ACR, American College of Radiology; EU, European; K, Korean; ATA, American Thyroid Association.

Table 3. Management of 41 thyroid nodules according to the the ACR-TIRADS, EU-TIRADS, K-TIRADS, and ATA US RSS criteria in 36 patients in our cohort.

Management Per ACR TIRADS Criteria	Benign Nodules (n)	Malignant Nodules (n)	Total Nodules (n)	Cancer Prevalence (%)	Unnecessary FNA Prevalence (%)
• FNA	7	5	12	41.7	58.3
• Follow-up/no FNA	22	7	29	24.1	
Management per EU-TIRADS criteria					
• FNA	7	5	12	41.7	58.3
• Follow-up/no FNA	22	7	29	24.1	
Management per K-TIRADS criteria					
• FNA	19	6	25	24	76
• Follow-up/no FNA	10	6	16	37.5	
Management per ATA US RSS criteria					
• FNA	19	6	25	24	76
• Follow-up/no FNA	10	6	16	37.5	

TIRADS, Thyroid Imaging Reporting and Data System; US RSS, ultrasound-based risk stratification system; ACR, American College of Radiology; EU, European; K, Korean; ATA, American Thyroid Association; FNA, fine-needle aspiration. The unnecessary FNA prevalence for the diagnosis of thyroid cancer was defined as the number of benign nodules among the FNA-required nodules.

Table 4. Reliability of the ACR-TIRADS, EU-TIRADS, K-TIRADS, and ATA US RSS in correctly indicating FNA in 41 nodules of 36 patients in our cohort.

	Sensitivity (%) (CI)	Specificity (%) (CI)	PPV (%) (CI)	NPV (%) (CI)	Accuracy (%)
ACR TIRADS	41.7 (27–58)	75.9 (60–87)	41.7 (27–58)	75.9 (60–87)	65.9
EU-TIRADS	41.7 (27–58)	75.9 (60–87)	41.7 (60–87)	75.9 (60–87)	65.9
K-TIRADS	50.0 (32–68)	34.5 (0.3–14)	24.0 (11–43)	62.5 (0.3–14)	39.0
ATA US RSS	50.0 (32–68)	34.5 (0.3–14)	24.0 (11–43)	62.5 (0.3–14)	39.0

TIRADS, Thyroid Imaging Reporting and Data System; US RSS, ultrasound-based risk stratification system; ACR, American College of Radiology; EU, European; K, Korean; ATA, American Thyroid Association; FNA, fine-needle aspiration; PPV, positive predictive value; NPV, negative predictive value; CI, 95% confidence interval.

The clinical and US characteristics of malignant nodules that would not have undergone FNA according to the RSSs are presented in Table 5. Six nodules (ID 1, 2, 4, 5, 6, and 7) would not have been identified using the four RSSs at initial visit, while one nodule (ID 3) would have undergone FNA according to K-TIRADS and ATA US RSS but not according to ACR-TIRADS and EU-TIRADS criteria. The median maximal dimension of these seven malignant nodules was 10 mm (7–12 mm). Five of the seven nodules were solitary. These were papillary carcinoma in five cases (four with conventional variant, including one multifocal and one follicular variant) and follicular carcinoma in two cases.

Table 5. Clinical and US characteristics of proven malignancies not identified with the RSSs (ACR-TIRADS, EU-TIRADS, K-TIRADS, and ATA US RSS).

ID	Age (Years)	Gender	Number	Location	Composition	Echogenicity	Taller Than Wide	Margin	Echogenic Foci	Maximum Dimension (mm)	TI-RADS Risk Level	Cytology	Histology	Preexisting Thyroid Disease
1	17	F	single	lower left pole	solid	hypoechoic	no	ill-defined	punctate	7	TR5, EU5, K5, High	TIR4	mCPTC	no
2	15	M	multiple	mid right lobe	solid	isoechoic	no	smooth	no	10	TR3, EU3, K3, Low	TIR5	CPTC	no
3	18	F	single	isthmus	solid	hypoechoic	no	smooth	no	13	TR4, EU4	TIR3A	FV-PTC	ACT
4	17	F	single	upper right lobe	mixed cystic and solid	isoechoic	no	smooth	no	7	TR2, EU2, K2, Low	TIR5	CPTC	GD
5	7	M	multiple	mid right lobe	solid	isoechoic	no	smooth	no	10	TR3, EU3, K3, Low	TIR3B	FTC	ACT
6	12	M	single	upper left lobe	solid	isoechoic	no	smooth	no	12	TR3, EU3, K3, Low	TIR3B	FTC	ACT
7	13	F	single	upper right lobe	solid	hypoechoic	no	ill-defined	punctate	7	TR5, EU5, K5, High	TIR5	CPTC	ACT

TIRADS, Thyroid Imaging Reporting and Data System; US RSS, ultrasound-based risk stratification system; ACR, American College of Radiology; EU, European; K, Korean; ATA, American Thyroid Association; FNA, fine-needle aspiration; mCPTC, multifocal conventional papillary thyroid cancer; CPTC, conventional papillary thyroid cancer; ACT, autoimmune chronic thyroiditis; FV-PTC, follicular variant of papillary thyroid cancer; GD, Graves' disease; FTC, follicular thyroid cancer.

4. Discussion

4.1. Principal Findings

In our final pediatric cohort, we found a malignancy rate (nearly 30%) similar to that reported in previous studies of children and higher than that associated with thyroid nodules in adults [1,6,7]. The risk of malignancy was highest for the high-risk levels of all four RSSs (i.e., TR5, EU-TIRADS 5, K-TIRADS 5, high suspicion) with 100% concordance between the US-based high-risk level and cancer. This finding was roughly in line with the adult-based estimated risk of malignancy reported in the four RSSs (i.e., >20% ACR-TIRADS, 26–87% EU-TIRADS, >60% K-TIRADS, and >20% ATA US RSS) [26–29]. Likewise, regarding the intermediate-risk level (i.e., TR4, EU-TIRADS 4, K-TIRADS 4, intermediate suspiscion), we found that the malignancy rate of 12.5% for all four RSSs was comparable to that reported in adults (i.e., 5–20% ACR-TIRADS, 6–17% EU-TIRADS, 15–50% K-TIRADS, and 10–20% ATA US RSS) [26–29]. Conversely, we found a risk of malignancy of about 30% associated with low-risk levels of all four RSSs (i.e., TR3, EU-TIRADS 3, K-TIRADS 3, low suspicion), which was relevant to and higher than that reported in adults (i.e., 5% ACR-TIRADS, 2–4% EU-TIRADS, 3–15% K-TIRADS, and 5–10% ATA US RSS) [26–29]. Moreover, a non-negligible risk of malignancy of 12.5–20% was associated with not suspicious/benign risk levels for ACR-TIRADS, EU-TIRADS, and K-TIRADS (i.e., TR2, EU-TIRADS 2, K-TIRADS 2), which was higher than the rates of adults (i.e., <2% ACR-TIRADS, 0% EU-TIRADS, and 1–3% K-TIRADS) [26–29]. All this means that, compared to thyroid nodules in adults, the probability of finding cancer in high- and intermediate-risk levels of the four RSSs (i.e., ACR-TIRADS, EU-TIRADS, K-TIRADS, and ATA US RSS) remains high and is not negligible for not suspicious/benign risk levels per ACR-TIRADS, EU-TIRADS, and K-TIRADS. These results are in line with what emerged in large studies by Richman et al. [34], Lee et al. [35], and Martinez-Rios et al. [36], where a significant number of malignant nodules fell in low-risk RSS categories.

While the majority of cancers (8/12, 66.7%) in our study fell within high- and intermediate-risk categories per all the four RSSs, as resumed in Table 5, six of the 12 cancers (50%) would not have undergone FNA at the initial visit according to all the four RSSs. One more cancer (ID 3) with a maximum dimension of 13 mm and intermediate-risk category would not have undergone FNA according to ACR-TIRADS and EU-TIRADS criteria. Two PTCs scored as high-risk lesions per all four RSSs would not have undergone FNA since they were 7 mm of maximum dimension. One PTC (ID 2) and the two FTCs (ID 5, ID 6) of the present cohort were scored as low-risk lesions, and, because of their size (<15 mm), FNA would have not been indicated per all four RSSs. The remaining PTC (ID 4) with maximum dimension <20 mm (i.e., 7 mm) fell within the not suspicious/benign risk categories per ACR-TIRADS, EU-TIRADS, and K-TIRADS (i.e., TR2, EU-TIRADS 2, K-TIRADS 2) and low-risk category per ATA US RSS; thus, it would not have undergone FNA.

Therefore, a high missed malignancy rate (~50%) was found in our study when using ACR-TIRADS, EU-TIRADS, K-TIRADS, and ATA US RSS. This result is conceptually comparable to what was reported by the largest study by Richman et al. [34], who found a 22.1% of missed malignancy rate applying ACR-TIRADS, and by Lee et al. [35], who found a 19.2% of missed malignancy rate applying K-TIRADS in the group without risk factors. This issue likely implies that the current RSSs (i.e., ACR-TIRADS, EU-TIRADS, K-TIRADS, and ATA US RSS) are likely inadequate for guiding FNA of thyroid nodules in patients younger than 19 years old. In this regard, as already shown for thyroid nodules in adults [19,20], we can hypothesize that the presence of two FTC cases in our pediatric cohort would also have increased the missed malignancy rate and, thus, decreased the overall ability of the four RSSs in detecting malignant nodules. Although a direct comparison with the adult population is somewhat difficult because the missed malignancy rate is largely influenced by the proportion of malignant nodules, we found the missed malignancy rate for the four RSSs to be significantly higher than that reported in the literature relative to adult patients (i.e., 2.2–9.5%) [24,37]. While this evidence may be acceptable for adult with thyroid nodules where US-based risk stratification systems are now mainly applied to detect clinically important cancers and to avoid waste of resources (conservative approach), this may not be applied in children and adolescents where the first aim should consist of early detection of malignant nodules.

One other parameter underlying the diagnostic performance of RSSs is represented by the unnecessary FNA rate. For management of thyroid nodules in children and adolescents, this parameter could be less important to improve, as the primary objective is detecting malignancy. However, we found higher unnecessary FNA rates (i.e., almost 60% for ACR-TIRADS and EU-TIRADS, and almost 80% for K-TIRADS and ATA US RSS) than recently reported by Kim et al. [38] for adults (pooled unnecessary FNA rates of ACR-TIRADS, EU-TIRADS, K-TIRADS, and ATA were 25%, 38%, 55%, and 51%, respectively). The higher unnecessary FNA rates of K-TIRADS/ATA US RSS than ACR-TIRADS/EU-TIRADS could also be due to the lower cutoffs for FNA associated with intermediate- and low-risk categories (i.e., 10 mm and 15 mm, respectively, compared to 15 and 20–25 mm of ACR-TIRADS and EU-TIRADS) [26–29].

In our cohort, the overall accuracy of the four RSSs in correctly indicating FNA was quite poor (i.e., ~66% for ACR-TIRADS and EU-TIRADS, ~40% for K-TIRADS and ATA US RSS). In particular, sensitivity values (i.e., 40–50%), although slightly higher for K-TIRADS and ATA US RSS, were inadequate to properly detect malignancy in this context, and they were significantly lower than that reported in adults (74% ACR-TIRADS, 54% EU-TIRADS, 86% K-TIRADS, and 87% ATA US RSS) [23].

All this suggests that, on the one hand, the four RSSs had an excellent yield in high-risk US nodules but, on the other hand, they should be appropriately modified to detect the best number of malignancies in children.

4.2. Strengths and Weaknesses

The strengths of our study are the following: (1) to our knowledge, this is the first comparative study regarding diagnostic performance of the four most used RSSs for detecting malignant thyroid lesions in pediatric patients; (2) in comparison with the largest study to date by Richman et al. [31], this study mainly provides data for the management of small thyroid nodules and cancers (the median nodule's maximal dimension was 13 mm, and the median maximal dimension of malignant thyroid nodules was 10 mm). The limitations of our study should also be discussed. This was a small and monocentric cohort. However, we strictly selected the cohort by excluding patients with apparent risk factors of malignancy, so that our results could be mainly applied to the majority of children and adolescents with sporadic thyroid cancer. Although we included patients with preexisting autoimmune thyroid disease, the putative role of the autoimmune background in the development of thyroid cancer in childhood is inconclusive to date [39,40]. This is a retrospective review of static US images which could result in inherent selection bias by the reviewers. However, interobserver agreement in scoring nodules according to all four RSSs was good. Patients with benign cytology could undergo surgical resection in the future, altering the current results of the current study. However, one-fifth of our benign cases received surgery and had histological confirmation. Since we did not have complete data on nUS relative to the vascularity of thyroid nodules, we could not assess this feature and score our nodules according to AACE/ACE/AME US RSS [41]. Our results mainly refer to PTC without apparent risk factors.

5. Conclusions

Our findings suggest that the four US-based RSSs (i.e., ACR-TIRADS, EU-TIRADS, K-TIRADS, and ATA US RSS) have suboptimal performance in managing pediatric patients with thyroid nodules, with one-half of cancers being without indication for FNA according to their recommendations. All thyroidologists, endocrinologists, and radiologists, as well as panelists of later TIRADSs, should be aware of these findings [42].

Author Contributions: Conceptualization, P.T. and L.S.; methodology, L.S. and P.T.; validation, L.S., M.L., C.L., A.P., P.T., G.B. and M.I.M.; formal analysis, L.S. and P.T.; investigation, L.S., resources, S.I., L.S., G.B., A.G. and I.C.; data curation, L.S.; writing—original draft preparation, L.S., P.T., G.B. and M.I.M.; writing—review and editing, L.S., P.T., G.B. and M.I.M.; supervision, G.D., E.M.D.G. and K.E.; project administration, L.S.; funding acquisition, K.E. All authors have read and agreed to the published version of the manuscript.

Funding: This research received no external funding.

Institutional Review Board Statement: The study was conducted according to the guidelines of the Declaration of Helsinki and approved by the Institutional Review Board (or Ethics Committee) of University Hospital "L. Vanvitelli" (Naples, Italy) (ethic code: 0028728/i approved date: 7 October 2021).

Informed Consent Statement: Informed consent was obtained from all subjects involved in the study.

Data Availability Statement: The data presented in this study are available on request from the corresponding author.

Conflicts of Interest: The authors declare no conflict of interest.

References

1. Francis, G.L.; Waguespack, S.G.; Bauer, A.J.; Angelos, P.; Benvenga, S.; Cerutti, J.M.; Dinauer, C.A.; Hamilton, J.; Hay, I.D.; Luster, M.; et al. Management guidelines for children with thyroid nodules and differentiated thyroid cancer. *Thyroid* **2015**, *25*, 716–759. [CrossRef]
2. Lebbink, C.A.; Dekker, B.L.; Bocca, G.; Braat, A.; Derikx, J.; Dierselhuis, M.P.; de Keizer, B.; Kruijff, S.; Kwast, A.; van Nederveen, F.; et al. New national recommendations for the treatment of pediatric differentiated thyroid carcinoma in The Netherlands. *Eur. J. Endocrinol.* **2020**, *183*, P11–P18. [CrossRef] [PubMed]
3. Niedziela, M.; Handkiewicz-Junak, D.; Małecka-Tendera, E.; Czarniecka, A.; Dedecjus, M.; Lange, D.; Kucharska, A.; Gawlik, A.; Pomorski, L.; Włoch, J. Diagnostics and treatment of differentiated thyroid carcinoma in children—Guidelines of Polish National Societies. *Endokrynol. Polska* **2016**, *67*, 628–642. [CrossRef] [PubMed]
4. Aghini-Lombardi, F.; Antonangeli, L.; Martino, E.; Vitti, P.; Maccherini, D.; Leoli, F.; Rago, T.; Grasso, L.; Valeriano, R.; Balestrieri, A.; et al. The spectrum of thyroid disorders in an iodine-deficient community: The Pescopagano survey. *J. Clin. Endocrinol. Metab.* **1999**, *84*, 561–566. [CrossRef]
5. Taniguchi, N.; Hayashida, N.; Shimura, H.; Okubo, N.; Asari, Y.; Nigawara, T.; Midorikawa, S.; Kotani, K.; Nakaji, S.; Imaizumi, M.; et al. Ultrasonographic thyroid nodular findings in Japanese children. *J. Med. Ultrason.* **2001**, *40*, 219–224. [CrossRef]
6. Bauer, A.J. Thyroid nodules in children and adolescents. *Curr. Opin. Endocrinol. Diabetes Obes.* **2019**, *26*, 266–274. [CrossRef] [PubMed]
7. Cherella, C.E.; Angell, T.E.; Richman, D.M.; Frates, M.C.; Benson, C.B.; Moore, F.D.; Barletta, J.A.; Hollowell, M.; Smith, J.R.; Alexander, E.K.; et al. Differences in thyroid nodule cytology and malignancy risk between children and adults. *Thyroid* **2019**, *29*, 1097–1104. [CrossRef] [PubMed]
8. Al Nofal, A.; Gionfriddo, M.R.; Javed, A.; Haydour, Q.; Brito, J.P.; Prokop, L.J.; Pittock, S.T.; Murad, M.H. Accuracy of thyroid nodule sonography for the detection of thyroid cancer in children: Systematic review and meta-analysis. *Clin. Endocrinol.* **2016**, *84*, 423–430. [CrossRef]
9. Essenmacher, A.C.; Joyce, P.H., Jr.; Kao, S.C.; Epelman, M.; Pesce, L.M.; D'Alessandro, M.P.; Sato, Y.; Johnson, C.M.; Podberesky, D.J. Sonographic evaluation of pediatric thyroid nodules. *Radiographics* **2017**, *37*, 1731–1752. [CrossRef]
10. Ogle, S.; Merz, A.; Parina, R.; Alsayed, M.; Milas, M. Ultrasound and the evaluation of pediatric thyroid malignancy: Current recommendations for diagnosis and follow-up. *J. Ultrasound Med.* **2018**, *37*, 2311–2324. [CrossRef] [PubMed]
11. Lim-Dunham, J.E. Ultrasound guidelines for pediatric thyroid nodules: Proceeding with caution. *Pediatr. Radiol.* **2019**, *49*, 851–853. [CrossRef] [PubMed]
12. Iakovou, I.; Giannoula, E.; Sachpekidis, C. Imaging and imaging-based management of pediatric thyroid nodules. *J. Clin. Med.* **2020**, *9*, 384. [CrossRef]
13. Cooper, D.S.; Doherty, G.M.; Haugen, B.R.; Kloos, R.T.; Lee, S.L.; Mandel, S.J.; Mazzaferri, E.L.; McIver, B.; Pacini, F.; American Thyroid Association (ATA) Guidelines Taskforce on Thyroid Nodules and Differentiated Thyroid Cancer; et al. Revised American Thyroid Association management guidelines for patients with thyroid nodules and differentiated thyroid cancer. *Thyroid* **2009**, *19*, 1167–1214. [CrossRef] [PubMed]
14. Corrias, A.; Mussa, A.; Baronio, F.; Arrigo, T.; Salerno, M.; Segni, M.; Vigone, M.C.; Gastaldi, R.; Zirilli, G.; Tuli, G.; et al. Diagnostic features of thyroid nodules in pediatrics. *Arch. Pediatr. Adolesc. Med.* **2010**, *164*, 714–719. [CrossRef] [PubMed]
15. Clement, S.C.; Lebbink, C.A.; Klein Hesselink, M.S.; Teepen, J.C.; Links, T.P.; Ronckers, C.M.; van Santen, H.M. Presentation and outcome of subsequent thyroid cancer among childhood cancer survivors compared to sporadic thyroid cancer: A matched national study. *Eur. J. Endocrinol.* **2020**, *183*, 169–180. [CrossRef] [PubMed]

16. Trimboli, P. Ultrasound: The extension of our hands to improve the management of thyroid patients. *Cancers* **2021**, *13*, 567. [CrossRef] [PubMed]
17. Trimboli, P.; Castellana, M.; Piccardo, A.; Romanelli, F.; Grani, G.; Giovanella, L.; Durante, C. The ultrasound risk stratification systems for thyroid nodule have been evaluated against papillary carcinoma. A meta-analysis. *Rev. Endocr. Metab. Disord.* **2021**, *22*, 453–460. [CrossRef] [PubMed]
18. Castellana, M.; Piccardo, A.; Virili, C.; Scappaticcio, L.; Grani, G.; Durante, C.; Giovanella, L.; Trimboli, P. Can ultrasound systems for risk stratification of thyroid nodules identify follicular carcinoma? *Cancer Cytopathol.* **2020**, *128*, 250–259. [CrossRef] [PubMed]
19. Li, J.; Li, H.; Yang, Y.; Zhang, X.; Qian, L. The KWAK TI-RADS and 2015 ATA guidelines for medullary thyroid carcinoma: Combined with cell block-assisted ultrasound-guided thyroid fine-needle aspiration. *Clin. Endocrinol.* **2020**, *92*, 450–460. [CrossRef]
20. Matrone, A.; Gambale, C.; Biagini, M.; Prete, A.; Vitti, P.; Elisei, R. Ultrasound features and risk stratification systems to identify medullary thyroid carcinoma. *Eur. J. Endocrinol.* **2021**, *185*, 193–200. [CrossRef] [PubMed]
21. Scappaticcio, L.; Virili, C.; Castellana, M.; Paone, G.; Centanni, M.; Trimboli, P.; Giovanella, L. An unsuspicious thyroid nodule with fatal outcome. *Hormones* **2019**, *18*, 321–324. [CrossRef]
22. Castellana, M.; Virili, C.; Paone, G.; Scappaticcio, L.; Piccardo, A.; Giovanella, L.; Trimboli, P. Ultrasound systems for risk stratification of thyroid nodules prompt inappropriate biopsy in autonomously functioning thyroid nodules. *Clin. Endocrinol.* **2020**, *93*, 67–75. [CrossRef]
23. Castellana, M.; Castellana, C.; Treglia, G.; Giorgino, F.; Giovanella, L.; Russ, G.; Trimboli, P. Performance of five ultrasound risk stratification systems in selecting thyroid nodules for FNA. *J. Clin. Endocrinol. Metab.* **2020**, *105*, 1659–1669. [CrossRef] [PubMed]
24. Kim, P.H.; Yoon, H.M.; Hwang, J.; Lee, J.S.; Jung, A.Y.; Cho, Y.A.; Baek, J.H. Diagnostic performance of adult-based ATA and ACR-TIRADS ultrasound risk stratification systems in pediatric thyroid nodules: A systematic review and meta-analysis. *Eur. Radiol.* **2021**, *31*, 7450–7463. [CrossRef]
25. Grani, G.; Brenta, G.; Trimboli, P.; Falcone, R.; Ramundo, V.; Maranghi, M.; Lucia, P.; Filetti, S.; Durante, C. Sonographic risk stratification systems for thyroid nodules as rule-out tests in older adults. *Cancers* **2020**, *12*, 2458. [CrossRef] [PubMed]
26. Tessler, F.N.; Middleton, W.D.; Grant, E.G.; Hoang, J.K.; Berland, L.L.; Teefey, S.A.; Cronan, J.J.; Beland, M.D.; Desser, T.S.; Frates, M.C.; et al. ACR thyroid imaging, reporting and data system (TI-RADS): White paper of the ACR TI-RADS committee. *JACR* **2017**, *14*, 587–595. [CrossRef]
27. Russ, G.; Bonnema, S.J.; Erdogan, M.F.; Durante, C.; Ngu, R.; Leenhardt, L. European thyroid association guidelines for ultrasound malignancy risk stratification of thyroid nodules in adults: The EU-TIRADS. *Eur. Thyroid J.* **2017**, *6*, 225–237. [CrossRef]
28. Shin, J.H.; Baek, J.H.; Chung, J.; Ha, E.J.; Kim, J.H.; Lee, Y.H.; Lim, H.K.; Moon, W.J.; Na, D.G.; Park, J.S.; et al. Ultrasonography diagnosis and imaging-based management of thyroid nodules: Revised korean society of thyroid radiology consensus statement and recommendations. *Korean J. Radiol.* **2016**, *17*, 370–395. [CrossRef] [PubMed]
29. Haugen, B.R.; Alexander, E.K.; Bible, K.C.; Doherty, G.M.; Mandel, S.J.; Nikiforov, Y.E.; Pacini, F.; Randolph, G.W.; Sawka, A.M.; Schlumberger, M.; et al. 2015 American Thyroid Association Management Guidelines for Adult Patients with Thyroid Nodules and Differentiated Thyroid Cancer: The American Thyroid Association Guidelines Task Force on Thyroid Nodules and Differentiated Thyroid Cancer. *Thyroid* **2016**, *26*, 1–133. [CrossRef]
30. Bossuyt, P.M.; Reitsma, J.B.; Bruns, D.E.; Gatsonis, C.A.; Glasziou, P.P.; Irwig, L.; Lijmer, J.G.; Moher, D.; Rennie, D.; de Vet, H.C.; et al. STARD 2015: An updated list of essential items for reporting diagnostic accuracy studies. *BMJ* **2015**, *351*, h5527. [CrossRef]
31. Nardi, F.; Basolo, F.; Crescenzi, A.; Fadda, G.; Frasoldati, A.; Orlandi, F.; Palombini, L.; Papini, E.; Zini, M.; Pontecorvi, A.; et al. Italian consensus for the classification and reporting of thyroid cytology. *J. Endocrinol. Investig.* **2014**, *37*, 593–599. [CrossRef]
32. Lloyd, R.V.; Osamura, R.Y.; Klöppel, G.; Rosai, J.; World Health Organization. International Agency for Research on Cancer. WHO Classification of Tumours of Endocrine Organs. 2017. Available online: https://www.iarc.who.int/news-events/who-classification-of-tumours-of-endocrine-organs/ (accessed on 28 August 2021).
33. Galen, R.S.; Gambino, S.R. *Beyond Normality: The Predictive Value and Efficiency of Medical Diagnoses*; John and Wiley and Sons: New York, NY, USA, 1975.
34. Richman, D.M.; Benson, C.B.; Doubilet, P.M.; Wassner, A.J.; Asch, E.; Cherella, C.E.; Smith, J.R.; Frates, M.C. Assessment of American College of Radiology Thyroid Imaging Reporting and Data System (TI-RADS) for pediatric thyroid nodules. *Radiology* **2020**, *294*, 415–420. [CrossRef] [PubMed]
35. Bi Lee, S.; Jin Cho, Y.; Lee, S.; Hun Choi, Y.; Cheon, J.E.; Sun Kim, W. Korean Society of Thyroid Radiology Guidelines for the Management of Pediatric Thyroid Nodules: Suitability and Risk Factors. *Thyroid* **2021**. [CrossRef]
36. Martinez-Rios, C.; Daneman, A.; Bajno, L.; van der Kaay, D.; Moineddin, R.; Wasserman, J.D. Utility of adult-based ultrasound malignancy risk stratifications in pediatric thyroid nodules. *Pediatr. Radiol.* **2018**, *48*, 74–84. [CrossRef] [PubMed]
37. Ha, S.M.; Baek, J.H.; Na, D.G.; Suh, C.H.; Chung, S.R.; Choi, Y.J.; Lee, J.H. Diagnostic performance of practice guidelines for thyroid nodules: Thyroid nodule size versus biopsy rates. *Radiology* **2019**, *291*, 92–99. [CrossRef]
38. Kim, P.H.; Suh, C.H.; Baek, J.H.; Chung, S.R.; Choi, Y.J.; Lee, J.H. Unnecessary thyroid nodule biopsy rates under four ultrasound risk stratification systems: A systematic review and meta-analysis. *Eur. Radiol.* **2021**, *31*, 2877–2885. [CrossRef]
39. Radetti, G.; Loche, S.; D'Antonio, V.; Salerno, M.; Guzzetti, C.; Aversa, T.; Cassio, A.; Cappa, M.; Gastaldi, R.; Deluca, F.; et al. Influence of hashimoto thyroiditis on the development of thyroid nodules and cancer in children and adolescents. *J. Endocr. Soc.* **2019**, *3*, 607–616. [CrossRef] [PubMed]

40. MacFarland, S.P.; Bauer, A.J.; Adzick, N.S.; Surrey, L.F.; Noyes, J.; Kazahaya, K.; Mostoufi-Moab, S. Disease burden and outcome in children and young adults with concurrent graves disease and differentiated thyroid carcinoma. *J. Clin. Endocrinol. Metab.* **2018**, *103*, 2918–2925. [CrossRef]
41. Gharib, H.; Papini, E.; Garber, J.R.; Duick, D.S.; Harrell, R.M.; Hegedüs, L.; Paschke, R.; Valcavi, R.; Vitti, P.; AACE/ACE/AME Task Force on Thyroid Nodules. American Association of Clinical Endocrinologists, American College Of Endocrinology, and Associazione Medici Endocrinologi Medical Guidelines for Clinical Practice for the Diagnosis and Management of Thyroid Nodules–2016 update. *Endocr. Pract.* **2016**, *22*, 622–639. [CrossRef]
42. Russ, G.; Trimboli, P.; Buffet, C. The new era of TIRADSs to stratify the risk of malignancy of thyroid nodules: Strengths, weaknesses and pitfalls. *Cancers* **2021**, *13*, 4316. [CrossRef]

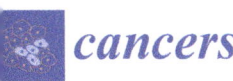

Article

Validation of Four Thyroid Ultrasound Risk Stratification Systems in Patients with Hashimoto's Thyroiditis; Impact of Changes in the Threshold for Nodule's Shape Criterion

Dorota Słowińska-Klencka [1,*], Mariusz Klencki [1,*], Martyna Wojtaszek-Nowicka [2], Kamila Wysocka-Konieczna [1], Ewa Woźniak-Osela [1] and Bożena Popowicz [1]

[1] Department of Morphometry of Endocrine Glands, Medical University of Lodz, Pomorska Street 251, 92-213 Łódź, Poland; kamilawysocka@tyreo.umed.lodz.pl (K.W.-K.); ewawozniak@tyreo.umed.lodz.pl (E.W.-O.); bozena.popowicz@umed.lodz.pl (B.P.)
[2] Department of Clinical Endocrinology, Medical University of Lodz, Pomorska Street 251, 92-213 Łódź, Poland; martyna.wojtaszek-nowicka@umed.lodz.pl
* Correspondence: dsk@tyreo.umed.lodz.pl (D.S.-K.); marklen@tyreo.umed.lodz.pl (M.K.)

Simple Summary: Thyroid Imaging Reporting and Data Systems (TIRADS) optimize the selection of thyroid nodules for cytological examination. There is a question: is the effectiveness of these systems affected by morphological changes to thyroid parenchyma that are visible in the course of Hashimoto's thyroiditis (HT)? This question is very important because of the increased risk of malignancy in thyroid nodules in patients with HT. We investigated widely accepted ultrasound malignancy risk features with a special consideration of the suspected nodule's shape in patients with and without HT. We also validated EU-TIRADS, K-TIRADS, ACR-TIRADS, and ATA guidelines in both groups and evaluated the impact of changes in the threshold for nodule's shape criterion on the diagnostic value of these TIRADS. The presence of Hashimoto's thyroiditis did not exert any significant adverse implications for the efficiency of examined TIRADS. The impact of changes in the threshold for nodule's shape criterion was the highest for EU-TIRADS.

Abstract: The aim of the study was to validate thyroid US malignancy features, especially the nodule's shape, and selected Thyroid Imaging Reporting and Data Systems (EU-TIRADS; K-TIRADS; ACR-TIRADS, ATA guidelines) in patients with or without Hashimoto's thyroiditis (HT and non-HT groups). The study included 1188 nodules (HT: 358, non-HT: 830) with known final diagnoses. We found that the strongest indications of nodule's malignancy were microcalcifications (OR: 22.7) in HT group and irregular margins (OR:13.8) in non-HT group. Solid echostructure and macrocalcifications were ineffective in patients with HT. The highest accuracy of nodule's shape criterion was noted on transverse section, with the cut-off value of anteroposterior to transverse dimension ratio (AP/T) close to 1.15 in both groups. When round nodules were regarded as suspicious in patients with HT (the cut-off value of AP/T set to ≥ 1), it led to a three-fold increase in sensitivity of this feature, with a disproportionally lower decrease in specificity and similar accuracy. Such a modification was effective also for cancers other than PTC. The diagnostic effectiveness of analyzed TIRADS in patients with HT and without HT was similar. Changes in the threshold for AP/T ratio influenced the number of nodules classified into the category of the highest risk, especially in the case of EU-TIRADS.

Keywords: thyroid; nodule; cancer; ultrasound; Thyroid Imaging Reporting and Data Systems (TIRADS)

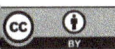

1. Introduction

Preoperative diagnostics of thyroid nodules is based on two main pillars—ultrasound imaging (US) and fine needle aspiration biopsy (FNA). The ultrasonographic examination is mainly used for the assessment of ultrasound malignancy risk features (US malignancy features), and subsequent qualification of nodules into particular categories of sonographic risk stratification systems (SRSs). These systems are usually called TIRADS (Thyroid Imaging Reporting and Data Systems) and they enable a more efficient estimation of the risk of malignancy (RoM) in nodules than the evaluation of separate US malignancy features. The most popular SRSs include EU-TIRADS—recommended by European Thyroid Association (ETA), K-TIRADS—recommended by Korean Society of Thyroid Radiology (KSThR), ACR-TIRADS—created by American College of Radiology (ACR), and the system recommended by American Thyroid Association (ATA guidelines) [1–4]. Our analyses, as well as many reports from other centers, indicate that all these systems not only optimize the selection of nodules for cytological examination but also help to make clinical decisions in patients with an equivocal FNA outcome [5–9]. There is, however, some disagreement between TIRADS systems about the precise definition of particular US malignancy features and their optimal association. One of the areas of notable difference refers to the definition of the nodule's suspicious shape, usually described as 'more taller than wide'. Not all SRSs include precise instructions on how to categorize nodules with the anterior-posterior (AP) dimension equal to the transverse (T) dimension or which thyroid plane should be used for the shape evaluation. Remarkably, there are reports that suggest a rationale for adopting a larger than 1.0 threshold for the AP to T ratio [10], and even studies indicating that the optimal threshold should be <1 [11,12]. There is another important question: is the effectiveness of the suspected nodule's shape and other US malignancy features affected by morphological changes to thyroid parenchyma that are visible in the course of Hashimoto's thyroiditis (HT).

HT is the most common autoimmune endocrine disease, as well as the most common cause of hypothyroidism. This inflammation is characterized by a progressive loss of thyroid follicular cells and lymphocytic infiltration of the thyroid parenchyma associated with fibrosis [13,14]. It is usually accompanied by a decrease in the gland's volume and several characteristic changes visible on US imaging. The thyroid may be hypoechoic, with a coarse, heterogeneous parenchymal echotexture, or have the presence of the marginal abnormality, echogenic septations, multiple discrete hypoechoic micronodules or pseudonodular structures. These features may be present separately or in different sets and make it difficult to differentiate between thyroid nodules and pseudonodules, and in the former case—between cancers and benign lesions [15–17]. The latter problem is of particular importance considering the increased risk of papillary thyroid carcinoma (PTC) in the case of nodules coexisting with HT [18,19].

Thus, we decided to validate US malignancy features, with a special consideration for the nodule's shape, and selected TIRADS systems in patients with or without coexisting HT (HT and non-HT groups).

2. Results

2.1. Effectiveness of the Assessment of Suspicious Nodule's Shape in Differentiation between Benign and Malignant Nodules in HT and non-HT Groups

The usefulness of AP/T ratio assessment in the differentiation between benign nodules and cancers, as measured with area under the receiver operating characteristic curve (AUC), was similar in both groups (transverse plane, Z: -0.1893, $p = 0.8498$; longitudinal plane, Z: 0.2837, $p = 0.7767$) (Table 1). When indexes of diagnostic effectiveness were calculated for the threshold AP > T they were found to be nearly the same in the case of transverse plane. However, in the case of longitudinal plane the AP > T threshold was ineffective in patients with HT.

Table 1. Data on the diagnostic effectiveness of particular thresholds for AP/T ratio in examined groups of nodules (HT and non-HT). Evaluation of AP/T ratio on transverse and longitudinal planes.

The Plane	AP/T Ratio	No./% of Nodules	Ben./Mal. p	SEN	SPC	ACC	PPV (RoM)	NPV	LR+	OR (95% CI) p	AUC (95% CI) p
							HT group				
transverse	AP ≥ T	76/21.2	42/34 <0.0000	39.1	84.5	73.5	44.7	81.2	2.5	3.5 (2.0–6.0) <0.0001	0.635 (0.565–0.704) <0.0001
transverse	AP > T	22/6.1	12/10 0.0170	11.5	95.6	74.7	46.6	76.6	2.6	2.8 (1.2–6.7) 0.0212	
transverse	AP/T ≥ 1.14 max ACC	11/3.1	4/7 0.0063	8.0	98.5	76.5	63.6	76.9	5.5	5.8 (1.8–5.4) <0.0001	
							non-HT group				
transverse	AP ≥ T	116/14.0	61/55 <0.000	26.4	90.2	74.2	47.4	78.6	2.7	3.3 (2.2–5.0) <0.0001	0.627 (0.582–0.671) <0.0001
transverse	AP > T	52/6.2	28/24 0.0003	11.5	95.5	74.5	46.2	76.3	2.6	2.8 (1.6–4.9) 0.0005	
transverse	AP/T ≥ 1.17 max ACC	28/3.4	10/18 <0.0000	8.7	98.4	75.9	64.3	76.3	5.4	5.8 (1.8–5.4) <0.0001	
							HT group				
longitudinal	AP ≥ T max ACC	24/6.7	12/12 0.0024	13.8	95.6	75.7	50.0	77.5	3.1	3.5 (1.5–8.0) <0.0038	0.635 (0.572–0.699) <0.0001
longitudinal	AP > T	9/2.5	7/2 0.8055	2.3	97.4	74.3	22.29	75.6	0.9	0.9 (0.2–4.4) 0.8830	
							non-HT group				
longitudinal	AP ≥ T max ACC	43/5.2	20/23 <0.0000	11.1	96.8	75.3	53.5	76.5	3.4	3.7 (2.0–7.0) <0.0001	0.647 (0.603–0.690) <0.0001
longitudinal	AP > T	15/1.8	7/8 0.0108	3.8	98.9	75.1	53.3	75.5	3.1	3.5 (1.3–9.8) <0.0164	

ACC—accuracy, AP—anteroposterior diameter, AUC—area under the receiver operating characteristic curve, Ben.—benign lesion in histopathological outcome, CI—confidence intervals, HT—Hashimoto's thyroiditis, LR+—positive likelihood ratio, Mal.—thyroid malignancy in histopathological outcome, NPV—negative predictive value, OR—odds ratio, PPV—positive predictive value, RoM—risk of malignancy, SEN—sensitivity, SPC—specificity, T—transverse diameter.

When AP > T threshold was replaced with AP ≥ T one, a significant increase in sensitivity (SEN) was observed in both groups, and that increase was higher in HT group than in non-HT group. More pronounced changes in HT group were a consequence of the higher incidence of round nodules with AP = T in that group in comparison with non-HT group (Table S1). On the transverse plane it was the case for both benign nodules and cancers. On the longitudinal plane the differences were smaller, insignificant and they were observed only for cancers. The higher incidence of round cancers on transverse plane was observed not only for PTC (HT: 27.6% vs. non-HT: 16.3%, p = 0.0408), but also for other malignant nodules, although insignificantly (HT: 27.3% vs. non-HT: 10.4%, p = 0.1408). Consequently, the threshold AP ≥ T on transverse plane was the only effective threshold in HT group for revealing cancers other than PTC, odds ratio (OR): 4.5, CI 95%: 1.3–15.6, p = 0.0160.

The highest accuracy (ACC) values for the differentiation between benign and malignant nodules were noted in both groups in the case of transverse plane. Maximal accuracy was reached in HT group with the cut-off value of AP/T ratio set to 1.14, while in non-HT group—to 1.17 (Figure S1). With those thresholds changes in SEN and specificity (SPC) did not exceed 4% in both groups when compared with the threshold AP > T, while risk of malignancy (RoM) of nodules was about 20% higher, and positive likelihood ratio (LR+) and OR increased twofold (Table 1). There were no significant differences between examined groups in indexes of diagnostic effectiveness of the suspicious shape when thresholds optimized for ACC were used.

When the longitudinal plane was used for measurements, the maximal ACC values were slightly lower than in the case of transverse plane and the optimal cut-off value of AP/T ratio was found to be AP ≥ T in both groups (Figure S2). Regardless of the adopted cut-off value, no improvement in ACC values was observed in any of the groups when the assessment of nodule's shape was performed on both planes (with positive nodules defined as those reaching the threshold on any plane) in comparison with the assessment on a single plane (Table S2).

There was no significant difference in AUC for nodules <1 cm and larger ones in either group (Z: 1.0524, p = 0.2926; non-HT: Z: −0.6656, p = 0.5056), but in HT group the assessment of suspicious shape feature was ineffective in nodules <1 cm (Table S3). In non-HT group significant differences in the frequency of nodules <1 cm with suspicious shape between cancers and benign nodules were observed only for the threshold AP ≥ T.

2.2. Effectiveness of the Assessment of Other US Malignancy Features

In non-HT group almost all other US malignancy features, except for pathological vascularization and rim calcifications, were observed significantly more often in cancers than in benign nodules (Tables 1 and 2). In the case of HT group, the list of insignificant features included also solid echostructure, more solid than cystic echostructure, and macrocalcifications. The logistic regression analysis showed that in HT group the presence of microcalcifications was the strongest indication of nodule's malignancy (OR: 22.7), and that the presence of suspicious margins or marked hypoechogenicity increased the risk of malignancy at least tenfold. In non-HT group, the strongest index of nodule's malignancy was the presence of irregular margins (OR: 13.8).

Table 2. Comparison of the incidence of sonographic features other than suspicious nodule's shape in HT and non-HT nodules in relation to the histopathological outcome: benign lesion vs. thyroid malignancy. Results of univariate logistic regression analysis in both groups.

Sonographic Feature	HT Group				Non-HT Group			
	Ben. (271) No/%	Mal. (87) No/%	p	OR (95% CI) p	Ben. (622) No/%	Mal. (208) No/%	p	OR (95% CI) p
marked hypoechogenicity *	14/5.2	31/35.6	<0.0001	10.2 (5.1–20.3) <0.0001	33/5.3	60/28.9	<0.0001	7.2 (4.6–11.5) 0.0001
Hypoechogenicity *	148/54.6	75/86.2	<0.0001	5.2 (2.7–10.0) <0.0001	365/58.7	178/85.8	<0.0001	4.2 (2.7–6.3) 0.0001
solid echostructure	247/91.1	84/96.6	0.0965	2.7 (0.8–9.3) 0.1094	436/70.1	188/90.4	<0.0001	4.0 (2.5–6.6) 0.0001
more solid than cystic echostructure	264/97.4	87/100.0	0.2021	-	533/85.7	204/98.1	<0.0001	8.5 (3.1–23.5) <0.0001
suspicious margins	14/5.2	38/43.7	<0.0001	14.2 (7.2–28.2) <0.0001	23/3.7	72/34.6	<0.0001	13.8 (8.3–22.8) <0.0001
microcalcifications	5/1.9	26/29.9	<0.0001	22.7 (8.4–61.4) <0.0001	17/2.7	38/18.3	<0.0001	8.0 (4.4–14.4) 0.0001
macrocalcifications	19/7.0	5/5.8	0.6817	0.8 (0.3–2.2) 0.6822	43/6.9	40/19.2	<0.0001	3.2 (2.0–5.1) <0.0001
rim calcifications	7/2.6	4/4.6	0.5549	1.8 (0.5–6.4) 0.3500	20/3.2	8/3.9	0.6627	1.2 (0.5–2.8) 0.6631
pathological vascularization	37/13.7	13/14.9	0.7628	1.1 (0.6–2.2) 0.7628	119/19.1	48/23.1	0.2192	1.3 (0.9–1.9) 0.2199

*—in the case of nodules with mixed echogenicity the presence of any hypoechoic tissue was considered; Ben.—benign lesion in histopathological outcome, CI—confidence intervals, OR—odds ratio, HT—Hashimoto's thyroiditis, Mal.—thyroid malignancy in histopathological outcome. Data on nodule's shape criterion are presented in Table 1.

Microcalcifications, irregular margins, marked hypoechogenicity, suspicious shape and hypoechogenicity were independent features in the differentiation between benign and malignant nodules in both groups (Table S4). Macrocalcifications and solid echostructure were such features only in non-HT group.

Benign nodules of HT group were solid significantly more often than those of non-HT group (91.1% vs. 70.1%, p < 0.0001) and more solid than cystic (97.4% vs. 85.7%,

$p < 0.0001$), but they showed pathological vascularization less frequently (13.7% vs. 19.1%, $p < 0.0474$). Malignant nodules of HT group contained microcalcifications more often than cancers of non-HT group (29.9% vs. 18.3%, $p < 0.0273$), while macrocalcifications were less frequent (5.8% vs. 19.2%, $p < 0.0033$). Spongiform echostructure was observed only in benign nodules of both groups, but it was less common in HT group than in non-HT group (5/1.9% vs. 46/7.4% respectively, $p = 0.0018$).

2.3. Comparison of the Effectiveness of Analyzed SRSs

Table 3 shows the distribution of benign and malignant nodules among particular categories of the examined SRSs for each of previously analyzed thresholds of AP/T ratio with measurements on transverse plane. In the majority of cases, calculated RoM for particular categories of analyzed TIRADSs corresponded to expected RoM or differed by less than 5%. Larger differences (up to 10%) were observed in the case of lower than expected RoM for category 5 of EU-TIRADS with the threshold $AP \geq T$ in both groups as well as higher than expected RoM for category 4 of K-TIRADS, ACR-TIRADS and ATA guidelines SRS in non-HT group.

All analyzed SRSs showed the highest ACC of distinguishing between benign and malignant nodules when category 5 was used as a cut-off level, irrespectively of the adopted threshold of AP/T ratio. Table 4 shows values of indexes describing the effectiveness of that distinction. System EU-TIRADS, with any of analyzed thresholds of AP/T ratio, showed the highest SEN and negative predictive value (NPV), but the lowest SPC and positive predictive value (PPV) (see Table 3). On the other hand, ACR-TIRADS system was characterized by the lowest SEN and the highest SPC. Generally, we did not find significant differences in AUC between analyzed SRSs at the same AP/T ratio thresholds. The only exception was observed in non-HT group, where AUC for ACR-TIRADS was significantly lower than for other SRSs when the threshold was $AP/T \geq 1.17$. No significant differences were found in the effectiveness any of SRSs between HT and non-HT groups when the comparison was made at the same AP/T ratio threshold.

When $AP > T$ threshold was replaced with $AP \geq T$ one, the numbers of nodules classified into category 5 increased in all SRSs. Accordingly, there was an increase in SEN of that category (when it was used as a threshold for malignancy) and a decrease in its SPC and RoM (Tables 3 and 4). In the case of EU-TIRADS that effect was stronger in HT group than non-HT group. In the former group the number of nodules in category 5 increased by 32.6%, SEN increased by 11.2%, SPC decreased by 11.2% and RoM decreased by 16.1%. In non-HT group analogous changes were 15.7%, 7.0%, 4.7% and 7.4%, respectively. In other SRSs the resultant changes in SEN, SPC, RoM and the percentage of nodules classified into category 5 were similar in both groups (Table S5).

When the AP/T ratio threshold was optimized to obtain the maximal ACC (HT group: $AP/T \geq 1.14$; non-HT group: $AP/T \geq 1.17$) the most distinct effects in comparison to $AP > T$ threshold were observed again in the case of EU-TIRADS. They were especially visible in non-HT group, where RoM increased by 7.2% and SEN decreased by only 0.8%. AUC value in non-HT group for EU-TIRADS with the threshold $AP/T \geq 1.17$ was significantly higher than for $AP > T$ threshold. No significant difference in AUC was observed in any other SRSs when AP/T ratio threshold was changed in either group.

Table 3. Distribution of benign and malignant nodules between particular categories of TIRADS, the comparison of expected RoM with calculated RoM for each category (TIRADS categories corresponding to the lack of nodules have been omitted, nodule's shape evaluated on the transverse plane).

Category of TIRADS/Guideline	Expected RoM (PPV)	Calculated RoM (PPV)					
		HT Group			Non-HT Group		
		AP ≥ T	AP > T	AP/T ≥ 1.14	AP ≥ T	AP > T	AP/T ≥ 1.17
EU-TIRADS							
2—benign	<3	0.0	0.0	0.0	0.0	0.0	0.0
3—low risk	3–15	4.0	5.1	5.0	7.0	7.5	7.3
4—intermediate risk	15–50	11.8	14.1	15.9	18.2	19.1	19.0
5—high risk	>60	51.5	61.4	62.1	54.6	58.5	62.7
K-TIRADS							
2—benign	0	0.0	0.0	0.0	0.0	0.0	0.0
3—low suspicion	2–4	5.7	6.5	6.2	7,6	8,3	8,1
4—intermediate	6–17	16.0	17.8	19.9	26.1	27.0	27.8
5—high suspicion	26–87	65.5	74.6	74.6	61.6	67.2	69.7
ACR-TIRADS							
1—benign	-	0.0	0.0	0.0	0.0	0.0	0.0
2—not suspicious	<2	0.0	0.0	0.0	3.3	4.8	4.8
3—mildly suspicious	5	5.5	6.7	7.1	9.5	10.0	9.6
4—moderately suspicious	5–20	17.7	20.2	21.2	26.1	27.8	28.7
5—highly suspicious	>20	65.4	76.8	77.4	63.4	69.7	73.9
ATA guidelines							
1—benign	<1	0.0	0.0	0.0	0.0	0.0	0.0
2—very low suspicion	<3	0.0	0.0	0.0	2.5	2.5	2.5
3- low suspicion	5–10	5.6	6.5	6.2	9.4	9.4	9.1
4—intermediate suspicion *	10–20	15.7	18.1	19.8	24.9	26.3	26.9
5—high suspicion	70–90	65.9	74.6	75.0	61.0	66.7	69.9

*—included 71 non-hypoechoic nodules with high risk features (including 22 cancers, 8 in HT group and 14 in non-HT group). AP—anteroposterior diameter, HT—Hashimoto's thyroiditis, PPV—positive predictive value, RoM—risk of malignancy, T—transverse diameter, TIRADS—Thyroid Imaging Reporting and Data Systems.

Table 4. Data on the diagnostic effectiveness of analyzed SRSs in HT and non-HT groups for the high risk category (nodule's shape evaluated on the transverse plane).

Index of Effectiveness	HT Group			Non-HT Group		
	AP ≥ T	AP > T	AP/T ≥ 1.14	AP ≥ T	AP > T	AP/T ≥ 1.17
	EU-TIRADS					
% of nodules	37.4	28.2	25.7	30.2	26.1	24.2
SEN	79.3	71.3	67.8	65.4	61.1	60.6
SPC	76.0	85.6	87.8	81.5	85.5	87.9
ACC	76.8	82.1	83.0	77.5	79.4	81.1
NPV	92.0	90.3	89.5	87.6	86.8	87.0
AUC (CI 95%)	0.798 (0.747–0.849)	0.817 (0.765–0.869)	0.814 (0.762–0.866)	0.779 (0.744–0.814)	0.782 (0.716–0.818)	0.794 [a] (0.759–0.830)
	K-TIRADS					
% of nodules	23.5	18.7	17.6	19.2	15.8	14.7
SEN	63.2	57.5	54.0	47.1	42.3	40.9
SPC	89.3	93.7	94.1	90.2	93.1	94.1
ACC	83.0	84.9	84.4	79.4	80.4	80.7
NPV	88.3	87.3	86.4	83.6	82.8	82.6
AUC (CI 95%)	0.804 (0.749–0.858)	0.808 (0.752–0.764)	0.805 (0.750–0.860)	0.775 (0.740–0.811)	0.775 (0.739–0.811)	0.779 (0.744–0.815)

Table 4. Cont.

Index of Effectiveness	HT Group			Non-HT Group		
	AP ≥ T	AP > T	AP/T ≥ 1.14	AP ≥ T	AP > T	AP/T ≥ 1.17
	ACR-TIRADS					
% of nodules	21.8	15.6	14.8	16.1	11.9	10.7
SEN	58.6	49.4	47.1	40.9	33.2	31.3
SPC	90.0	95.2	95.6	92.1	95.2	96.1
ACC	82.4	84.1	83.8	79.3	79.6	79.9
NPV	87.1	85.4	84.9	82.3	81.0	80.7
AUC (CI 95%)	0.795 (0.741–0.850)	0.791 (0.735–0.848)	0.787 (0.731–0.844)	0.760 (0.724–0.796)	0.752 [c] (0.715–0.788)	0.757 [b] (0.070–0.793)
	ATA guidelines					
% of nodules	23.7	18.7	17.6	20.0	15.9	14.8
SEN	64.4	57.5	54.0	48.1	42.3	41.3
SPC	89.3	93.7	94.1	89.4	92.9	94.1
ACC	83.2	84.9	84.4	79.0	80.2	80.8
NPV	88.6	87.3	86.4	83.7	82.8	82.7
AUC (CI 95%)	0.809 (0.756–0.863)	0.811 (0.756–0.866)	0.811 (0.757–0.865)	0.768 (0.731–0.804)	0.769 (0.732–0.806)	0.776 (0.740–0.812)

[a]—$p < 0.01$ vs. EU-TIRADS threshold AP > T. [b]—$p < 0.05$ vs. EU-TIRADS, K-TIRADS and ATA guidelines (threshold AP/T ≥ 1.17 all).
[c]—$p < 0.05$ vs. EU-TIRADS and K-TIRADS (threshold AP > T all). ACC—accuracy, AP—anteroposterior diameter, AUC—area under the receiver operating characteristic curve, Ben.—benign lesion in histopathological outcome, CI—confidence intervals, HT—Hashimoto's thyroiditis, LR+—positive likelihood ratio, Mal.—thyroid malignancy in histopathological outcome, NPV—negative predictive value, SEN—sensitivity, SPC—specificity, T—transverse diameter, TIRADS—Thyroid Imaging Reporting and Data Systems.

3. Discussion

Hashimoto's thyroiditis is a common thyroid disease, especially in areas of high iodine supply. It is usually accompanied by significant changes in the morphology of the gland that impair the identification of thyroid nodules and the assessment of a nodule's US malignancy features. These difficulties are commonly aggravated by the small size of nodules. Despite these complications, our analysis shows that all four of the most recognized and strongest US malignancy features (i.e., marked hypoechogenicity, irregular margins, microcalcifications, and suspicious shape) are effective in distinguishing benign nodules from cancers in the case of coexisting HT. Other investigators also indicate that the majority of US malignancy features present similar efficiency in patients with or without HT [16,20–26]. However, there are some differences. In our study, microcalcifications were an almost three times stronger indication of malignancy in a nodule in patients with HT than in those without HT. We believe that this difference is a consequence of increased prevalence of PTC among cancers in patients with HT. In addition, it is PTC that microcalcifications are particularly characteristic of. However, there is no full agreement on the incidence of various types of calcifications in patients with HT. As with our observations, Baser et al. (2015) found that macrocalcifications were observed less often in HT than non-HT patients [22]. Durfee et al. (2014) and Gul et al. (2010) did not find any significant differences in calcification types between HT and non-HT groups [20,25]. In addition, Ohmori et al. (2007) even noted an increased incidence of dense calcifications and decreased incidence of psammoma bodies in thyroid cancer associated with HT compared to cancers without HT [27]. More concordant is the opinion that the assessment of solid structure of nodules is not useful in patients with HT [16,23,24,26], as can also be concluded from our study. That is a consequence of the fact that almost all nodules which accompany HT are solid, even the benign ones. This may result from their smaller sizes; an influence of morphological changes induced by HT cannot be excluded either. Observations regarding suspicious margins are less concordant [16,20,28]. In our study, their assessment was effective regardless of the presence of HT. Such results can be achieved only if the assessment is performed by an experienced ultrasonographer. Experience is necessary to avoid the interpretation of ill-defined pseudonodules as true nodules. Our team is fully aware of that danger due to our previous studies on the relation between FNA outcomes in patients with HT and different ultrasonographic images of thyroid parenchyma, including variants with pseudonodules [29]. All systems analyzed in our study regard irregular margins as suspicious. The authors of K-TIRADS underline that ill-defined margins are visible not only in thyroiditis, but also in infiltrative malignant tumors, but in our opinion the latter almost always present irregularity in their margins. The problem arises because that irregularity is frequently very fine, which gives an impression of ill-defined margins.

The most complicated issue related to US malignancy features is the assessment of the suspicious shape of a nodule. We have shown that thyroid nodules in patients with HT are round (their AP = T) more often than nodules in patients without HT. When the transverse plane is used for measurements the above is equally true for benign nodules and cancers, and in the latter case, not only PTCs but other cancers too. When the longitudinal plane is used, only cancers are more often round. Consequently, in patients with HT the assessment of the suspicious shape of a nodule on the transverse plane is effective with both thresholds: AP > T and AP $\geq$ T, while on the longitudinal plane only AP $\geq$ T threshold is effective. Interestingly, when AP $\geq$ T threshold is used on the transverse plane the assessment of the suspicious shape becomes also effective in diagnosis of cancers other than PTC. Previously, other authors did not find the assessment of suspicious shape to be useful for diagnosing patients with FTC [30], so that issue should be investigated further. However, the key question is an equivocal definition of the suspicious shape of a nodule. It is usually described as 'more taller than wide', which in practice in the majority of studies translates into AP > T threshold, but in some of them into the AP $\geq$ T one [31]. In the guidelines and in many reports, there are no precise indications as how to categorize round nodules or such indications are contradictory. Among SRSs analyzed in our study, EU-TIRADS identifies the suspicious shape of a nodule as non-oval or round [1]. In contrast, K-TIRADS defines the suspicious shape as neither round nor oval [2]. Similarly, in ACR-TIRADS the threshold of AP/T ratio >1, and ATA guidelines use the description 'more taller than wide shape' [3,4]. There is also some controversy over the plane of measurements. K-TIRADS specifies that AP > T should be observed on a transverse or longitudinal plane, while ACR-TIRADS and ATA guidelines limit that condition to the transverse plane only. In addition, EU-TIRADS does not specify the plane of measurements in regard to non-oval shape, but indicates that the definition of round shape and oval shape demands the respective conditions (AP = T or AP < T) to be satisfied on both the transverse and longitudinal planes. One could argue that a nodule that is non-oval on any plane is suspicious according to EU-TIRADS. However, that way there would be two different regimens of measurements for non-oval and round shaped nodules, both types regarded as suspicious in EU-TIRADS.

Irrespectively of these differences, our analyzes, like reports from many other centers, indicate that the assessment of nodule's suspicious shape is characterized by a very high SPC [10,30,32,33], with lower SEN, especially on the longitudinal plane [30]. SEN of that feature on the longitudinal plane reaches values similar to those on the transverse plane when round nodules are regarded as suspicious too. The inclusion of round nodules into suspicious category improves SEN on the transverse plane by several times, especially in patients with HT. It is noteworthy that the effectiveness of the shape assessment is not improved when the conditions AP > T or AP $\geq$ T are evaluated on both planes (with positive feature defined as the condition satisfied on any plane) when compared with the measurements performed on a single plane. Both our study and other reports [34] indicate that the assessment on the transverse plane and the longitudinal plane have similar ACC. However, the nodule's suspicious shape is very rarely identified on the longitudinal plane only. Thus, like Kim et al. (2021) we believe that there is no need for the assessment of a nodule's shape on both planes and measurements on the transverse plane are satisfactory [32]. There are some earlier contradictory reports in this regard [35].

The highest ACC of the assessment could be obtained with measurements on the transverse plane when the threshold for AP/T ratio is close to 1.15 (1.14 in HT group and 1.17 in non-HT group). If such a threshold is used there are moderate changes in SEN and SPC, but a twofold increase in OR and LR+ is observed when compared to the threshold

AP > T. A further increase of AP/T threshold to values proposed by Grani et al. (2020) (AP/T ratio = 1.2) in patients without HT would not improve OR (OR: 4.2 vs. 5.8), and in patients with HT there would even be a loss of discrimination power of the suspicious shape feature (incidence of benign nodules with AP/T $\geq$ 1.2 did not differ significantly from the incidence of such cancers: 1.1% vs. 3.5%, $p = 0.1602$) [10]. It is possible that these differences between our data and the study by Grani are a consequence of the lack of nodules with indeterminate cytology in the Italian study. In such nodules, US malignancy features generally have lower effectiveness, due to a lower percentage of PTC among cancers. On the other hand, Topaloglu et al. (2016) examined patients with nodules of category III of the Bethesda System for Reporting Thyroid Cytology (BSRTC) and proposed the threshold for AP/T ratio below one (0.81) [11]. A lower threshold was even proposed by Huang et al. (2018) while diagnosing papillary microcarcinomas (0.7) [12]. However, those thresholds were established in a different way. They were optimized to produce maximal SEN and SPC at the same time, but not ACC. When we followed the same priorities then the threshold (as determined with ROC curve analysis) was 0.92 in patients with HT (SEN: 43.7%, SPC: 80.1%, ACC: 71.2%, PPV: 41.3%, NPV: 81.6%, OR: 3.1) and 0.87 in patients without HT: 0.87 (SEN: 46.6%, SPC: 72.5%, ACC: 66.0, PPV: 36.2%, NPV: 80.2%, OR: 2.3). In HT group these values did not differ significantly from those obtained for the threshold AP $\geq$ T. However, in a non-HT group such a low threshold was unsatisfactory, leading to low SPC and PPV as almost 1/3 of nodules (32.3%) reached that threshold. This is an important weakness in the case of a US malignancy feature that is key in assigning nodules into the highest risk category of SRS. In the studies by Topaloglu and Huang reported SPC values for proposed thresholds were even lower (61.6% and 66.7%, respectively), and PPV did not exceed 30% (Topaloglu et al.: 29.1%, Huang et al.: missing data on PPV) [11,12].

We found that in patients with HT the assessment of nodule's suspicious shape has low effectiveness in the case of nodules <1 cm. Fukushima et al. (2021) did not find differences in the effectiveness of that feature between small and larger nodules [30]. Ren et al. (2015) found it to be even higher in nodules <1 cm, but they did not analyze the possible influence of HT on that effectiveness [33]. In our group of patients without HT the AUC value for nodules < 1 cm was also slightly higher than for larger nodules.

For obvious reasons, the use of a precise threshold for AP/T ratio in practice demands an additional effort from the ultrasonographer. The authors of some reports admitted that the suspicious shape was determined based on ultrasonographer's impression instead of the measurements of nodules' diameters. Such an assessment makes it difficult to detect fine abnormalities in a nodule's shape. As our data indicate, it is worthwhile to perform proper measurements because even a minor modification of the threshold for nodule's suspicious shape may lead to a several-fold change in SEN of that feature and marked changes in its SPC and RoM. The local experience of a center is especially valuable in this case, because the reproducibility of the assessment of nodule's suspicious shape, like other US malignancy features, is not high [36]. It results not only from technical differences in measurements (e.g., caused by different positions of a patient, or different pressure exerted by a probe on the examined area), but also from differences in the epidemiology of thyroid diseases in examined patients (different incidence of HT, other profile of cancers). Thus, in our opinion, it could be advisable to determine the optimal threshold for AP/T ratio in each center individually, to adjust it to its specific situation. It should be noted that while the discussed changes in the AP/T ratio threshold may lead to a several-fold increase in SEN, the resultant SEN is still far from satisfactory, similarly to other high risk features of malignancy.

The results of our study indicate that changes in the threshold of AP/T ratio have a different impact on the effectiveness of particular SRSs in classification of benign and malignant nodules. The impact is bigger for EU-TIRADS than for other SRSs. This is a result of the particular definition of high risk category in EU-TIRADS which is different from other systems based on similar rules: K-TIRADS and ATA guidelines (ACR-TIRADS uses points for US malignancy features unlike all other SRSs). In EU-TIRADS a nodule with strong risk features does not need to be hypoechoic to be classified into category 5 [1]. Consequently, category 5 of that system directly reflects all effects of categorization of all round nodules as suspicious. In addition, these effects are larger in HT group than non-HT group. Similarly, the change of AP > T threshold to a threshold that gives maximal ACC of the nodule's shape assessment produces more pronounced effects on category 5 in EU-TIRADS than in other SRSs. This effect is advantageous as it leads to larger increase in RoM and SPC of that category. Therefore, in the case of EU-TIRADS there is the greatest possibility of selecting various thresholds of AP/T ratio in order to optimize SPC (the threshold close to 1.15) or SEN (AP $\geq$ T threshold) of that system.

Despite these differences it should be emphasized that all SRSs showed similar effectiveness in distinguishing benign nodules from cancers in patients with HT at the same thresholds of AP/T ratio. Additionally, there were no significant differences in the effectiveness of those systems in patients with or without HT. Likewise, Wang et al. (2015) did not find any significant influence of HT on the effectiveness of SRSs (they evaluated the system proposed by Kwak, ACR-TIRADS and ATA guidelines) [37]. We showed that EU-TIRADS had the highest SEN with the lowest SPC and ACR-TIRADS had the highest SPC with the lowest SEN irrespectively of the threshold used for AP/T ratio or the presence of HT, which is concordant with other reports [5,37–40]. In both HT and non-HT patients the calculated RoM of nodules in particular categories of SRSs was generally close to the expected one. Differences over 5% were observed for category 4 of K-TIRADS, ACR-TIRADS and ATA guidelines systems, where the risk in non-HT group was higher than expected. That could be the consequence of a notable fraction of cancers other than PTC in our material, amounting to 23.1% in non-HT group. These cancers were mainly FTC and HTC and were usually classified into category 4 of those SRSs (56.3% cancers other than PTC for K-TIRADS and ATA guidelines, 64.6% for ACR-TIRADS). The higher percentage of cancers other than PTC was also a probable cause of slightly lower AUC of those SRSs in non-HT group than in patients with HT. It should be kept in mind that US malignancy features and SRSs were established mainly on the basis of the ultrasound image of the most common PTCs [41]. Effectiveness of SRSs could potentially be improved by the inclusion of elastographic measurements [42,43]. Promising results in this respect were also obtained in patients with HT [21,44,45].

A limitation of our study is the difference in mean sizes of nodules in patients with and without HT. The size might affect the US characteristics of thyroid nodules, but small nodules are typical of HT. The advantage of our study is performing US malignancy feature evaluation directly prior to biopsy. Therefore, the result of FNA did not influence the evaluation. The majority of final diagnoses were based on postoperative histopathological examination. It is an advantage because of the certainty of the final diagnosis but on the other hand it could be a source of a bias in patient selection. In clinical practice, patients with HT are usually not referred to surgical treatment. Despite this way of including patients in the study the distribution of nodules among equivocal and unequivocal categories of BSRTC was similar in both groups. That is advantageous because there are significant differences in the usefulness of the assessment of US malignancy features in relation to nodule's category of FNA outcome [6]. The adopted way of confirmation of HT diagnosis may also be regarded as advantageous because of rather rigorous criteria. However, it may be seen as a limitation in relation to seronegative cases of HT. In our study, patients with a positive TPOab test dominated, and seronegative patients, in whom HT was confirmed by its characteristic features in the cytological examination, constituted a very small percentage of HT group.

4. Materials and Methods

4.1. Examined Patients

Ultrasound imaging and FNA examinations were performed in a single center, in the years 2012–2020, in patients referred by endocrinologists from outpatient clinics. The study included all nodules classified into the categories II–VI of BSRTC with full ultrasound imaging data, a known result of the postoperative histopathological examination and a known status of HT presence. The exclusion criteria consisted of previous surgical or radioiodine treatment, as well as positive neck irradiation history. Because of relatively small number of nodules assigned to category II in BSRTC with a known result of histopathological examination in patients with HT, in that group we additionally included all nodules with full ultrasound imaging data and category II of BSRTC confirmed in at least three FNAs. The study included 1188 nodules (revealed in 1022 patients), i.e., 358 nodules in patients with HT (HT group) and 830 nodules in patients without HT (non-HT group) (Table 5). The differences in the incidence of particular categories of the Bethesda system between groups HT and non-HT did not exceed 5%. Frequencies of nodules with an equivocal (categories III–V) FNA outcome were similar in both groups (HT: 50.8% vs. non-HT: 54.1%, $p = 0.3018$).

Table 5. Data on the diagnostic effectiveness of analyzed SRSs in HT and non-HT groups for the high risk category (nodule's shape evaluated on the transverse plane).

Parameter	HT Group	Non-HT Group	p
Number of nodules	358	830	
Number of patients	310	712	
Age, mean ± SD (years)	55.1 ± 14.0	53.7 ± 13.3	0.1113
No/% of males	12/3.9	94/13.2	<0.0001
Volume of nodules mean ± SD (cm^3)	3.17 ± 7.4	7.61 ± 16.2	<0.0001
No/% of nodules < 1 cm #	58/16.2%	77/9.3%	0.0006
No/% of cancers	87/24.3	208/25.1	0.7813
No/% of PTCs among cancers	76/87.4	160/76.9	0.0411
Other cancers (No/%)	FTC (4/4.6) HTC (1/1.1) MTC (5/5.7) ST (1/1.1)	FTC (13/6.3), HTC (13/6.3) MTC (14/6.7), PDTC (2/1.0) AC (2/1.0), ST (2/1.0) ANG (1/0.5), FT-UMP (1/0.5)	
category of BSRTC (No/%)	II: 124/34.6 * III: 121/33.8 IV: 40/11.2 V: 21/5.9 VI: 52/14.5	II: 253/30.5 III: 277/33.4 IV: 135/16.2 V: 37/4.5 VI: 128/15.4	0.1580 0.8867 0.0203 0.2580 0.6925

*—including 78 nodules, without the surgical treatment but after three FNAs with all outcomes classified into category II of BSRTC. #—both cancers and benign nodules <1 cm were more frequent in HT group than non-HT one (34.5% vs. 19.7%, $p = 0.0068$ and 10.3% vs. 5.8%, $p = 0.0155$, respectively). PTC—papillary thyroid carcinoma, MTC—medullary thyroid carcinoma, FTC follicular thyroid carcinoma, HTC—Hurthle cell thyroid carcinoma, PDTC—poorly differentiated thyroid carcinoma, AC—anaplastic carcinoma, ST—secondary tumor, ANG—angiosarcoma, FT-UMP—follicular tumor of uncertain malignant potential.

In all patients, the clinical diagnosis of HT was established by an endocrinologist in the endocrine outpatient clinic on the basis of clinical symptoms, serological tests (measurement of anti-thyroid antibodies), assessment of serum concentrations of thyroid stimulating hormone and thyroid hormones, ultrasound examination, as well as cytological examinations. Because fewer than 30% of patients with HT present all the above-mentioned HT features [13,14,46], we decided to adopt minimal conditions for the diagnosis of HT. We assumed that all patients in HT group had to have a clinical diagnosis of HT confirmed with elevated levels of serum anti-thyroid peroxidase antibodies (TPOab) or characteristic features of HT in the microscopic examination. On the other hand, patients included in the non-HT group did not have any hormonal, morphological, or ultrasound features of HT and they had normal TPOab.

4.2. Analysis of US Malignancy Features

The analysis of US malignancy features was done prospectively. The presence of particular US malignancy features was assessed by experienced sonographers (four physicians with over ten years' experience) directly before FNA, according to a unified pattern that had been used at our department for many years. We used a computer system dedicated for collecting detailed information on examined nodules in a database. The system was created by one of the authors of the study—MK. On the basis of those data, three diameters of biopsied nodules were determined as well as the presence of: (1) marked hypoechogenicity (compared to the echogenicity of the strap muscles); (2) hypoechogenicity (as compared to the normal thyroid); (3) solid echostructure (>90% solid) (4) more solid than cystic echostructure (>50% solid); (5) suspicious shape/orientation, assessed on the transverse and longitudinal planes, interpreted in two variants: $AP \geq T$ and $AP > T$; (6) suspicious margins—irregular (including microlobulated, spiculated, and suggesting extrathyroidal extension); (7) microcalcifications; (8) macrocalcifications; (9) rim calcifications; (10) pathological vascularization (marked intranodular vascular spots). The presence of spongiform echostructure (>50% of nodule, without obvious solid areas) was also assessed. The US examinations were performed with the use of the Aloka Prosound Alpha 7 ultrasound system, ALOKA co. Ltd., Tokyo, Japan with a 7.5–14 MHz linear transducer.

With the use of the set of features specified above, all thyroid nodules were classified into specific categories of four SRSs: EU-TIRADS [1], K-TIRADS [2], ACR-TIRADS [3], and the system recommended by ATA [4]. The differences in the interpretation of nodules with mixed echogenicity between particular SRSs were considered (the presence of any hypoechoic tissue assessed in EU-TIRADS or predominant echogenicity in other SRSs). In the case of the ATA guidelines, a modification was applied, because this system does not cover all nodule's ultrasound patterns; in particular it lacks patterns in which iso- or hyperechoic nodules show high malignancy risk features. In total, 71 (6.0%) nodules did not satisfy the criteria of ATA classification and those nodules corresponded to 22 cancers (8/9.2% in HT group and 14/6.7% in non-HT group, $p = 0.4625$). We decided to classify such nodules into the intermediate suspicion category. That allowed us to compare how all systems worked in the evaluation of the same set of nodules. We did not identify disrupted rim calcifications with small extrusive soft tissue component as a separate feature (which is included in ATA guidelines), but the nodules presenting such an image were treated as ones with irregular margins which resulted in the same output of the categorization. Two researchers (DSK and MK) independently assigned all the ultrasound features for TIRADS score calculation. In the case of discrepancy, the US report was jointly reevaluated and discussed to confirm its categorization.

4.3. Analyses, Statistical Evaluation

At the first step of the evaluation, receiver operating characteristic (ROC) curves were determined in both groups and both thyroid planes for AP/T ratio describing nodule's shape. The Z test was used to compare the area under the ROC (AUC) value between HT and non-HT groups. The cut-off values of AP/T ratio that showed the highest accuracy (ACC) in the classification of benign and malignant lesions were also identified. Odds ratios (OR) with relative 95% confidence intervals (95% CI) for the established cut-off values were assessed with the use of logistic regression analysis. The effectiveness of the determined thresholds as well as the 'standard' thresholds: $AP > T$ and $AP \geq T$ was described with the use of sensitivity (SEN), specificity (SPC), ACC, positive likelihood ratio (LR+) and the percentage of nodules reaching given threshold. The RoM of those nodules (the proportion of cancers among all positive nodules, i.e., the positive predictive value—PPV) and the negative predictive value (NPV) were calculated. Additionally, the effectiveness of all examined thresholds of AP/T ratio was assessed for nodules <1 cm and larger as well as for cancers other than PTC.

Next, the incidence of other US malignancy features was assessed in the nodules classified into HT and non-HT groups in respect to the division of the nodules into benign lesions and cancers according to the final diagnosis. In the case of nodules of mixed echogenicity the presence of any hypoechoic tissue was regarded as hypoechogenicity. The associations between individual US malignancy features and malignancy were evaluated with the use of logistic regression analysis in both groups. The OR were calculated to determine the relevance of all potential predictors of the outcome. The incidence of all

US malignancy features was also compared between benign nodules of HT and non-HT groups and between malignant nodules in both groups.

Then the distribution of benign and malignant nodules among particular categories of the examined SRSs was assessed. The efficiency of the systems was compared analyzing ROC curves and cut-off categories with the highest ACC were identified for each of the SRSs. Using those cut-off categories SEN, SPC ACC, RoM/PPV, NPV were calculated, as well as the percentage of positive nodules in both groups. Those analyzes were performed separately for three variants of AP/T ratio interpretation described above.

The statistical analysis was performed with the Dell Statistica (data analysis software system), version 13, Dell Inc. (2016), Round Rock, TX, USA. The comparison of frequency distributions was performed with chi2 test (with modifications appropriate for the number of analyzed cases). The Kruskal–Wallis test was used for comparing continuous variables between groups. The value of 0.05 was assumed as the level of significance.

4.4. Microscopic Examination

Biopsies were performed following regular procedures, on nodules with a diameter of at least 5 mm (and usually over 1 cm) and at least one malignancy risk factor (ultrasonographic or clinical). In most cases, two aspirations of a nodule were done. Smears were fixed with a 95% ethanol solution and stained with haematoxylin and eosin. The FNA outcome of each nodule was classified into one of six categories in the BSRTC—category I: non-diagnostic/unsatisfactory biopsies, category II: benign lesions (BL), category III: follicular lesion of undetermined significance (FLUS)/atypia of undetermined significance (AUS), category IV: suspicious for a follicular neoplasm (SFN), category V: suspicious for malignancy (SM) and category VI: malignant neoplasm (MN) [47,48]. Patients with a FNA outcome of category IV, V, or VI were routinely referred for thyroid surgery. In the case of a diagnosis of BL or FLUS/AUS, surgical treatment was performed based on the patient's preference or due to the large size of the goiter as well as the presence of other clinical, ultrasonographic or cytological risk features (especially in the case of AUS diagnosis).

5. Conclusions

The optimal usage of US malignancy features in patients with HT is very important because of the increased risk of malignancy in thyroid nodules in that group. To reach this goal, it may be helpful to adjust the threshold for AP/T ratio to the specific characteristics of nodules found in patients with HT. This specificity consists in more frequent occurrence of round nodules. In patients with HT, a slight modification of the threshold for AP/T ratio and regarding round nodules as suspicious leads to a three-fold increase in SEN of the suspected nodule's shape feature, with a disproportionally lower decrease in SPC and similar ACC. Importantly, such a modification is effective also for cancers other than PTC. In patients without HT there are analogical, yet less marked changes. Thus, the use of AP $\geq$ T threshold instead AP > T is justified, especially in patients with HT and in centers that intend to improve SEN. On the other hand, in centers where, due to the epidemiology of thyroid diseases, the priority is not an improvement of SEN but maximization of SPC and PPV, it is rational to use threshold for the AP/T ratio over 1, close to 1.15. It enables a twofold increase in OR of nodules that reach such a threshold in comparison to the classic AP > T threshold, with a very low loss of SEN and maximization of ACC. It also could lead to an even twofold reduction of the number of performed FNA. The assessment of a nodule's shape on the transverse plane is sufficient for the effective use of that feature with any of the analyzed thresholds. The diagnostic effectiveness of EU-TIRADS, K-TIRADS, ACR-TIRADS, and ATA guidelines in patients with HT and without HT is similar. Changes in the threshold for AP/T ratio modify that effectiveness, and their influence on the number of nodules classified into the category of the highest risk is the greatest in the case of EU-TIRADS.

Supplementary Materials: The following are available online at https://www.mdpi.com/article/10.3390/cancers13194900/s1, Figure S1: ROC curve analysis of the evaluation of AP/T ratio on transverse plane in HT and non-HT groups; points of maximal ACC indicated on both curves, Figure S2: ROC curve analysis of the evaluation of AP/T ratio on longitudinal plane in HT and non-HT groups; points of maximal ACC indicated on both curves, Table S1: Incidence of round nodules (with anteroposterior diameter equal to transverse diameter) in HT and non-HT group, Table S2: Data on the diagnostic effectiveness of AP/T ratio evaluation in examined groups of nodules (HT and non-HT), with the threshold AP $\geq$ T or AP > T satisfied on any plane (transverse or longitudinal), Table S3: Data on the diagnostic effectiveness of AP/T ratio evaluation (on transverse plane) in examined groups of nodules (HT and non-HT), in relation to nodule's size (largest diameter <1 cm and $\geq$1 cm), Table S4: Results of multivariate logistic regression analysis in HT and non-HT groups, Table S5: Influence of modifications of the threshold for suspicious nodule's shape (from AP > T to AP $\geq$ T and AP/T $\geq$ 1.14 in HT group or AP/T $\geq$ 1.17 in non-HT group) on values of SEN, SPC, RoM and the percentage of nodules in the high risk category (changes expressed as percentage of values for AP > T threshold).

Author Contributions: Conceptualization, D.S.-K.; Methodology, D.S.-K., M.K., K.W.-K., M.W.-N. and B.P.; Project administration, D.S.-K., K.W.-K. and B.P.; Software: M.K.; Supervision, D.S.-K. and M.K.; Validation, D.S.-K. and M.K.; Formal analysis, M.K.; Investigation, D.S.-K., K.W.-K., M.W.-N., B.P., E.W.-O. and M.K.; Data curation, D.S.-K., K.W.-K., M.W.-N., E.W.-O. and M.K.; Writing—original draft preparation, D.S.-K. and M.K.; Writing—review and editing, M.K., M.W.-N. and D.S.-K. All authors have read and agreed to the published version of the manuscript.

Funding: This research was funded by the Medical University of Lodz, grant number 503/1-153-05/503-11-001.

Institutional Review Board Statement: The study was conducted according to the guidelines of the Declaration of Helsinki, and approved by the Institutional Ethics Committee of Medical University of Lodz (protocol code RNN/151/17/KE approved on 16 May 2017).

Informed Consent Statement: Informed consent was obtained from all subjects involved in the study.

Data Availability Statement: The data presented in this study are available on request from the corresponding authors. The data are not publicly available due to patient privacy restrictions.

Conflicts of Interest: The authors declare no conflict of interest. The funders had no role in the design of the study; in the collection, analyses, or interpretation of data; in the writing of the manuscript, or in the decision to publish the results.

References

1. Russ, G.; Bonnema, S.J.; Erdogan, M.F.; Durante, C.; Ngu, R.; Leenhardt, L. European Thyroid Association Guidelines for Ultrasound Malignancy Risk Stratification of Thyroid Nodules in Adults: The EU-TIRADS. *Eur. Thyroid J.* **2017**, *6*, 225–237. [CrossRef]
2. Shin, J.H.; Baek, J.H.; Chung, J.; Ha, E.J.; Kim, J.H.; Lee, Y.H.; Lim, H.K.; Moon, W.J.; Na, D.G.; Park, J.S.; et al. Korean Society of Thyroid Radiology (KSThR) and Korean Society of Radiology. Ultrasonography Diagnosis and Imaging-Based Management of Thyroid Nodules: Revised Korean Society of Thyroid Radiology Consensus Statement and Recommendations. *Korean J. Radiol.* **2016**, *17*, 370–395. [CrossRef] [PubMed]
3. Tessler, F.N.; Middleton, W.D.; Grant, E.G.; Hoang, J.K.; Berland, L.L.; Teefey, S.A.; Cronan, J.J.; Beland, M.D.; Desser, T.S.; Frates, M.C.; et al. ACR Thyroid Imaging, Reporting and Data System (TI-RADS): White Paper of the ACR TI-RADS Committee. *J. Am. Coll. Radiol.* **2017**, *14*, 587–595. [CrossRef]
4. Haugen, B.R.; Alexander, E.K.; Bible, K.C.; Doherty, G.M.; Mandelm, S.J.; Nikiforov, Y.E.; Pacini, F.; Randolph, G.W.; Sawka, A.M.; Schlumberger, M.; et al. 2015 American Thyroid Association Management Guidelines for Adult Patients with Thyroid Nodules and Differentiated Thyroid Cancer: The American Thyroid Association Guidelines Task Force on Thyroid Nodules and Differentiated Thyroid Cancer. *Thyroid* **2016**, *26*, 1–133. [CrossRef]
5. Kim, P.H.; Suh, C.H.; Baek, J.H.; Chung, S.R.; Choi, Y.J.; Lee, J.H. Diagnostic Performance of Four Ultrasound Risk Stratification Systems: A Systematic Review and Meta-Analysis. *Thyroid* **2020**, *30*, 1159–1168. [CrossRef]
6. Słowińska-Klencka, D.; Wysocka-Konieczna, K.; Klencki, M.; Popowicz, B. Diagnostic Value of Six Thyroid Imaging Reporting and Data Systems (TIRADS) in Cytologically Equivocal Thyroid Nodules. *J. Clin. Med.* **2020**, *9*, 2281. [CrossRef]
7. Hong, M.J.; Na, D.G.; Baek, J.H.; Sung, J.Y.; Kim, J.H. Cytology-Ultrasonography Risk-Stratification Scoring System Based on Fine-Needle Aspiration Cytology and the Korean-Thyroid Imaging Reporting and Data System. *Thyroid* **2017**, *27*, 953–959. [CrossRef]

8. Ahmadi, S.; Herbst, R.; Oyekunle, T.; Jiang, X.; Strickland, K.; Roman, S.; Sosa, J.A. Using the ATA and ACR TI-RADS sonographic classifications as adjunctive predictors of malignancy for indeterminate thyroid nodules. *Endocr. Pract.* **2019**, *25*, 908–917. [CrossRef] [PubMed]
9. Barbosa, T.L.M.; Junior, C.O.M.; Graf, H.; Cavalvanti, T.; Trippia, M.A.; da Silveira Ugino, R.T.; de Oliveira, G.L.; Granella, V.H.; de Carvalho, G.A. ACR TI-RADS and ATA US scores are helpful for the management of thyroid nodules with indeterminate cytology. *BMC Endocr. Disord.* **2019**, *19*, 112. [CrossRef] [PubMed]
10. Grani, G.; Lamartina, L.; Ramundo, V.; Falcone, R.; Lomonaco, C.; Ciotti, L.; Barone, M.; Maranghi, M.; Cantisani, V.; Filetti, S.; et al. Taller-Than-Wide Shape: A New Definition Improves the Specificity of TIRADS Systems. *Eur. Thyroid J.* **2020**, *9*, 85–91. [CrossRef]
11. Topaloglu, O.; Baser, H.; Cuhaci, F.N.; Sungu, N.; Yalcin, A.; Ersoy, R.; Cakir, B. Malignancy is associated with microcalcification and higher AP/T ratio in ultrasonography, but not with Hashimoto's thyroiditis in histopathology in patients with thyroid nodules evaluated as Bethesda Category III (AUS/FLUS) in cytology. *Endocrine* **2016**, *54*, 156–168. [CrossRef]
12. Huang, K.; Gao, N.; Zhai, Q.; Bian, D.; Wang, D.; Wang, X. The anteroposterior diameter of nodules in the risk assessment of papillary thyroid microcarcinoma. *Medicine* **2018**, *97*, e9712. [CrossRef]
13. Ragusa, F.; Fallahi, P.; Elia, G.; Gonnella, D.; Paparo, S.R.; Giusti, C.; Churilov, L.P.; Ferrari, S.M.; Antonelli, A. Hashimotos' thyroiditis: Epidemiology, pathogenesis, clinic and therapy. *Best Pract Res. Clin. Endocrinol. Metab.* **2019**, *33*, 101367. [CrossRef]
14. Caturegli, P.; De Remigis, A.; Rose, N.R. Hashimoto thyroiditis: Clinical and diagnostic criteria. *Autoimmun Rev.* **2014**, *13*, 391–397. [CrossRef] [PubMed]
15. Anderson, L.; Middleton, W.D.; Teefey, S.A.; Reading, C.C.; Langer, J.E.; Desser, T.; Szabunio, M.M.; Hildebolt, C.F.; Mandel, S.J.; Cronan, J.J. Hashimoto thyroiditis: Part 1, sonographic analysis of the nodular form of Hashimoto thyroiditis. *AJR Am. J. Roentgenol.* **2010**, *195*, 208–215. [CrossRef]
16. Anderson, L.; Middleton, W.D.; Teefey, S.A.; Reading, C.C.; Langer, J.E.; Desserm, T.; Szabunio, M.M.; Mandel, S.J.; Hildebolt, C.F.; Cronan, J.J. Hashimoto thyroiditis: Part 2, sonographic analysis of benign and malignant nodules in patients with diffuse Hashimoto thyroiditis. *AJR Am. J. Roentgenol.* **2010**, *195*, 216–222. [CrossRef] [PubMed]
17. Oppenheimer, D.C.; Giampoli, E.; Montoya, S.; Patel, S.; Dogra, V. Sonographic Features of Nodular Hashimoto Thyroiditis. *Ultrasound Q.* **2016**, *32*, 271–276. [CrossRef] [PubMed]
18. Boi, F.; Pani, F.; Calò, P.G.; Lai, M.L.; Mariotti, S. High prevalence of papillary thyroid carcinoma in nodular Hashimoto's thyroiditis at the first diagnosis and during the follow-up. *J. Endocrinol Invest.* **2018**, *41*, 395–402. [CrossRef]
19. Resende de Paiva, C.; Grønhøj, C.; Feldt-Rasmussen, U.; von Buchwald, C. Association between Hashimoto's Thyroiditis and Thyroid Cancer in 64,628 Patients. *Front. Oncol.* **2017**, *7*, 53. [CrossRef] [PubMed]
20. Durfee, S.M.; Benson, C.B.; Arthaud, D.M.; Alexander, E.K.; Frates, M.C. Sonographic appearance of thyroid cancer in patients with Hashimoto thyroiditis. *J. Ultrasound Med.* **2015**, *34*, 697–704. [CrossRef]
21. Han, R.; Li, F.; Wang, Y.; Ying, Z.; Zhang, Y. Virtual touch tissue quantification (VTQ) in the diagnosis of thyroid nodules with coexistent chronic autoimmune Hashimoto's thyroiditis: A preliminary study. *Eur. J. Radiol.* **2015**, *84*, 327–331. [CrossRef] [PubMed]
22. Baser, H.; Ozdemir, D.; Cuhaci, N.; Aydin, C.; Ersoy, R.; Kilicarslan, A.; Cakir, B. Hashimoto's Thyroiditis Does Not Affect Ultrasonographical, Cytological, and Histopathological Features in Patients with Papillary Thyroid Carcinoma. *Endocr. Pathol.* **2015**, *26*, 356–364. [CrossRef]
23. Zhou, H.; Yue, W.W.; Du, L.Y.; Xu, J.M.; Liu, B.J.; Li, X.L.; Wang, D.; Zhou, X.L.; Xu, H.X. A Modified Thyroid Imaging Reporting and Data System (mTI-RADS) For Thyroid Nodules in Coexisting Hashimoto's Thyroiditis. *Sci. Rep.* **2016**, *6*, 26410. [CrossRef] [PubMed]
24. Zhang, J.W.; Chen, Z.J.; Gopinathan, A. Focal Nodular Hashimoto's Thyroiditis: Comparison of Ultrasonographic Features with Malignant and Other Benign Nodules. *Ann. Acad Med. Singap.* **2016**, *45*, 357–363.
25. Gul, K.; Dirikoc, A.; Kiyak, G.; Ersoy, P.; Ugras, N.S.; Ersoy, R.; Cakir, B. The association between thyroid carcinoma and Hashimoto's thyroiditis: The ultrasonographic and histopathologic characteristics of malignant nodules. *Thyroid* **2010**, *20*, 873–878. [CrossRef] [PubMed]
26. Peng, Q.; Niu, C.; Zhang, M.; Peng, Q.; Chen, S. Sonographic Characteristics of Papillary Thyroid Carcinoma with Coexistent Hashimoto's Thyroiditis: Conventional Ultrasound, Acoustic Radiation Force Impulse Imaging and Contrast-Enhanced Ultrasound. *Ultrasound Med. Biol.* **2019**, *45*, 471–480. [CrossRef] [PubMed]
27. Ohmori, N.; Miyakawa, M.; Ohmori, K.; Takano, K. Ultrasonographic findings of papillary thyroid carcinoma with Hashimoto's thyroiditis. *Intern. Med.* **2007**, *46*, 547–550. [CrossRef]
28. Park, M.; Park, S.H.; Kim, E.K.; Yoon, J.H.; Moon, H.J.; Lee, H.S.; Kwak, J.Y. Heterogeneous echogenicity of the underlying thyroid parenchyma: How does this affect the analysis of a thyroid nodule? *BMC Cancer* **2013**, *13*, 550. [CrossRef]
29. Słowińska-Klencka, D.; Wojtaszek-Nowicka, M.; Klencki, M.; Wysocka-Konieczna, K.; Popowicz, B. The Presence of Hypoechoic Micronodules in Patients with Hashimoto's Thyroiditis Increases the Risk of an Alarming Cytological Outcome. *J. Clin. Med.* **2021**, *10*, 638. [CrossRef]
30. Fukushima, M.; Fukunari, N.; Murakami, T.; Kunii, Y.; Suzuki, S.; Kitaoka, M. Reconfirmation of the accuracy of the taller-than-wide sign in multicenter collaborative research in Japan. *Endocr. J.* **2021**, *68*, 897–904. [CrossRef]
31. Cappelli, C.; Castellano, M.; Pirola, I.; Gandossi, E.; De Martino, E.; Cumetti, D.; Agosti, B.; Rosei, E.A. Thyroid nodule shape suggests malignancy. *Eur. J. Endocrinol.* **2006**, *155*, 27–31. [CrossRef] [PubMed]

32. Kim, S.Y.; Na, D.G.; Paik, W. Which ultrasound image plane is appropriate for evaluating the taller-than-wide sign in the risk stratification of thyroid nodules? *Eur. Radiol.* **2021**, *8*, 1–9. [CrossRef]
33. Ren, J.; Liu, B.; Zhang, L.L.; Li, H.Y.; Zhang, F.; Li, S.; Zhao, L.R. A taller-than-wide shape is a good predictor of papillary thyroid carcinoma in small solid nodules. *J. Ultrasound Med.* **2015**, *34*, 19–26. [CrossRef]
34. Chen, S.P.; Hu, Y.P.; Chen, B. Taller-than-wide sign for predicting thyroid microcarcinoma: Comparison and combination of two ultrasonographic planes. *Ultrasound Med. Biol.* **2014**, *40*, 2004–2011. [CrossRef] [PubMed]
35. Moon, H.J.; Kwak, J.Y.; Kim, E.K.; Kim, M.J. A taller-than-wide shape in thyroid nodules in transverse and longitudinal ultrasonographic planes and the prediction of malignancy. *Thyroid* **2011**, *21*, 1249–1253. [CrossRef]
36. Wildman-Tobriner, B.; Ahmed, S.; Erkanli, A.; Mazurowski, M.A.; Hoang, J.K. Using the American College of Radiology Thyroid Imaging Reporting and Data System at the Point of Care: Sonographer Performance and Interobserver Variability. *Ultrasound Med. Biol.* **2020**, *46*, 1928–1933. [CrossRef]
37. Wang, J.; Li, P.; Sun, L.; Sun, Y.; Fang, S.; Liu, X. Diagnostic value of strain ratio measurement in differential diagnosis of thyroid nodules coexisted with Hashimoto thyroiditis. *Int. J. Clin. Exp. Med.* **2015**, *8*, 6420–6426.
38. Gao, L.; Xi, X.; Jiang, Y.; Yang, X.; Wang, Y.; Zhu, S.; Lai, X.; Zhang, X.; Zhao, R.; Zhang, B. Comparison among TIRADS (ACR TI-RADS and KWAK- TI-RADS) and 2015 ATA Guidelines in the diagnostic efficiency of thyroid nodules. *Endocrine* **2019**, *64*, 90–96. [CrossRef]
39. Shen, Y.; Liu, M.; He, J.; Wu, S.; Chen, M.; Wan, Y.; Gao, L.; Cai, X.; Ding, J.; Fu, X. Comparison of Different Risk-Stratification Systems for the Diagnosis of Benign and Malignant Thyroid Nodules. *Front. Oncol.* **2019**, *9*, 378. [CrossRef]
40. Castellana, M.; Piccardo, A.; Virili, C.; Scappaticcio, L.; Grani, G.; Durante, C.; Giovanella, L.; Trimboli, P. Can ultrasound systems for risk stratification of thyroid nodules identify follicular carcinoma? *Cancer Cytopathol.* **2020**, *128*, 250–259. [CrossRef] [PubMed]
41. Trimboli, P.; Castellana, M.; Piccardo, A.; Romanelli, F.; Grani, G.; Giovanella, L.; Durante, C. The ultrasound risk stratification systems for thyroid nodule have been evaluated against papillary carcinoma. A meta-analysis. *Rev. Endocr. Metab. Disord.* **2021**, *22*, 453–460. [CrossRef] [PubMed]
42. Borlea, A.; Borcan, F.; Sporea, I.; Dehelean, C.A.; Negrea, R.; Cotoi, L.; Stoian, D. TI-RADS Diagnostic Performance: Which Algorithm is Superior and How Elastography and 4D Vascularity Improve the Malignancy Risk Assessment. *Diagnostics* **2020**, *10*, 180. [CrossRef]
43. Russ, G. Risk stratification of thyroid nodules on ultrasonography with the French TI-RADS: Description and reflections. *Ultrasonography* **2016**, *35*, 25–38. [CrossRef] [PubMed]
44. Li, Y.; Wang, Y.; Wu, Q.; Hu, B. Papillary thyroid microcarcinoma co-exists with Hashimoto's thyroiditis: Is strain elastography still useful? *Ultrasonics* **2016**, *68*, 127–133. [CrossRef] [PubMed]
45. Liu, B.; Liang, J.; Zhou, L.; Lu, Y.; Zheng, Y.; Tian, W.; Xie, X. Shear Wave Elastography in the Diagnosis of Thyroid Nodules with Coexistent Chronic Autoimmune Hashimoto's Thyroiditis. *Otolaryngol. Head Neck Surg.* **2015**, *153*, 779–785. [CrossRef] [PubMed]
46. Guan, H.; de Morais, N.S.; Stuart, J.; Ahmadi, S.; Marqusee, E.; Kimm, M.I.; Alexander, E.K. Discordance of serological and sonographic markers for Hashimoto's thyroiditis with gold standard histopathology. *Eur. J. Endocrinol.* **2019**, *181*, 539–544. [CrossRef]
47. Cibas, E.S.; Ali, S.Z. The Bethesda System for Reporting Thyroid Cytopathology. *Thyroid* **2009**, *19*, 1159–1165. [CrossRef]
48. Cibas, E.S.; Ali, S.Z. The 2017 Bethesda System for Reporting Thyroid Cytopathology. *Thyroid* **2017**, *27*, 1341–1346. [CrossRef]

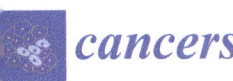

Review

Artificial Intelligence in Thyroid Field—A Comprehensive Review

Fabiano Bini [1,*], Andrada Pica [1], Laura Azzimonti [2], Alessandro Giusti [2], Lorenzo Ruinelli [3,4], Franco Marinozzi [1] and Pierpaolo Trimboli [5,6]

1. Department of Mechanical and Aerospace Engineering, Sapienza-University of Rome, 00184 Rome, Italy; andrada.pica@uniroma1.it (A.P.); franco.marinozzi@uniroma1.it (F.M.)
2. Dalle Molle Institute for Artificial Intelligence (IDSIA), Università della Svizzera Italiana (USI), Scuola Universitaria Professionale della Svizzera Italiana (SUPSI), Polo Universitario Lugano-Campus Est, 6962 Lugano-Viganello, Switzerland; laura.azzimonti@idsia.ch (L.A.); alessandro.giusti@idsia.ch (A.G.)
3. Information and Communications Technology, Ente Ospedaliero Cantonale, 6500 Bellinzona, Switzerland; lorenzo.ruinelli@eoc.ch
4. Clinical Trial Unit, Ente Ospedaliero Cantonale, 6500 Bellinzona, Switzerland
5. Servizio di Endocrinologia e Diabetologia, Ospedale Regionale di Lugano e Mendrisio, Ente Ospedaliero Cantonale, 6900 Lugano, Switzerland; Pierpaolo.Trimboli@eoc.ch
6. Faculty of Biomedical Sciences, Università della Svizzera Italiana (USI), 6900 Lugano, Switzerland
* Correspondence: fabiano.bini@uniroma1.it

Citation: Bini, F.; Pica, A.; Azzimonti, L.; Giusti, A.; Ruinelli, L.; Marinozzi, F.; Trimboli, P. Artificial Intelligence in Thyroid Field—A Comprehensive Review. *Cancers* **2021**, *13*, 4740. https://doi.org/10.3390/cancers13194740

Academic Editor: Kennichi Kakudo

Received: 31 August 2021
Accepted: 20 September 2021
Published: 22 September 2021

Publisher's Note: MDPI stays neutral with regard to jurisdictional claims in published maps and institutional affiliations.

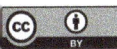

Copyright: © 2021 by the authors. Licensee MDPI, Basel, Switzerland. This article is an open access article distributed under the terms and conditions of the Creative Commons Attribution (CC BY) license (https://creativecommons.org/licenses/by/4.0/).

Simple Summary: The incidence of thyroid pathologies has been increasing worldwide. Historically, the detection of thyroid neoplasms relies on medical imaging analysis, depending mainly on the experience of clinicians. The advent of artificial intelligence (AI) techniques led to a remarkable progress in image-recognition tasks. AI represents a powerful tool that may facilitate understanding of thyroid pathologies, but actually, the diagnostic accuracy is uncertain. This article aims to provide an overview of the basic aspects, limitations and open issues of the AI methods applied to thyroid images. Medical experts should be familiar with the workflow of AI techniques in order to avoid misleading outcomes.

Abstract: Artificial intelligence (AI) uses mathematical algorithms to perform tasks that require human cognitive abilities. AI-based methodologies, e.g., machine learning and deep learning, as well as the recently developed research field of radiomics have noticeable potential to transform medical diagnostics. AI-based techniques applied to medical imaging allow to detect biological abnormalities, to diagnostic neoplasms or to predict the response to treatment. Nonetheless, the diagnostic accuracy of these methods is still a matter of debate. In this article, we first illustrate the key concepts and workflow characteristics of machine learning, deep learning and radiomics. We outline considerations regarding data input requirements, differences among these methodologies and their limitations. Subsequently, a concise overview is presented regarding the application of AI methods to the evaluation of thyroid images. We developed a critical discussion concerning limits and open challenges that should be addressed before the translation of AI techniques to the broad clinical use. Clarification of the pitfalls of AI-based techniques results crucial in order to ensure the optimal application for each patient.

Keywords: thyroid neoplasm; medical imaging; artificial intelligence; machine learning; deep learning; radiomics; prediction; diagnosis

1. Introduction

The role of medical imaging in the clinical workflow has noticeably increased from a mainly diagnostic tool up to a central contribution in early detection, diagnosis, treatment planning and monitoring of diseases [1–4]. Medical imaging provides information concerning the characteristics of human tissues in a non-invasive, repeatable manner and became a routine practice in clinical care [2]. In recent decades, the innovations in this field concerned both devices, i.e., hardware, and analysis tools used in medical imaging. In the clinical practice, the main use of medical images corresponds with qualitative assessment of the anatomical area. Images, in addition, are characterized also by a high quantity of numerical information and recently, a quantitative evaluation has been developed in order to identify possible correlations between the numerical data contained in the digital images and the pathophysiology of the tissue [3]. The quantitative analysis has the aim to achieve information from standard-of-care images, e.g., ultrasound imaging (US), computer tomography (CT), magnetic resonance imaging (MRI) and positron emission tomography (PET), which are not easily quantifiable by means of naked-eye observations for clinical outcomes [5,6].

Analysis of image features in the context of medical imaging is an emerging field of study but extensive literature already exists [7–9]. In the majority of earlier works, the image features are analyzed with the aim of detection and diagnosis of abnormal regions within human tissues [10–12]. These applications are often referred as computer-aided detection (CADe) and computer-aided diagnosis (CADx) systems [3]. The output of the CAD analysis is used by the expert clinicians as a second opinion in detecting lesions or making diagnosis and aims at improving the accuracy of the diagnosis and reducing the time for image interpretation [6].

Recently, a further detailed extension associated with quantitative analysis of medical imagines has led to the emergence of radiomics as a new field of medical research [1,2]. Radiomics aims at extracting numerous quantitative descriptors with the purpose of achieving more useful information of tissue lesion and response of treatment in order to be used for personalized medicine [1,2,13]. It is worth noticing that standardization of the procedure is still under development, as thoroughly discussed in [14].

The above-mentioned approaches apply methodologies from the artificial intelligence (AI) field to achieve a partial or full automation of various steps of the process concerning the analysis of medical images [6]. Thorough understanding of their working principle is necessary in order to develop efficient predictive models and personalization treatment. This review article aims to highlight strengths and limitations of the different AI-based techniques applied for the evaluation of the pathophysiological state of the thyroid.

2. Artificial Intelligence in Medical Imaging

Artificial intelligence (AI) is a term coined by McCarthy and colleagues [15,16] in 1950s referring to a branch of computer sciences in which mathematical algorithms attempt to perform tasks that normally require human cognitive abilities [8]. Applications of AI have witnessed unprecedented growth in recent decades due to the enhancement of computational power and availability of large dataset. In the medical field, AI can use complex algorithms to develop models with the scope of improving diagnostic accuracy, prognosis, and medical image interpretation [17]. We discuss in the following two different machine learning (ML) methodologies adopted to perform medical imaging analysis.

2.1. Machine Learning

Machine learning (ML), a term first coined by Arthur Samuel [18], is a field of AI in which the computer is trained to perform tasks by learning from example data and make predictions based on its exposition to previous samples [4]. In medical imaging analysis, ML algorithms are crucial components of both CAD systems and radiomics studies.

ML algorithms are generally divided into supervised and unsupervised learning methods. Supervised learning requires a labelled dataset, i.e., a set of input data with their corresponding output (labels) that is used to identify a function linking inputs to outputs [19]. Unsupervised learning operates on an input dataset without the need of labels. This ML algorithm searches for patterns that can separate input data into subsets with similar characteristics [7]. In this review article, we focus on supervised learning since it is the most common approach applied to medical images analysis [20].

In medical applications, input data include medical images or clinical data, while the output label can be the differentiation of malignant from benign nodules, the classification of images into diagnostic categories or the response treatment, e.g., recurrence, survival. The output of the predictive model leads to a subsequent distinction of ML problems: classification and regression. In classification tasks, the model performs a decision among a small and discrete set of choices, i.e., binary classification, e.g., identifying a tumor as malignant or benign. Regression models refers to the estimation of continuous output variables, e.g., assessment of disease severity [20].

Historically, ML algorithms were applied in CAD systems for classifications purposes [20]. Subsequently, this method was used as a step of radiomics analysis. In this section we describe the workflow of the ML algorithm with classification task frequently encountered in the CAD framework [10,21,22] (Figure 1). A supervised ML model is composed of two phases, i.e., training and application phase (Figure 1a). In the training phase, a set of input images with their corresponding class labels are used to train the predicting model. From the input image, a region of interest (ROI) is delineated manually or semi-automatically by expert clinicians. Subsequently, a set of image features, e.g., morphological and grey level-based features, are extracted. Differently from other methods that will be discussed subsequently in this work, in ML algorithms of CAD systems, the extraction and selection of image features are performed manually by the expert. It represents a crucial step in order to identify the significant variables that can be correlated with the medical endpoint. In CAD applications, the features used in the analysis are those closely associated with what clinicians use in their diagnosis of the lesions [4]. Subsequently, the features are entered as input to the ML algorithm to train the model.

Examples of typical feature-based supervised learning algorithms are logistic regressions, support vector machine, random forests and neural networks [23]. As an example of these feature-based ML algorithms, we focus here on the support vector machine (SVM) method, which is commonly used in biomedical binary classification problems [17,24]. Overall, SVM (Figure 1b) is a binary classifier that aims to identify the decision boundary, or hyperplane, that maximizes the separating margin between two classes [4,25].

For instance, let consider N training samples $\{(x_i, y_i)\}_{n=1}^{N}$ of input features x and their corresponding class or label $y_i \in \{-1; +1\}$ where $y_i = -1$ indicates the class with malignant samples and $y_i = 1$ indicates the class with benign samples. In the simplest case, there exists a function $f(x)$:

$$f(x) = \beta \cdot x + \beta_0, \qquad (1)$$

with β and β_0—decision boundary parameters such that $f(x) \geq 0$ for $y_i = +1$ and $f(x) < 0$ for $y_i = -1$.

This means that the training samples from the two classes are separated by the hyperplane $f(x) = \beta \cdot x + \beta_0 = 0$. The margin m, i.e., the distance between a class and the decision boundary, is set to be inversely proportional to the decision boundary parameter, i.e., $m = \frac{1}{\|\beta\|}$.

In order to identify the hyperplane that maximizes the separating margin between the two classes, SVM solves the following optimization problem that aims to minimize the cost function $J(\beta, \xi)$ with respect to β, ξ [24,26]:

$$\min_{\beta, \xi} J(\beta, \xi) = \min_{\beta, \xi} \frac{1}{2}\|\beta\|^2 + C \sum_{i=1}^{N} \xi_i \qquad (2)$$

subject to the constraints $y_i (\beta \cdot x + \beta_0) \geq 1 - \xi_i$, $\xi_i \geq 0$, $i = 1, \ldots, N$. In Equation (2), $C > 0$ is a penalty parameter to control the tolerance error ξ_i allowed for each sample being on the wrong side of the margin.

From Equation (2), it can be noticed that the minimization of the parameter β increases the separation between the two classes and improves generalizability of the classifier, while minimization of second term of Equation (1) improves fitting accuracy [4].

Subsequently, in the testing phase, the trained classifier is used to characterize new input data with unknown label (test set).

It is worth pointing out that the decision function of the classifier is fully specified by the training set, while the test set is only used to evaluate the performance of the model. On one hand, to obtain a model that well-performs when applied to new data, the training dataset should be sufficiently large. On the other hand, to obtain robust and reliable evaluation of the performance of the model, the test set should be sufficiently large. Frequently, since this condition is difficult to achieve in the medical field by simply splitting the available data in training and test set, a k-fold cross-validation framework [7] is usually adopted. K-fold cross validation consists of partitioning the dataset into k subsets of equal size. The model is trained on (k − 1) datasets while one subset is retained for model test. The process is repeated k times with each subset used once as test dataset [20]. The overall performance of the model is then assessed for example as the average performance over the k repetitions.

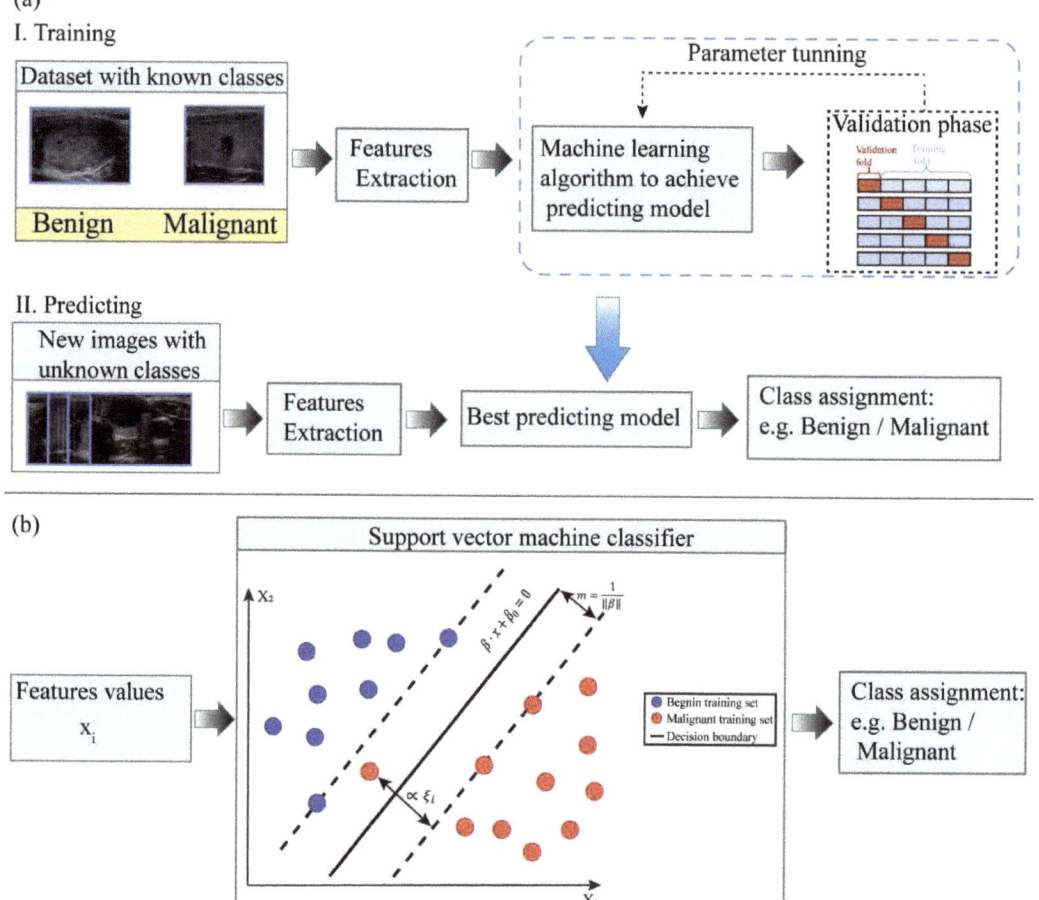

Figure 1. (a) Schematic flowchart of the machine learning model implementation and application for medical images classification purposes. (b) Example of the support vector machine (SVM) classification with a hyperplane that maximizes the separating margin m between the two classes.

Feature-based ML algorithms are suitable for medical image analysis since predictive models can be developed from small datasets [7]. Moreover, these methods are usually interpretable and can provide insights on the reasons why a certain class is predicted. Nonetheless, some initial steps of the process, as the definition of the features to be extracted from images and the selection of the medical region of interest has to be performed by experts. In addition, it should be taken into account that all supervised ML methods could be affected by overfitting, i.e., the predicting model learns exactly the training set but fails to fit new data from the test set [20]. However, it is possible to mitigate this issue by adopting a cross-validation set-up and by reducing the number of features used by the model by means of feature selection methods.

2.2. Deep Learning

Deep learning (DL), a term coined in 1986 by Rina Dechter [27], is a new class of ML methods developed through the advancement of artificial neural networks which were considered as artificial representations of the human neural architecture [23]. DL relies on networks of computational units, i.e., neural units arranged in layers that gradually extract higher level features from input data, e.g., image. These structures learn discriminative features from data automatically, allowing to approximate complex nonlinear relationship with outstanding performance [27,28]. Differently from traditional feature-based ML approaches, DL is able to achieve diagnosis automation, avoiding human intervention [29]. In medical applications, DL algorithms are implemented for detection and characterization of tissue lesions as well as for the analysis of disease progression [27,28].

While several DL architectures have been developed, this article focuses on convolutional neural networks (CNNs), introduced by LeCun [30]. CNNs are typically applied for image recognition and computer vision applications because they preserve spatial relationships in 2D data, and therefore outperform other architectures on image pattern recognition. More specifically, the input of a CNN is arranged in a grid structure and processed through convolution and pooling layers that preserve these relationships. The final layers are typically fully connected and can be conceived as a multi-layer perceptron classifier on the features automatically extracted by the convolutional part. The network is trained to identify patterns in a set of labelled training data and the outputs are compared with the actual labels. During training the network parameters are tuned until the patterns identified by the network represent good predictions for training data. The network is then used to make predictions on new data in the test set [31].

Figure 2 shows a typical architecture of CNN developed to perform classification tasks. The input of the CNN algorithm is represented by numerical data of the selected ROI from the medical image. Firstly, a convolutional step is considered which contains a set of filters, e.g., k_1 in Figure 2. Thus, a convolution is performed between each filter and the input of the layer, e.g., image data. A convolution is a space-invariant linear operation on 2D grids and is equivalent to applying a filter to an image. The filter slides over the input image, its values are multiplied with the image pixel values and then summed to determine the value in the corresponding position of the output feature map. An example of a convolution operation is reported in Figure 3a. The number and size of filters are CNN hyperparameters and are typically not optimized during training. More and larger filters lead to more powerful network with more parameters to optimize, which increases the risk of overfitting [32]. The convolutional process in every convolutional layer is expressed mathematically as follows:

$$X_k^\ell = \sigma\left(W_k^{\ell-1} * X^{\ell-1} + b_k^\ell\right) \qquad (3)$$

where X_k^ℓ is the new feature map, $\sigma(\cdot)$ is an element-wise nonlinear activation function, W is the filter values, b_k^ℓ is a bias parameter and the symbol $*$ indicates a convolutional operator.

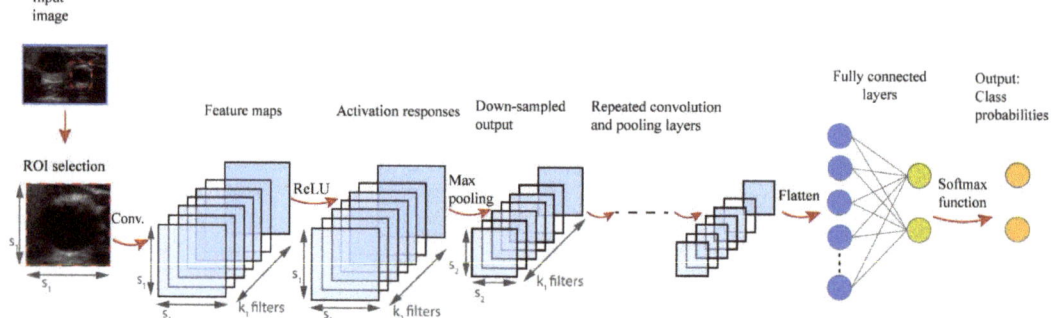

Figure 2. Schematic flowchart of the deep learning model implementation and application for medical images classification purposes.

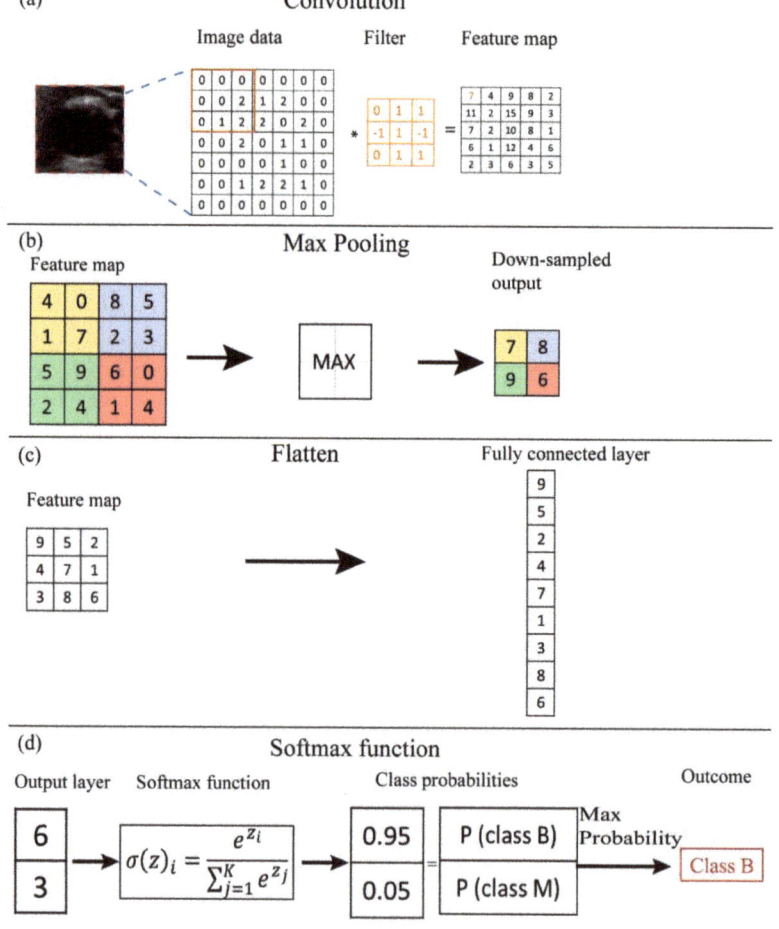

Figure 3. (a) Numerical example of the functions that compose the CNN architecture: (a) convolution, (b) max pooling, (c) flattening, (d) softmax function.

Subsequently, an activation function is applied element-by-element to the calculated output of the convolution prior to using the map as an input to the next layer of the network. Rectified linear unit (ReLU) is one of the most used activation functions, and has been empirically found to accelerate the convergence of the learning procedure [28]. It is linear for positive inputs, mapping them unchanged to the next layer, while it blocks negative values. Mathematically, ReLU is expressed as follows [28]:

$$f(x) = \max(0, x) \qquad (4)$$

where x is an activation value achieved from the previous layer.

Some CNN architectures also consider pooling operations, whose effect is to down-sample the feature maps. This operation considers small regions of the input map and outputs a single number for each region, e.g., the maximum value as illustrated in Figure 3b. It reduces the dimensions of the feature map and decreases the number of pixels to be processed in the next layers of the network [33]. Conceptually, as we progress deeper in the network, neuron activation values represent progressively higher-level and larger-scale visual patterns in the input, and therefore require lower spatial resolution.

The final part of the CNN architecture is characterized by a fully connected layer, i.e., each neural unit of the actual layer is connected to every neural unit in the successive layer (Figure 2). Firstly, the feature map is flattened into a column vector (Figure 3c) and then connected to one or more fully connected layers. The output nodes of the last fully connected layer can be regarded as a vector of unnormalized probabilities [28].

The softmax function is a function applied to the last fully connected layer of the CNN in order to transform the k real values of the vector into values in the range (0;1) so that can be assumed as probabilities (Figure 3d). The relation is as follows [28,33]:

$$\sigma(z)_i = \frac{e^{z_i}}{\sum_{j=1}^{K} e^{z_j}} \qquad (5)$$

where the z_i values are the elements of the fully connected layer and the denominator represents the normalization term.

The output layer of the CNN considered is constituted by neural units which indicate the probabilities for each class.

The analysis of the available literature shows an increasing interest on applying DL architecture for medical image analysis. It is worth mentioning that for systems in which the set of visual features is well defined, simpler feature-based ML techniques, such as SVM algorithms, are easier, more interpretable and more effective [28].

The main limitation to the use of DL consists of the large datasets required to train the model [34]. Compared with publicly available datasets in other areas, the current availability of medical US datasets is still limited [34]. To face the data requirements, several studies [33,35] considered pre-trained CNN architectures developed with trainings on ImageNet, a large labelled collection of low-resolution color photographs. To date, DL architectures pre-trained on high resolution medical images are not available. Therefore, a large dataset of medical images is a mandatory step to enhance CNNs performance [34].

3. Radiomics

Radiomics is an emerging field that uses automated high-throughput extraction algorithms to achieve large amounts (200+) of quantitative features from medical images [1,2]. Radiomics is also indicated as quantitative imaging [36] which can be applied to any image generated in the clinical setting. It can be performed on subregions of a tumor, metastatic lesions and in normal tissues. The term feature represents a descriptor of an image, of tumor or healthy tissue, such as parameters derived from image grayscale intensity or shape [37].

Radiomics has its roots on computer-aided diagnosis systems [38], although methodological workflow and applications are distinct [2]. It concerns the extraction of quantitative features from medical images that subsequently are related to biological endpoints and clinical outcomes [39]. Radiomics makes use of digital data stored in those images to develop diagnostic, predictive or prognostic models to support clinical decisions and optimize personalized treatment planning. The main difference with CAD systems consists of the relationship that radiomics has to identify between the current characteristics of the tissue lesion and its temporal evolution in the perspective of a personalization of the therapy [38].

Radiomics involves several processes, each with its own critical aspects that need to be taken into account. Two workflows can be implemented to perform radiomic studies in function of the AI technique adopted (Figure 4): (i) conventional or ML-based radiomics where the features to be extracted are predefined and (ii) DL-based radiomics where the features are not predefined but automatically extracted from the underlying data [6,7].

I. Conventional radiomics

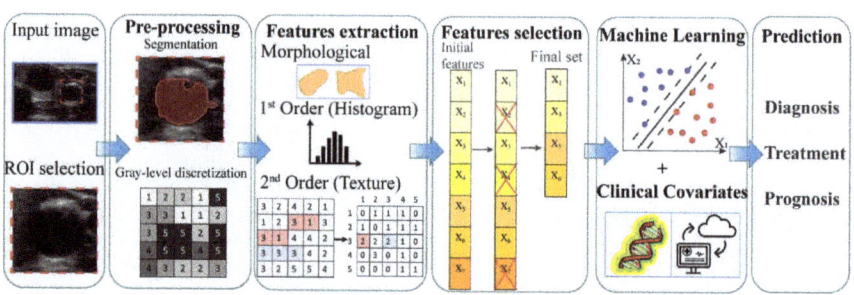

II. Deep Learning based radiomics

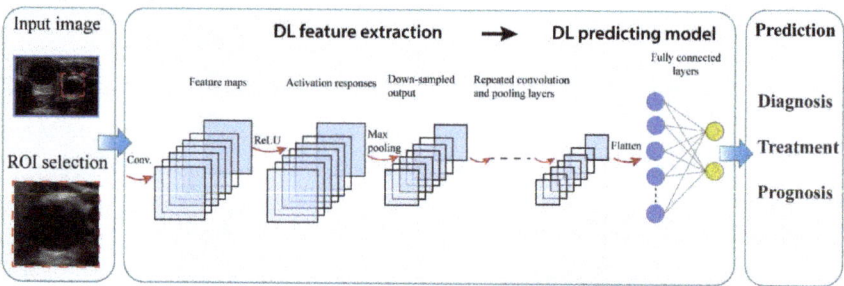

Figure 4. Schematic flowchart of radiomics approach. X_i represent the feature extracted from the image data.

The main aspects of the conventional radiomics workflow concerns: image acquisition, data selection, feature extraction and selection and the development of predictive model [1,36]. From medical image such as US, CT, MR and/or PET images, the region of interest (ROI) is selected and subsequently the lesion is manually segmented, i.e., delineated with computer-assisted contouring, by an experienced clinician [7]. Subsequently, image data undergoes preprocessing operations, e.g., gray-level discretization, which enable a higher reproducibility of results [6]. The extraction of quantitative imaging features involves descriptors of spatial relationships between the various intensity level, heterogeneity patterns, shape and relations of the tissue lesion with surrounding tissues. A feature selection procedure is then performed to identify the most relevant predictive features [7,24]. The collection of features which hold prognostic or predictive value represent a feature signature, frequently indicated also as quantitative imaging biomarkers. The selected features are then analyzed to develop classified models to predict outcomes either alone or in combination with additional information, such as demographic, clinical, comorbidity or genomic data [1,3].

Segmentation represents a crucial subprocess of radiomics since many extracted features may depend on the segmented region. In several radiomics studies the ROI is manually delineated by experts [21,40–42]. A number of algorithms has been developed for semi-automatic segmentation [22]. Region growing-based algorithm and grey-scale threshold-based methods are frequent techniques applied for ROI definition. However, manual delineation by an expert is considered the gold standard though is subjected to inter-observer variability and is a time-consuming task [37]. To avoid possible bias, evaluation by multiple clinicians or a combination of multiple algorithms could be considered [43].

Typically, radiomics features are divided into [2,6,44]:

1. Morphological, that are based on the geometric properties of the ROI, e.g.: volume, maximum surface area, maximum diameter.
2. First-order statistics or histogram based, which describe, through histograms, the distribution of grayscale intensity without concern for spatial relationships within the ROI. For instance, calculated features are grey level mean, maximum, minimum and percentiles.
3. Second-order statistics or textural features, that represent statistical relationship between the intensity levels of neighboring pixels within the ROI that allow to quantify image heterogeneity, e.g., absolute gradient, grey level co-occurrence matrix (GLCM) grey level run-length matrix (GLRLM), grey level size zone matrix (GLSZM) and grey level distance zone matrix (GLDZM). For instance, GLCM indicates the number of times the same combination of intensity occurs in two pixels separated by a specific distance δ in a known direction.
4. Higher-order statistics features, which are computed after the application of mathematical transformation and filters that lead to highlighting repeated patterns, histogram-oriented patterns or local binary patterns, e.g., wavelet or Fourier transforms.

Accurate definitions of radiomics features are provided in the image biomarker standardization initiative (IBSI) [14].

The radiomic features are subjected to a subsequent feature selection to prevent overfitting, improve learning accuracy and reduce computation time. The selection process should eliminate unreliable, not informative or redundant features. The selection methods can be divided into three classes: (i) filter methods which asses the usefulness of a given feature with various statistical tests for their correlation with the outcome variable [2,7]; (ii) wrapper method which uses an external classifier algorithm to score different subsets of features based on their classification performance; (iii) embedded method where the selection is intrinsic to the model training, i.e., features are selected to optimize the performance of the implemented learning algorithm. Filter methods are simple and computationally efficient, but consider features as independent and any interaction between them is ignored [24]. Wrapper methods reduce the risk of overfitting but are computationally intensive [7,24]. Embedded methods are computationally more efficient since the selection procedure is part of the training process [7,24]. A frequent embedded algorithm with good performance used in radiomics studies is the least absolute shrinkage and selection operator (LASSO) [7,24].

Subsequently, the selected features are used to implement a mathematical model in order to predict the established medical endpoints. Regarding the choice of modelling methodology, the identification of a suitable method depends on several factors as sample size or study endpoint [36]. It is advantageous to include in the model information beyond radiomics, e.g., clinical data and/or other "-omic" information, e.g., genomic data [45]. The integration of data from multiple sources, e.g., medical imaging, disease risk factors, therapy procedures and follow up data, in the mathematical model will facilitate the development of a personalized treatment.

As previously mentioned, the target of the radiomics studies can be either a present characteristic, e.g., tumor phenotype, or a future prediction, e.g., treatment response. Usually, radiomics studies make use of the feature-based ML algorithms that are also considered in CAD systems. By means of feature-based ML methods, the relationship between input data, e.g., selected radiomics features and target outcome, is determined by means of training examples. SVM is one of the most successfully applied algorithms.

DL-based radiomics allows to automatically extract imaging features and achieve the predicted outcome. In fact, the different components of the DL architecture perform all the processing steps described in the ML-based model, including feature extraction, selection and predicting model implementation. CNNs is the most common architecture used in radiomics studies and its characteristics have been previously described in Section 2.2.

Validation is a crucial component of the workflow of both conventional and DL-based radiomics. Ideally, the trained model should be tested in cross-validation or on an external, independent dataset before being applied on the new dataset [38].

4. AI and Radiomics in Thyroid Diseases

Ultrasound imaging is the recommended method for early detection and diagnosis of thyroid lesions due to its economy, effectivity and absence of radiation [46–49]. It is widely accepted as the first imaging modality for thyroid disease, for instance by American and European associations of endocrinology [50]. AI applications in the medical field are of increasing interest since they represent a possible approach to reduce the number of invasive clinical procedures [36].

Mainly, AI algorithms have been implemented for the classification of thyroid nodules, i.e., differentiating among benign or malignant state [9,10,21,22,33,41,51–56]. The outcomes of these studies are compared with the diagnosis of radiologists with different levels of experience. Research comparing the diagnostic ability between feature-based ML and DL algorithms is limited in the literature, but interesting outcomes are provided in [22]. Overall, an improvement emerged in terms of both specificity and accuracy in DL studies [57,58] with respect to feature-based ML classical applications [22], mostly determined by the capacity of DL of capturing complex patterns. In some studies [57–59], DL algorithms show accuracy values in line with those of radiologists. In addition, Jin et al. [20] also pointed out that the use of AI algorithms was useful to junior radiologists allowing a noticeable improvement of their diagnostic performance, reaching values of accuracy similar to those of intermediate-level radiologists. Studies of interest concerning the application of feature-based ML methods and DL algorithms are described in Tables 1 and 2, respectively. Tables were organized according to the publication time, in a decreasing order.

Table 1. Machine learning (ML)-based studies.

Study	Description	Cohort	Method	Performance
Zhao et al., 2021 [21]	Classification Benign/malignant thyroid nodules US	106 patients	SVM	Accuracy: 82% Sensitivity: 91% Specificity: 78%
Park et al., 2019 [22]	Classification Benign/malignant thyroid nodules US	286 patients	SVM	Accuracy: 75.9% Sensitivity: 90.4% Specificity: 58.8%
Zhang et al., 2019 [51]	Classification Benign/malignant thyroid nodules US	826 patients	SVM	Accuracy: 83% Sensitivity: 86.1% Specificity: 82.7%
Yoo et al., 2018 [41]	Classification Benign/malignant thyroid nodules US	50 patients	SVM	Accuracy: 84.6% Sensitivity: 80% Specificity: 88.1%
Chang et al., 2016 [10]	Classification Benign/malignant thyroid nodules US	118 patients	SVM	Accuracy: 98.3% Sensitivity: N/A Specificity: N/A

Abbreviations: US—ultrasound; SVM—support vector machine; N/A—not available.

Table 2. Deep learning (DL) studies.

Study	Description	Cohort	Method	Performance
Kim et al., 2021 [59]	Malignancy risk thyroid modules	757 patients	CNN	Accuracy: 85.1% Sensitivity: 81.8% Specificity: 86.1%
Wu et al., 2021 [52]	Classification Benign/malignant thyroid nodules US	1396 patients	CNN	Accuracy: 82% Sensitivity: 85% Specificity: 78%
Jin et al., 2020 [11]	Classification Benign/malignant thyroid nodules US	695 patients	CNN	Accuracy: 80.3% Sensitivity: 80.6% Specificity: 80.1%
Liang et al., 2020 [9]	Classification Benign/malignant thyroid nodules US	221 patients	CNN	Accuracy: 75% Sensitivity: 84.9% Specificity: 69%
Buda et al., 2019 [57]	Nodule detection Predict malignancy Risk level stratification	1230 patients	CNN	Accuracy: N/A Sensitivity: 87% Specificity: 52%
Ko et al., 2019 [54]	Classification Benign/malignant thyroid nodules US	519 patients	CNN	Accuracy: 87.3% Sensitivity: 90% Specificity: 82%
Park et al., 2019 [22]	Classification Benign/malignant thyroid nodules US	286 patients	CNN	Accuracy: 86% Sensitivity: 91% Specificity: 80%
Wang et al., 2019 [33]	Classification Benign/malignant thyroid nodules US	276 patients	CNN	Accuracy: 90.3% Sensitivity: 90.5% Specificity: 89.91%
Li et al., 2018 [55]	Classification Benign/malignant thyroid nodules US	17 627 patients	CNN	Accuracy: 86% Sensitivity: 84% Specificity: 87%
Chi et al., 2017 [58]	Classification Benign/malignant thyroid nodules US	592 patients	CNN	Accuracy: 96.3% Sensitivity: 82.8% Specificity: 99.3%
Ma et al., 2017 [56]	Classification Benign/malignant thyroid nodules US	4782 patients	CNN	Accuracy: 83% Sensitivity: 82.4% Specificity: 84.9%

Abbreviations: US—ultrasound; CNN—convolutional neural network; N/A—not available.

Radiomics is considered a promising method to be encompassed in the pipeline of precision medicine on the basis of specific characteristics of the patient [2]. Whilst the first AI approach to the medical imaging, i.e., CAD system, is focused on the differentiation among benign and malignant thyroid lesions, radiomics extends the analysis to prognosis and response to treatment evaluation [1]. In fact, [42,60,61] implemented radiomics models that analyze the risk stratification and predict the aggressiveness of the thyroid carcinoma with high values of accuracy, i.e., roughly 85 percent. Radiomics analysis has the potential to determine tumor phenotypes or the presence of gene mutations [62,63]. Furthermore, several studies have investigated by means of radiomic features the occurrence of metastases [64] or disease-free survival [65]. It also emerged that radiomics studies aimed at performing classification tasks regarding the nature of thyroid nodules are characterized by minor accuracy with respect to classical ML approach [66]. It is worth pointing out that although radiomics has been applied for several anatomical areas, research concerning thyroid lesions is relatively limited. Studies of interest concerning radiomics applications for thyroid lesions are described in Table 3, organized according to the publication time, in a decreasing order.

Table 3. Radiomics studies.

Study	Description	Cohort	Method	Performance
Park et al., 2021 [60]	Classification: Benign/malignant thyroid nodules 730 features extracted and 66 selected US	1609 patients	ML-based radiomics	Accuracy: 77.8% Sensitivity: 70.6% Specificity: 79.8%
Peng et al., 2021 [67]	Classification: Benign/malignant thyroid nodules US	8339 patients	DL-based radiomics	Accuracy: 89.1% Sensitivity: 94.9% Specificity: 81.2%
Wang et al., 2021 [42]	Evaluation of extrathyroidal extension (ETE) in patients with papillary thyroid carcinoma; 479 features extracted; 10 features selected US	132 patients	ML-based radiomics	Accuracy: 83% Sensitivity: 65% Specificity: 74%
Wei et al., 2021 [61]	Evaluation of extrathyroidal extension (ETE) in patients with papillary thyroid carcinoma MRI	102 patients	ML-based radiomics	Accuracy: 79% Sensitivity: 75% Specificity: 80%
Zhao et al., 2021 [21]	Classification: Benign/malignant thyroid nodules US	106 patients	ML-based radiomics	Accuracy: 75.5% Sensitivity: 69.7% Specificity: 78.1%
Guo et al., 2020 [64]	Prediction of thyroid cartilage invasion from Laryngeal and hypopharyngeal squamous cell carcinoma; 1029 features extracted; 30 features selected CT images	265 patients	ML-based radiomics	Accuracy: 90% Sensitivity: 80.2% Specificity: 88.3%
Kwon et al., 2020 [62]	Predict the presence or absence of BRAF proto-oncogene, serine/threonine kinase (BRAF) mutation in papillary thyroid cancer US	96 patients	ML-based radiomics	Accuracy: 64.3% Sensitivity: 66.8% Specificity: 61.8%
Wang et al., 2020 [66]	Classification: Benign/malignant thyroid nodules US	1040 patients	ML-based radiomics	Accuracy: 66.8% Sensitivity: 51.2% Specificity: 75.8%
Zhou et al., 2020 [40]	Classification: Benign/malignant thyroid nodules US	1734 patients	DL-based radiomics	Accuracy: 97% Sensitivity: 89.5% Specificity: 84.1%
Gu et al., 2019 [63]	Evaluating immunohistochemical characteristics in patients with suspected thyroid nodules CT images	103 patients	ML-based radiomics	Accuracy: 84% Sensitivity: 93% Specificity: 73%
Park et al., 2019 [65]	Estimate disease free survival rate in patients with papillary thyroid carcinoma; 730 features extracted and 40 selected US	768 patients	ML-based radiomics	Accuracy: 77% Sensitivity: N/A Specificity: N/A

Abbreviations: US—ultrasound; MRI—magnetic resonance imaging; CT—computer tomography; ML—machine learning; DL—deep learning; N/A—not available.

5. Discussion

Medical images provide a comprehensive view of the tumor and its environment, and they can be used to improve the diagnostic accuracy of early lesions, to classify benign from malignant tissues and to define risk and improve therapy [43,68]. Imaging is a non-invasive method and with no risk of the infections or the complications that accompany biopsies [2]. In recent decades, images have been converted into quantitative data and subsequently analyzed with AI tools.

Intratumoral heterogeneity and modifications over time are common features of neoplasms [43]. Samples of tumor acquired through biopsy may fail to represent the variations within the tumor. In addition, AI methods, analyzing the overall image of the lesion, have the potential to capture tumor heterogeneity and could represent an intermediate step between imaging and biopsy [28,36]. Nonetheless, it is worth pointing out that AI systems learn on a case-by-case basis. AI algorithms are implemented considering gold standards of pathological diagnosis that are hard to identify in every patient, due to inter-variability among subjects. Moreover, as it emerged from the overview of the AI methods, the predicting model is developed on the basis of a finite training dataset. Thus, since human tissues are characterized by high heterogeneity and variability inter- and intra-subjects, no finite training set can fully represent the variety of cases that might occur in the clinical practice. Extensive research is still required to improve the generalizability and accuracy of AI-based models. From this perspective, the standalone use of AI applications for diagnosis should be still avoided in the clinical practice. In fact, to this date, several studies [7,20,28,43] recommend that the lesion evaluation should be achieved from a combination between the clinician evaluation and ML or DL outcome. Moreover, it is worth noticing that most AI-based studies focused on thyroid pathologies are performed using retrospectively collected data [9,11,33,40,42,51,55,60–63,65–67]. Conversely, studies that prospectively evaluate AI predictive models concerning thyroid disease diagnosis are limited in the literature [22,41]. In retrospective studies, cohorts are selected among patients with definitive diagnosis achieved mainly through histopathological examination. As highlighted by Wu et al. [69], evaluations should include more prospective studies on medical AI models to reduce risk of overfitting and enhance accuracy of the clinical outcomes.

AI methods are based on the analysis of image features in order to develop predictive models. Differentiating benign and malignant thyroid nodule is mainly achieved from ML-based studies. The most used US features adopted by ML algorithms for thyroid investigations were size, shape, margin, composition echogenicity, as defined by the thyroid imaging reporting and data system (TI-RADS) classification [10,21,22,51]. According to an analysis of the available literature, the TI-RADS approach allows a good discrimination among benign and malignant thyroid nodules. However, the inclusion of additional features, e.g., calcifications, internal content, can represent a factor that improves accuracy [70].

Radiomics studies were applied also to other thyroid pathologies, e.g., extrathyroidal extension (ETE) in patients with papillary thyroid carcinoma (PTC) [42,61], thyroid cartilage invasion from laryngeal and hypopharyngeal squamous cell carcinoma [64]. In these studies, the extracted features derive from morphological, first order statistics, textural and higher order statistics groups. Wang and colleagues [42] highlighted that improvement of ETE diagnosis is achieved when features related to PTC heterogeneity are taken into account. Similarly, in [64] Guo et al. studied thyroid cartilage invasion from laryngeal and hypopharyngeal squamous cell carcinoma and showed that tumor invasiveness can be investigated considering features related to tumor heterogeneity. Furthermore, Kwon et al. [62] highlight that BRAF mutation may be investigated with histogram-based and textural features that reflect echogenicity and heterogeneity of the region of interest, respectively.

Several studies also performed comparison between the performance of AI-based models and that of expert clinicians. The available data in literature mostly report that the performance of DL algorithms is similar to that of healthcare professionals. As discussed by [20,67], AI applications may improve the accuracy of thyroid diagnosis diseases, especially for junior radiologists. In fact, interpretation of medical images highly depends on the experience level of clinicians. For instance, for junior radiologists the sensitivity is reported in a range between 40 percent and 100 percent while the specificity spans between 50 percent and 100 percent. It was observed that the use of AI algorithms to achieve a second opinion on the characterization of thyroid lesions can improve the accuracy of junior radiologists from roughly 82 percent to 87 percent [67]. Moreover, Peng and coworkers [67] highlighted that taking into account the outcomes of AI as a second opinion has reduced fine needle aspiration procedures by 27 percent and the number of missed malignancies of roughly 2 percent.

Furthermore, the experience level of the clinicians has an important impact also on the performance of the AI-based methods. The input data of the AI algorithms is the ROI selected by the expert. It is commonly accepted that image acquisition and segmentation are critical subprocesses due to inter-operator variability. Recent studies [8,28] suggest that semi- or fully automated methods could improve algorithm performance, but currently the manual segmentation performed by experts continues to be the main method adopted. For instance, most of the ML-based studies applied to the thyroid are performed considering a manual segmentation of the ROI [21,41]. In addition, the ML-based investigations reported in [10,22] have introduced a semi-automatic method that is characterized by an initial automatic selection of a box region and subsequently by a manual contouring performed by expert clinicians. Conversely, the studies that applied DL algorithms to thyroid imaging considered a manual selected box around the region under investigation [9,11,52,54]. Furthermore, it is worth pointing out that radiomics studies are based on a manual contouring along the borders of the thyroid tumor [60–62] or slightly within the borders of the tumor to avoid artifacts [64].

To date, most studies highlight that the main limitation of AI algorithms is the reduced dataset used for predictive model development and validation. Ideally, independent training and validation datasets, composed of data images achieved with different US equipment and from multiple centers, i.e., multicenter training cohorts, allow to optimally develop the predicting model, avoiding overfitting and enhancing generalizability and model performance [67].

For instance, in radiomics studies, Gilies and coworkers [43] provide an empirical rule concerning the size of the dataset in order to avoid overfitting. It is suggested that almost 10–15 patients are needed for each examined radiomic feature. Thus, also features selection represents a crucial step during the evaluation.

AI methods represent a powerful approach that in future may assist clinicians in diagnostic decisions [22,71], while combined with other "-omic" data as occur in radiomics analysis may improve the risk factor analysis for personalized estimation of disease-free survival. As mentioned, AI methods could be also applied to contribute to treatment planning. For instance, radiomics combined with other clinical parameters may help to predict which patients are likely to have a satisfactory response to emerging therapies as high-intensity focused ultrasound (HIFU), that allows the thermal tissue treatment and the consequent reduction in thyroid nodule volume by directing energy inside the target zone with non-invasive instruments [72–74].

Several efforts are performed to increase the availability of open access database of labeled medical images that will help to train the predictive models developed with AI techniques. However, pitfalls and limitations associated with the AI approach should be considered, especially related to the difficulty to achieve a generalizable model in order to ensure optimal application for each patient.

With regard to the application of the AI in the daily practice of the clinical medicine, beyond the hype around these technologies, the financial investment is pouring and brand-new products started flowing into the market. As of early 2020, there were 64 FDA-approved AI-ML medical device and algorithms, many of which are already integrated into clinical care. Remarkably, 21 were related to Radiology [75]. Nonetheless, recent literature reviews report that the impact is still minimal as the majority of the AI-ML studies are retrospective in nature, deviate from existing reporting standards and often outline proof-of-concept approach [76].

From the pure clinical standpoint, all these findings should be interpreted according to the routine clinical practice. In fact, US is recognized as the most relevant imaging procedure for the assessment of thyroid nodule and almost all thyroid patients are managed according to US features of their thyroid gland. This worldwide diffused approach is based on the high sensitivity and specificity of US in discriminating malignant from benign thyroid lesions. Further improvement of US performance by AI remains however desirable [77,78]. In addition, a not negligible number of thyroid goiters are incidentally discovered during other imaging evaluations (i.e., CT, MR, PET/CT) of patients with non-thyroid indication [79]. While the performance of these imaging procedures is poor or suboptimal to identify malignant and benign nodules among adrenal thyroid incidentalomas, a significant effort should be made in the future to improve their capability to initially select patients requiring an urgent or not endocrinological evaluation combined with in-office US examination.

6. Conclusions

The evaluation of images has a central role in the clinical workflow. It is worth highlighting that image interpretation requires deductive reasoning, using knowledge of pathological processes, integration from prior examination and investigations and consultation with other physicians. To date, AI techniques can be an integral part of the procedure, but cannot emulate the overall process.

A further approach to improve the assessment of medical images can be represented by the integration of AI-based models with mixed reality tools. The authors retain that in-depth analysis should be performed to analyze the potential of mixed reality within the diagnostic workflow.

Author Contributions: Conceptualization, F.B. and P.T.; methodology, F.B., A.P., L.A., A.G., L.R., F.M. and P.T.; software, A.P.; validation, F.B., A.P., L.A., A.G., L.R., F.M. and P.T.; formal analysis, F.B. and A.P.; investigation, F.B., A.P., L.A., A.G., L.R. and P.T.; resources, P.T.; data curation, F.B. and A.P.; writing—original draft preparation, F.B. and A.P.; writing—review and editing, F.B., A.P., L.A., A.G., L.R., F.M. and P.T.; visualization, F.B. and A.P.; supervision, F.B., F.M. and P.T.; project administration, P.T.; funding acquisition, P.T. All authors have read and agreed to the published version of the manuscript.

Funding: This research received no external funding.

Conflicts of Interest: The authors declare no conflict of interest.

References

1. Lambin, P.; Rios-Velazquez, E.; Leijenaar, R.; Carvalho, S.; van Stiphout, R.G.P.M.; Granton, P.; Zegers, C.M.L.; Gillies, R.; Boellard, R.; Dekker, A.; et al. Radiomics: Extracting more information from medical images using advanced feature analysis. *Eur. J. Cancer* **2012**, *48*, 441–446. [CrossRef] [PubMed]
2. Aerts, H.J.W.L.; Velazquez, E.R.; Leijenaar, R.T.H.; Parmar, C.; Grossmann, P.; Carvalho, S.; Bussink, J.; Monshouwer, R.; Haibe-Kains, B.; Rietveld, D.; et al. Decoding tumour phenotype by noninvasive imaging using a quantitative radiomics approach. *Nat. Commun.* **2014**, *5*, 4006. [CrossRef] [PubMed]
3. Gillies, R.J.; Kinahan, P.E.; Hricak, H. Radiomics: Images Are More than Pictures, They Are Data. *Radiology* **2016**, *278*, 563–577. [CrossRef]
4. *Machine Learning in Radiation Oncology*; El Naqa, I.; Li, R.; Murphy, M. (Eds.) Springer: Cham, Switzerland, 2015. [CrossRef]
5. Lohmann, P.; Bousabarah, K.; Hoevels, M.; Treuer, H. Radiomics in radiation oncology—basics, methods, and limitations. *Strahlenther. Onkol.* **2020**, *196*, 848–855. [CrossRef] [PubMed]
6. Frix, A.-N.; Cousin, F.; Refaee, T.; Bottari, F.; Vaidyanathan, A.; Desir, C.; Vos, W.; Walsh, S.; Occhipinti, M.; Lovinfosse, P.; et al. Radiomics in Lung Diseases Imaging: State-of-the-Art for Clinicians. *Pers. Med.* **2021**, *11*, 602. [CrossRef] [PubMed]

7. Castiglioni, I.; Rundo, L.; Codari, M.; Di Leo, G.; Salvatore, C.; Interlenghi, M.; Gallivanone, F.; Cozzi, A.; D'Amico, N.C.; Sardanelli, F. AI applications to medical images: From machine learning to deep learning. *Phys. Med.* **2021**, *83*, 9–24. [CrossRef]
8. Iqbal, M.J.; Javed, Z.; Sadia, H.; Qureshi, I.A.; Irshad, A.; Ahmed, R.; Malik, K.; Raza, S.; Abbas, A.; Pezzani, R.; et al. Clinical applications of artificial intelligence and machine learning in cancer diagnosis: Looking into the future. *Cancer Cell Int.* **2021**, *21*, 1–11. [CrossRef]
9. Liang, X.; Yu, J.; Liao, J.; Chen, Z. Convolutional Neural Network for Breast and Thyroid Nodules Diagnosis in Ultrasound Imaging. *BioMed Res. Int.* **2020**, *2020*, 1763803. [CrossRef]
10. Chang, Y.; Paul, A.K.; Kim, N.; Baek, J.H.; Choi, Y.J.; Ha, E.J.; Lee, K.D.; Lee, H.S.; Shin, D.; Kim, N. Computer-aided diagnosis for classifying benign versus malignant thyroid nodules based on ultrasound images: A comparison with radiologist-based assessments. *Med. Phys.* **2016**, *43*, 554–567. [CrossRef]
11. Jin, Z.; Zhu, Y.; Zhang, S.; Xie, F.; Zhang, M.; Zhang, Y.; Tian, X.; Zhang, J.; Luo, Y.; Cao, J. Ultrasound Computer-Aided Diagnosis (CAD) Based on the Thyroid Imaging Reporting and Data System (TI-RADS) to Distinguish Benign from Malignant Thyroid Nodules and the Diagnostic Performance of Radiologists with Different Diagnostic Experience. *Med. Sci. Monit.* **2020**, *26*, e918452. [CrossRef]
12. Fujita, H. AI-based computer-aided diagnosis (AI-CAD): The latest review to read first. *Radiol. Phys. Technol.* **2020**, *13*, 6–19. [CrossRef] [PubMed]
13. Parmar, C.; Grossmann, P.; Bussink, J.; Lambin, P.; Aerts, H.J.W.L. Machine Learning methods for Quantitative Radiomic Biomarkers. *Sci. Rep.* **2015**, *5*, 13087. [CrossRef] [PubMed]
14. Zwanenburg, A.; Vallières, M.; Abdalah, M.A.; Aerts, H.J.W.L.; Andrearczyk, V.; Apte, A.; Ashrafinia, S.; Bakas, S.; Beukinga, R.J.; Boellaard, R.; et al. The Image Biomarker Standardization Initiative: Standardized Quantitative Radiomics for High-Throughput Image-based Phenotyping. *Radiology* **2020**, *295*, 328–338. [CrossRef] [PubMed]
15. McCarthy, J.J.; Minsky, M.L.; Rochester, N. Artificial Intelligence. Research Laboratory of Electronics (RLE) at the Massachusetts Institute of Technology (MIT). 1959. Available online: https://dspace.mit.edu/handle/1721.1/52263 (accessed on 3 March 2010).
16. McCarthy, J.; Minsky, M.L.; Rochester, N.; Shannon, C.E. A proposal for the Dartmouth summer research project on artificial intelligence, August 31, 1955. *AI Mag.* **2006**, *27*, 12.
17. Jiang, F.; Jiang, Y.; Zhi, H.; Dong, Y.; Li, H.; Ma, S.; Wang, Y.; Dong, Q.; Shen, H.; Wang, Y. Artificial intelligence in healthcare: Past, present and future. *Stroke Vasc. Neurol.* **2017**, *2*, 230–243. [CrossRef] [PubMed]
18. Bera, K.; Schalper, K.A.; Rimm, D.L.; Velcheti, V.; Madabhushi, A. Artificial intelligence in digital pathology—New tools for diagnosis and precision oncology. *Nat. Rev. Clin. Oncol.* **2019**, *16*, 703–715. [CrossRef]
19. Wernick, M.N.; Yang, Y.; Brankov, J.G.; Yourganov, G.; Strother, S. Machine Learning in Medical Imaging. *IEEE Signal Process. Mag.* **2010**, *27*, 25–38. [CrossRef] [PubMed]
20. Erickson, B.J.; Korfiatis, P.; Akkus, Z.; Kline, T.L. Machine Learning for Medical Imaging. *RadioGraphics* **2017**, *37*, 505–515. [CrossRef]
21. Zhao, C.-K.; Ren, T.-T.; Yin, Y.-F.; Shi, H.; Wang, H.-X.; Zhou, B.-Y.; Wang, X.-R.; Li, X.; Zhang, Y.-F.; Liu, C.; et al. A Comparative Analysis of Two Machine Learning-Based Diagnostic Patterns with Thyroid Imaging Reporting and Data System for Thyroid Nodules: Diagnostic Performance and Unnecessary Biopsy Rate. *Thyroid* **2021**, *31*, 470–481. [CrossRef]
22. Park, V.; Han, K.; Seong, Y.K.; Park, M.H.; Kim, E.-K.; Moon, H.J.; Yoon, J.H.; Kwak, J.Y. Diagnosis of Thyroid Nodules: Performance of a Deep Learning Convolutional Neural Network Model vs. Radiologists. *Sci. Rep.* **2019**, *9*, 1–9. [CrossRef]
23. Cui, S.; Tseng, H.; Pakela, J.; Haken, R.K.T.; El Naqa, I. Introduction to machine and deep learning for medical physicists. *Med. Phys.* **2020**, *47*, e127–e147. [CrossRef]
24. Forghani, R.; Savadjiev, P.; Chatterjee, A.; Muthukrishnan, N.; Reinhold, C.; Forghani, B. Radiomics and Artificial Intelligence for Biomarker and Prediction Model Development in Oncology. *Comput. Struct. Biotechnol. J.* **2019**, *17*, 995–1008. [CrossRef] [PubMed]
25. Guorong, W.; Dinggang, S.; Mert, R.S. *Machine Learning and Medical Imaging*; Academic Press: London, UK, 2016. [CrossRef]
26. El-Naqa, I.; Yang, Y.; Wernick, M.N.; Galatsanos, N.P.; Nishikawa, R. A support vector machine approach for detection of microcalcifications. *IEEE Trans. Med. Imaging* **2002**, *21*, 1552–1563. [CrossRef] [PubMed]
27. Hosny, A.; Parmar, C.; Quackenbush, J.; Schwartz, L.H.; Aerts, H. Artificial intelligence in radiology. *Nat. Rev. Cancer* **2018**, *18*, 500–510. [CrossRef] [PubMed]
28. Chartrand, G.; Cheng, P.M.; Vorontsov, E.; Drozdzal, M.; Turcotte, S.; Pal, C.J.; Kadoury, S.; Tang, A. Deep Learning: A Primer for Radiologists. *RadioGraphics* **2017**, *37*, 2113–2131. [CrossRef]
29. Aggarwal, R.; Sounderajah, V.; Martin, G.; Ting, D.S.W.; Karthikesalingam, A.; King, D.; Ashrafian, H.; Darzi, A. Diagnostic accuracy of deep learning in medical imaging: A systematic review and meta-analysis. *NPJ Digit. Med.* **2021**, *4*, 65. [CrossRef]
30. LeCun, Y.; Bengio, Y.; Hinton, G. Deep learning. *Nature* **2015**, *521*, 436–444. [CrossRef] [PubMed]
31. Lundervold, A.S.; Lundervold, A. An overview of deep learning in medical imaging focusing on MRI. *Z Med. Phys.* **2019**, *29*, 102–127. [CrossRef]
32. Mazurowski, M.A.; Buda, M.; Saha, A.; Bashir, M.R. Deep learning in radiology: An overview of the concepts and a survey of the state of the art with focus on MRI. *J. Magn. Reson. Imaging* **2019**, *49*, 939–954. [CrossRef]
33. Wang, L.; Yang, S.; Yang, S.; Zhao, C.; Tian, G.; Gao, Y.; Chen, Y.; Lu, Y. Automatic thyroid nodule recognition and diagnosis in ultrasound imaging with the YOLOv2 neural network. *World J. Surg. Oncol.* **2019**, *17*, 1–9. [CrossRef] [PubMed]

4. Liu, S.; Wang, Y.; Yang, X.; Lei, B.; Liu, L.; Li, S.X.; Ni, D.; Wang, T. Deep Learning in Medical Ultrasound Analysis: A Review. *Engineering* **2019**, *5*, 261–275. [CrossRef]
5. Erickson, B.J.; Korfiatis, P.; Kline, T.L.; Akkus, Z.; Philbrick, K.; Weston, A.D. Deep Learning in Radiology: Does One Size Fit All? *J. Am. Coll. Radiol.* **2018**, *15*, 521–526. [CrossRef]
6. Lambin, P.; Leijenaar, R.T.H.; Deist, T.M.; Peerlings, J.; de Jong, E.E.C.; van Timmeren, J.; Sanduleanu, S.; Larue, R.T.H.M.; Even, A.J.G.; Jochems, A.; et al. Radiomics: The bridge between medical imaging and personalized medicine. *Nat. Rev. Clin. Oncol.* **2017**, *14*, 749–762. [CrossRef]
7. Avanzo, M.; Stancanello, J.; El Naqa, I. Beyond imaging: The promise of radiomics. *Phys. Med.* **2017**, *38*, 122–139. [CrossRef] [PubMed]
8. Avanzo, M.; Wei, L.; Stancanello, J.; Vallières, M.; Rao, A.; Morin, O.; Mattonen, S.A.; El Naqa, I. Machine and deep learning methods for radiomics. *Med. Phys.* **2020**, *47*, e185–e202. [CrossRef] [PubMed]
9. Tseng, H.-H.; Wei, L.; Cui, S.; Luo, Y.; Haken, R.K.T.; El Naqa, I. Machine Learning and Imaging Informatics in Oncology. *Oncology* **2020**, *98*, 344–362. [CrossRef] [PubMed]
10. Zhou, H.; Jin, Y.; Dai, L.; Zhang, M.; Qiu, Y.; Wang, K.; Tian, J.; Zheng, J. Differential Diagnosis of Benign and Malignant Thyroid Nodules Using Deep Learning Radiomics of Thyroid Ultrasound Images. *Eur. J. Radiol.* **2020**, *127*, 108992. [CrossRef]
11. Yoo, Y.J.; Ha, E.J.; Cho, Y.J.; Kim, H.L.; Han, M.; Kang, S.Y. Computer-Aided Diagnosis of Thyroid Nodules via Ultrasonography: Initial Clinical Experience. *Korean J. Radiol.* **2018**, *19*, 665–672. [CrossRef] [PubMed]
12. Wang, X.; Agyekum, E.A.; Ren, Y.; Zhang, J.; Zhang, Q.; Sun, H.; Zhang, G.; Xu, F.; Bo, X.; Lv, W.; et al. A Radiomic Nomogram for the Ultrasound-Based Evaluation of Extrathyroidal Extension in Papillary Thyroid Carcinoma. *Front. Oncol.* **2021**, *11*, 625646. [CrossRef]
13. Gillies, R.J.; Schabath, M.B. Radiomics Improves Cancer Screening and Early Detection. *Cancer Epidemiol. Biomark. Prev.* **2020**, *29*, 2556–2567. [CrossRef]
14. Mayerhoefer, M.E.; Materka, A.; Langs, G.; Häggström, I.; Szczypiński, P.; Gibbs, P.; Cook, G. Introduction to Radiomics. *J. Nucl. Med.* **2020**, *61*, 488–495. [CrossRef]
15. Tunali, I.; Gillies, R.J.; Schabath, M.B. Application of Radiomics and Artificial Intelligence for Lung Cancer Precision Medicine. *Cold Spring Harb. Perspect. Med.* **2021**, *11*, a039537. [CrossRef] [PubMed]
16. Cao, Y.; Zhong, X.; Diao, W.; Mu, J.; Cheng, Y.; Jia, Z. Radiomics in Differentiated Thyroid Cancer and Nodules: Explorations; Application; and Limitations. *Cancers* **2021**, *13*, 2436. [CrossRef] [PubMed]
17. Araneo, R.; Bini, F.; Rinaldi, A.; Notargiacomo, A.; Pea, M.; Celozzi, S. Thermal-electric model for piezoelectric ZnO nanowires. *Nanotechnology* **2015**, *26*, 265402. [CrossRef] [PubMed]
18. Scorza, A.; Lupi, G.; Sciuto, S.A.; Bini, F.; Marinozzi, F. A novel approach to a phantom based method for maximum depth of penetration measurement in diagnostic ultrasound: A preliminary study. In Proceedings of the 2015 IEEE International Symposium on Medical Measurements and Applications (MeMeA), Turin, Italy, 7–9 May 2015; pp. 369–374. [CrossRef]
19. Marinozzi, F.; Branca, F.P.; Bini, F.; Scorza, A. Calibration procedure for performance evaluation of clinical Pulsed Doppler Systems. *Measurement* **2012**, *45*, 1334–1342. [CrossRef]
20. Shen, Y.-T.; Chen, L.; Yue, W.-W.; Xu, H.-X. Artificial intelligence in ultrasound. *Eur. J. Radiol.* **2021**, *139*. [CrossRef]
21. Zhang, B.; Tian, J.; Pei, S.; Chen, Y.; He, X.; Dong, Y.; Zhang, L.; Mo, X.; Huang, W.; Cong, S.; et al. Machine Learning-Assisted System for Thyroid Nodule Diagnosis. *Thyroid* **2019**, *29*, 858–867. [CrossRef]
22. Wu, G.G.; Lv, W.Z.; Yin, R.; Xu, J.W.; Yan, Y.J.; Chen, R.X.; Wang, J.Y.; Zhang, B.; Cui, X.W.; Dietrich, C.F. Deep Learning Based on ACR TI-RADS Can Improve the Differential Diagnosis of Thyroid Nodules. *Front. Oncol.* **2021**, *11*, 575166. [CrossRef]
23. Koh, J.; Lee, E.; Han, K.; Kim, E.-K.; Son, E.J.; Sohn, Y.-M.; Seo, M.; Kwon, M.-R.; Yoon, J.H.; Lee, J.H.; et al. Diagnosis of thyroid nodules on ultrasonography by a deep convolutional neural network. *Sci. Rep.* **2020**, *10*, 1–9. [CrossRef]
24. Ko, S.Y.; Lee, J.H.; Yoon, J.H.; Na, H.; Hong, E.; Han, K.; Jung, I.; Kim, E.K.; Moon, H.J.; Park, V.Y.; et al. Deep convolutional neural network for the diagnosis of thyroid nodules on ultrasound. *Head Neck* **2019**, *41*, 885–891. [CrossRef]
25. Li, X.; Zhang, S.; Zhang, Q.; Wei, X.; Pan, Y.; Zhao, J.; Xin, X.; Qin, C.; Wang, X.; Li, J.; et al. Diagnosis of thyroid cancer using deep convolutional neural network models applied to sonographic images: A retrospective; multicohort; diagnostic study. *Lancet Oncol.* **2019**, *20*, 193–201. [CrossRef]
26. Ma, J.; Wu, F.; Zhu, J.; Xu, D.; Kong, D. A pre-trained convolutional neural network based method for thyroid nodule diagnosis. *Ultrasonics* **2017**, *73*, 221–230. [CrossRef] [PubMed]
27. Buda, M.; Wildman-Tobriner, B.; Hoang, J.K.; Thayer, D.; Tessler, F.N.; Middleton, W.D.; Mazurowski, M.A. Management of Thyroid Nodules Seen on US Images: Deep Learning May Match Performance of Radiologists. *Radiology* **2019**, *292*, 695–701. [CrossRef] [PubMed]
28. Chi, J.; Walia, E.; Babyn, P.; Wang, J.; Groot, G.; Eramian, M. Thyroid Nodule Classification in Ultrasound Images by Fine-Tuning Deep Convolutional Neural Network. *J. Digit. Imaging.* **2017**, *30*, 477–486. [CrossRef] [PubMed]
29. Kim, G.R.; Lee, E.; Kim, H.R.; Yoon, J.H.; Park, V.Y.; Kwak, J.Y. Convolutional Neural Network to Stratify the Malignancy Risk of Thyroid Nodules: Diagnostic Performance Compared with the American College of Radiology Thyroid Imaging Reporting and Data System Implemented by Experienced Radiologists. *AJNR Am. J. Neuroradiol.* **2021**, *42*, 1513–1519. [CrossRef] [PubMed]

60. Park, V.Y.; Lee, E.; Lee, H.S.; Kim, H.J.; Yoon, J.; Son, J.; Song, K.; Moon, H.J.; Yoon, J.H.; Kim, G.R.; et al. Combining radiomics with ultrasound-based risk stratification systems for thyroid nodules: An approach for improving performance. *Eur. Radiol.* **2021**, *31*, 2405–2413. [CrossRef] [PubMed]
61. Wei, R.; Wang, H.; Wang, L.; Hu, W.; Sun, X.; Dai, Z.; Zhu, J.; Li, H.; Ge, Y.; Song, B. Radiomics based on multiparametric MRI for extrathyroidal extension feature prediction in papillary thyroid cancer. *BMC Med. Imaging* **2021**, *21*, 20. [CrossRef] [PubMed]
62. Kwon, M.-R.; Shin, J.; Park, H.; Cho, H.; Hahn, S.; Park, K. Radiomics Study of Thyroid Ultrasound for Predicting BRAF Mutation in Papillary Thyroid Carcinoma: Preliminary Results. *Am. J. Neuroradiol.* **2020**, *41*, 700–705. [CrossRef]
63. Gu, J.; Zhu, J.; Qiu, Q.; Wang, Y.; Bai, T.; Yin, Y. Prediction of Immunohistochemistry of Suspected Thyroid Nodules by Use of Machine Learning-Based Radiomics. *AJR Am. J. Roentgenol.* **2019**, *213*, 1348–1357. [CrossRef]
64. Guo, R.; Guo, J.; Zhang, L.; Qu, X.; Dai, S.; Peng, R.; Chong, V.F.H.; Xian, J. CT-based radiomics features in the prediction of thyroid cartilage invasion from laryngeal and hypopharyngeal squamous cell carcinoma. *Cancer Imaging* **2020**, *20*, 81. [CrossRef]
65. Park, V.; Han, K.; Lee, E.; Kim, E.-K.; Moon, H.J.; Yoon, J.H.; Kwak, J.Y. Association Between Radiomics Signature and Disease-Free Survival in Conventional Papillary Thyroid Carcinoma. *Sci. Rep.* **2019**, *9*, 1–7. [CrossRef]
66. Wang, Y.; Yue, W.; Li, X.; Liu, S.; Guo, L.; Xu, H.; Zhang, H.; Yang, G. Comparison Study of Radiomics and Deep Learning-Based Methods for Thyroid Nodules Classification Using Ultrasound Images. *IEEE Access* **2020**, *8*, 52010–52017. [CrossRef]
67. Peng, S.; Liu, Y.; Lv, W.; Liu, L.; Zhou, Q.; Yang, H.; Ren, J.; Liu, G.; Wang, X.; Zhang, X.; et al. Deep learning-based artificial intelligence model to assist thyroid nodule diagnosis and management: A multicentre diagnostic study. *Lancet Digit. Health* **2021**, *3*, e250–e259. [CrossRef]
68. Trimboli, P.; Bini, F.; Andrioli, M.; Giovanella, L.; Thorel, M.F.; Ceriani, L.; Valabrega, S.; Lenzi, A.; Drudi, F.M.; Marinozzi, F.; et al. Analysis of tissue surrounding thyroid nodules by ultrasound digital images. *Endocrine* **2015**, *48*, 434–438. [CrossRef] [PubMed]
69. Wu, E.; Wu, K.; Daneshjou, R.; Ouyang, D.; Ho, D.E.; Zou, J. How medical AI devices are evaluated: Limitations and recommendations from an analysis of FDA approvals. *Nat. Med.* **2021**, *27*, 582–584. [CrossRef] [PubMed]
70. Verburg, F.; Reiners, C. Sonographic diagnosis of thyroid cancer with support of AI. *Nat. Rev. Endocrinol.* **2019**, *15*, 319–321. [CrossRef]
71. Litjens, G.; Kooi, T.; Bejnordi, B.E.; Setio, A.A.A.; Ciompi, F.; Ghafoorian, M.; van der Laak, J.A.W.M.; van Ginneken, B.; Sánchez, C.I. A survey on deep learning in medical image analysis. *Med. Image Anal.* **2017**, *42*, 60–88. [CrossRef]
72. Bini, F.; Trimboli, P.; Marinozzi, F.; Giovanella, L. Treatment of benign thyroid nodules by high intensity focused ultrasound (HIFU) at different acoustic powers: A study on in-silico phantom. *Endocrine* **2018**, *59*, 506–509. [CrossRef]
73. Trimboli, P.; Bini, F.; Baek, J.H.; Marinozzi, F.; Giovanella, L. High intensity focused ultrasounds (HIFU) therapy for benign thyroid nodules without anesthesia or sedation. *Endocrine* **2018**, *61*, 210–215. [CrossRef]
74. Giovanella, L.; Piccardo, A.; Pezzoli, C.; Bini, F.; Ricci, R.; Ruberto, T.; Trimboli, P. Comparison of High Intensity Focused Ultrasound and radioiodine for treating toxic Thyroid nodules. *Clin. Endocrinol.* **2018**, *89*, 219–225. [CrossRef]
75. Benjamens, S.; Dhunnoo, P.; Mesko, B. The state of artificial intelligence-based FDA-approved medical devices and algorithms: An online database. *NPJ Digit. Med.* **2020**, *3*, 118. [CrossRef]
76. Ben-Israel, D.; Jacobs, W.B.; Casha, S.; Lang, S.; Ryu, W.H.A.; de Lotbiniere-Bassett, M.; Cadotte, D.W. The impact of machine learning on patient care: A systematic review. *Artif. Intell. Med.* **2020**, *103*, 101785. [CrossRef]
77. Russ, G.; Trimboli, P.; Buffet, C. The New Era of TIRADSs to Stratify the Risk of Malignancy of Thyroid Nodules: Strengths, Weaknesses and Pitfalls. *Cancers* **2021**, *13*, 4316. [CrossRef] [PubMed]
78. Trimboli, P. Ultrasound: The Extension of Our Hands to Improve the Management of Thyroid Patients. *Cancers* **2021**, *13*, 567. [CrossRef] [PubMed]
79. Scappaticcio, L.; Piccardo, A.; Treglia, G.; Poller, D.N.; Trimboli, P. The dilemma of 18F-FDG PET/CT thyroid incidentaloma: What we should expect from FNA. A systematic review and meta-analysis. *Endocrine* **2021**, *73*, 540–549. [CrossRef] [PubMed]

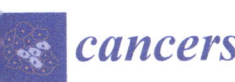

Article

Facing Thyroid Nodules in Paediatric Patients Previously Treated with Radiotherapy for Non-Thyroidal Cancers: Are Adult Ultrasound Risk Stratification Systems Reliable?

Arnoldo Piccardo [1], Francesco Fiz [1,*], Gianluca Bottoni [1], Camilla De Luca [2], Michela Massollo [1], Ugo Catrambone [3], Luca Foppiani [4], Monica Muraca [5], Alberto Garaventa [6] and Pierpaolo Trimboli [7,8]

1. Department of Nuclear Medicine, E.O. "Ospedali Galliera", 16128 Genoa, Italy; arnoldo.piccardo@galliera.it (A.P.); gianluca.bottoni@galliera.it (G.B.); michela.massollo@galliera.it (M.M.)
2. Department of Health Sciences (DISSAL), Università di Genova, 16132 Genoa, Italy; camilla.deluca93@gmail.com
3. Department of Surgery, E.O. "Ospedali Galliera", 16128 Genoa, Italy; ugo.catrambone@galliera.it
4. Department of Internal Medicine, E.O. "Ospedali Galliera", 16128 Genoa, Italy; luca.foppiani@galliera.it
5. Epidemiology and Biostatistic Unit and DOPO Clinic, IRCCS Istituto Giannina Gaslini, 16147 Genoa, Italy; monicamuraca@gaslini.org
6. Department of Oncology, IRCCS Istituto Giannina Gaslini, 16147 Genoa, Italy; albertogaraventa@gaslini.org
7. Clinic for Endocrinology and Diabetology, Regional Hospital of Lugano, Ente Ospedaliero Cantonale, 6900 Lugano, Switzerland; Pierpaolo.Trimboli@eoc.ch
8. Faculty of Biomedical Sciences, Università della Svizzera Italiana (USI), 6900 Lugano, Switzerland
* Correspondence: francesco.fiz@galliera.it; Tel.: +39-010-563-4530

Simple Summary: The risk of thyroid nodules harbouring cancer has been evaluated, in adults, using specific ultrasound criteria. However, it is unclear whether such evaluation can be translated in paediatric patients. In this study, we tested the effectiveness of three known risk evaluation systems in children with thyroid nodules and with a history of radiation exposure. We found that these systems are reliable in confirming or ruling out cancer in most cases, except when evaluating very small nodules (<1 cm). For these reasons, these risk criteria should be adopted to account for the reduced size of malignant lesions when evaluating paediatric subjects.

Abstract: Thyroid nodule ultrasound-based risk stratification systems (US-RSSs) have been successfully used in adults to predict the likelihood of malignancies. However, their applicability to the paediatric population is unclear, especially in children with a history of radiation exposure, who are at a higher cancer risk. We tested the efficacy of three US-RSSs in this setting by retrospectively applying three classification systems (ACR-TIRADS, ATA and EU-TIRADS) to all paediatric patients referred for thyroid nodules and with a radiation exposure history. We compared the results with a reference standard (pathology or 36-month follow-up); sensitivity, specificity, positive and negative predictive values (PPV and NPV) and accuracy were calculated. A total of 52 patients were included; fourteen of them (27%) had papillary thyroid cancer (PTC) at the final histology. No significant differences across the US-RSSs were detected; specificity (range 95–97%) and NPV (range 88–93%) were particularly elevated. However, ACR-TIRADS, ATA and EU-TIRADS did not indicate the need for a biopsy in six (42.8%), seven (50%) and eight (57%) cases of PTC; in five cases, this lack of indication was due to a small (<1 cm) nodule size. In conclusion, US-RSSs show a high NPV and specificity in paediatric patients, whereas the cytology indication could be improved by reconsidering the dimensional criterion.

Keywords: thyroid nodules; paediatrics; radiotherapy; risk assessment; ultrasonography; DTC

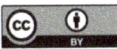

1. Introduction

Thyroid nodules are fairly uncommon among paediatric subjects [1]. However, whenever a thyroid lesion is identified in children and teenagers, it does bear a higher likelihood of malignancy, which can be as high as 20–25%, when compared with the adult counterpart (5%) [2,3]. Some risk factors may increase the probability of developing thyroid nodules in children, including iodine deficiency, prior radiation exposure and several genetic syndromes.

In particular, childhood cancer survivors who were treated for their non-thyroidal primary malignancy with radiation therapy (RT) represent a population at risk. This group includes survivors of Hodgkin lymphoma, leukaemia, neuroblastoma and central nervous system tumours [2,4,5]. In fact, the history of malignancy and the radiation exposure can represent synergic factors for the development of a second malignant neoplasm, particularly differentiated thyroid cancer (DTC) [6–8].

Neck ultrasonography is the first-line imaging procedure, which is able to identify and classify the risk of the thyroid nodules [9–11]. Adult-based neck US risk stratification systems (RSSs) have been developed in recent years to integrate the US features in an effort to improve diagnostic accuracy and as an aid in the stratification of the risk of malignancy [9,12,13].

However, few studies are available about the reliability of these systems in paediatric age, and conflicting results have been reported about the accuracy of the adult US-RSSs.

In particular, little can be said about the efficacy of US-RSSs when it comes to stratifying the risk of malignancy in patients with a history of previous radiotherapy for oncological reasons who need a strict follow-up after the identification of thyroid nodules [7,14]. This could bear particular relevance considering that an early identification of DTC could avoid a more advanced presentation that, in paediatric patients, can imply extrathyroidal extension and metastases.

The most recent guidelines seem to be concordant in considering those patients at high risk of developing DTCs with thyroid nodules and a previous history of irradiation regardless of the neck ultrasonography features and dimensions. Indeed, while fine-needle aspiration cytology (FNA) can be generally recommended in adults with nodules sized at least 1 cm, in the paediatric population, this procedure is indicated even for small nodules [9,15]. Current US-RSSs do not include young age and previous history of RT as risk factors [16]. Indeed, whether the RSS reliability is concordant with the one that is generally reported remains to be clarified [17].

The aim of our study was to: (1) evaluate the diagnostic performance of the principal neck US classification systems (ACR-TIRADS, ATA and EU-TIRADS) in a selected paediatric population of patients previously treated with radiotherapy, (2) test the malignancy prevalence of each category delineated by US-RSSs and (3) evaluate whether these neck US systems are able to correctly select nodules for FNA.

2. Materials and Methods

We retrospectively analysed all paediatric patients consecutively referred to our centre (Galliera Hospital) for FNA of a thyroid nodule between 1 January 2012 and 31 December 2017. Before FNA, all patients underwent thyroid US and were tested for TSH, free-T4, free-T3 and calcitonin. Additionally, thyroid scintigraphy (TS) was performed only in the case of suppressed TSH levels [2]. Patients were excluded only if US data had not been retrieved in the local picture archiving and communication system (PACS). Then, only patients with thyroid nodules and previously treated with radiotherapy (RT) for primary paediatric non-thyroidal tumours were included in our study. The institutional review board (Comitato Etico Regionale Liguria, Registration Number: 326/2020-DB id 10315) approved this retrospective study.

2.1. Neck Ultrasonography

Thyroid US was performed using a LOGIQ S8 (General Electric Medical Systems) with a 9 to 15 MHz linear probe. All imaging procedures were performed in combination with a clinical visit by 3 expert physicians (A.P., G.B., M.M.). For all patients, a greyscale and colour Doppler imaging data were acquired.

2.2. Ultrasound Risk Stratification Systems

All thyroid nodules were retrospectively risk stratified according to the principal US-RSSs (i.e., ACR-TIRADS, ATA and EU-TIRADS). Indications for FNA were ascertained depending on risk classes identified by each US-RSS. More in general, FNA could be indicated depending on US features and nodule dimensions.

2.3. Imaging Review and Interpretation

Neck US images we retrieved from the PACS and then visually analysed by 2 reviewers (AP, PT) unaware of patients' data and final outcome. The inter- and intra-reader variabilities in identifying the classes of each US-RSS were previously tested in a different set of 30 paediatric patients with thyroid nodules and showed excellent agreement (Cohen's κ, 0.82 [95% CI, 0.68–0.91]). In case of interpretation disagreement, the final diagnosis was achieved after a consensus meeting with a third expert (GB).

For statistical purposes, each thyroid nodule with US features corresponding to the last class of each US-RSS (i.e., EU-TIRADS 5, ACR-TIRAD5 and ATA High-risk) was regarded as positive. Prevalence of malignancy was calculated as the percent of nodules in each class that were confirmed as DTC at the final histology.

2.4. Reference Standard

Cytology according to the Italian consensus of cytopathology was adopted as the gold standard. The first edition, used until 2014, considered 5 classes, with a single indeterminate category, while the second edition included 6 classes, of which 2 were indeterminate [18,19]. However, for all these patients, a US follow-up of at least 36 months was available. In case of surgery, histopathology of the resected nodule represented the standard of trough.

2.5. Statistical Analysis

Sensitivity, specificity, positive and negative predictive values (PPV and NPV) and accuracy were calculated for each system. Differences in categorical variables between groups were analysed using the chi-square test or Fisher's exact test as appropriate.

The prevalence of malignancy was calculated as the ratio between the number of DTCs in each class and the total number of DTCs.

The proportion of FNA that would not have been indicated by the various systems in patients with a diagnosis of DTC was compared using the pairwise chi-square test.

3. Results

During the study period, we evaluated 259 paediatric patients with thyroid nodules who had undergone neck US at our department. Out of these patients, 52 were selected for the present study according to our inclusion criteria (Figure 1), and their principal characteristics are summarised in Table 1.

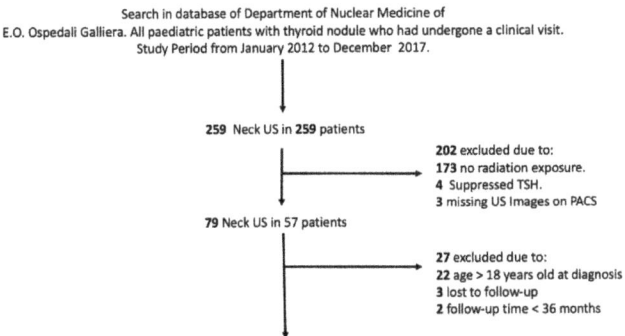

Figure 1. Flow chart illustrating the selection of the patients.

Table 1. Characteristics of the patients.

Variable	Subjects Included (n = 52)
Sex	
Female, n. (%)	32 (61.5)
Male, n. (%)	20 (38.5)
Age on nodule diagnosis, median (IQR), years	17 (15–18)
<15 years, n. (%)	11 (21.1)
≥15 years, n. (%)	41 (78.9)
Age on irradiation, median (IQR), year	5 (3–7)
<5 years, n. (%)	24 (46.1)
≥5 years, n. (%)	28 (53.9)
Time from RT to thyroid nodule diagnosis median (IQR), year	11 (8–14)
<10 years, n. (%)	16 (30.8)
≥10 years, n. (%)	36 (69.2)
Nodule dimensions, median (IQR), mm	13 (11–22)
<10 mm, n. (%)	7 (13.4)
10–15 mm, n. (%)	26 (50.0)
16–20 mm, n. (%)	5 (9.6)
>20 mm, n. (%)	16 (30.7)
Thyroid cytology *	
Tir 2, n. (%)	36 (69.2)
Tir 3, n. (%)	2 (3.8)
Tir 3b, n.(%)	2 (3.8)
Tir 4, n. (%)	3 (5.7)
Tir 5, n. (%)	9 (17.3)
Thyroidectomy	
Yes, n. (%)	19 (36.5)
No, n. (%)	33 (63.5)
Pathology	
Papillary thyroid carcinoma, n. (%)	14 (73.)
Follicular thyroid carcinoma, n. (%)	0 (0)
Follicular hyperplasia	4 (21.0)
Follicular adenoma	1 (5.3)
Age on DTC diagnosis, median (IQR), years	15 (14–18)
<15 years, no. (%)	4 (28.5)
≥15 years, no. (%)	10 (71.5)
Time from RT to DTC diagnosis, median (IQR), year	11 (10–12)
<10 years, no. (%)	3 (21.4)
≥10 years, no. (%)	10 (78.6)

Table 1. Cont.

Variable	Subjects Included (n = 52)
Clinico-pathological classification **	
T1, no. (%)	12 (85.7)
T2, no. (%)	2 (14.3)
N0, no. (%)	5 (35.7)
N1a, no. (%)	7 (50.0)
N1b, no. (%)	2 (14.3)
M0, no. (%)	14 (100)

Legend: * According to the Italian Consensus Working Group [reference]. ** This feature included all histopathological findings and pre-surgical imaging. IQR: Interquartile range, RT: radiation treatment, DTC: differentiated thyroid carcinoma.

Among these 52 patients, 19 underwent surgery because of a symptomatic nodular goitre (n = 3), indeterminate cytology (n = 4) and cytology suspicious (n = 3) or consistent with DTC (n = 9). Finally, 14 papillary cancers (27%) were histologically confirmed (Table 1).

The diagnostic performances of each US-RSS in terms of sensitivity, specificity, positive and negative predictive values (PPV and NPV) and accuracy in identifying DTCs are summarised in Table 2. No significant differences across these systems were observed.

Table 2. Diagnostic performances of the US-RSSs.

US-RSSs	ACR-TIRADS	EU-TIRADS	ATA	p-VALUE (ACR vs. EU TIRADS)	p-VALUE (ACR TIRADS vs. ATA)	p-VALUE (EU TIRADS vs. ATA)
Sensitivity	71%	71%	64%	0.66	0.4	0.68
Specificity	97%	95%	95%	0.56	0.56	1
NPV	91%	90%	88%	0.69	0.47	0.75
PPV	91%	83%	82%	0.53	0.47	0.92
Accuracy	91%	88%	87%	0.87	0.83	0.72

Legend US-RSSs: Ultra-sound risk stratification systems, ACR: American college of radiology. TI-RADS: Thyroid imaging reporting and data system, EU: European thyroid association, ATA: American thyroid association, NPV: negative predictive value, PPV: positive predictive value.

When benign nodules were evaluated according to the three US-RSSs, the principal classes in which they were included were EU-TIRADS 3 by EU-TIRADS, TR3 by ACR-TIRADS and "Low suspicion" by ATA.

When PTCs were considered, the most represented classes were EU-TIRADS 5 by EU-TIRADS (71.4%), TR5 by ACR-TIRADS (71.4%) and "High suspicion" by ATA (64.2%).

A statistical comparison showed no significant differences in the benign lesion and PTC distributions among the three systems (Figure 2).

At evaluation of the risk of malignancy of each category of the various US-RSSs, we found that EU-TIRADS 5, TR5 and ATA High suspicion presented a DTC percentage of 71, 71 and 64, respectively (Table 3). Conversely, no DTCs were found in the lowest categories.

When FNA indication in patients subsequently diagnosed with papillary thyroid cancer on histopathology was analysed according to the US-RSSs, EU-TIRADS missed eight cases (57%), ACR TIRADS six (42.8%) cases and ATA seven cases (50%) (Figure 3). The lack of indication for FNA was principally related (five patients) to the small dimensions (<1 cm) of the malignant thyroid nodules.

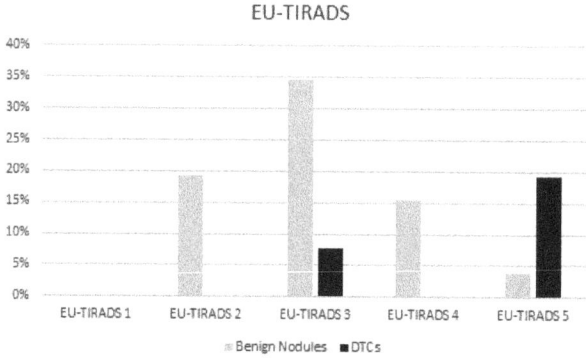

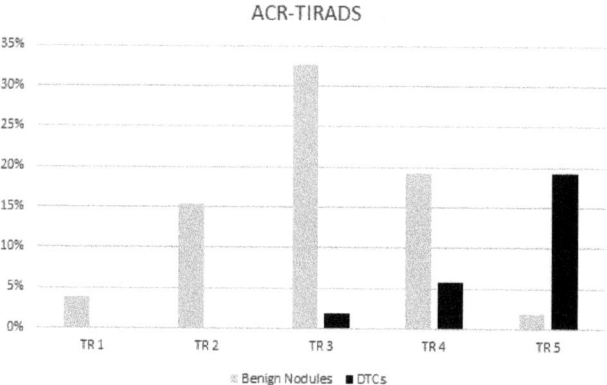

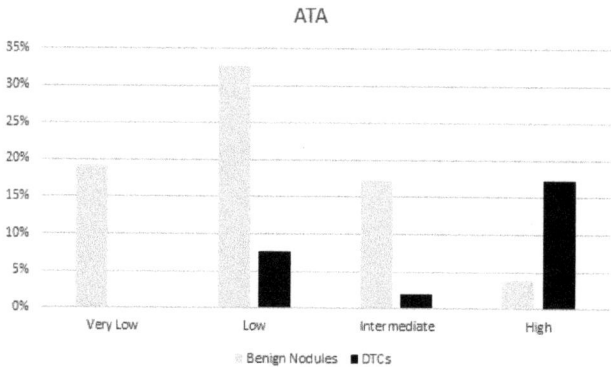

Figure 2. Distribution of benign and malignant thyroid nodules among the categories of the three US-RSSs.

Table 3. Frequency of malignancy according to the various US-RSSs.

Category	Prevalence of Malignancy
EU-TIRADS	
EU-TIRADS 2	0%
EU-TIRADS 3	4/14 (29%)
EU-TIRADS 4	0%
EU-TIRADS 4	10/14 (71%)
ACR TIRADS	
TR 1	0%
TR 2	0%
TR 3	1/14 (7%)
TR 4	3/14 (22%)
TR 5	10/14 (71%)
ATA	
Benign	0%
Very low	0%
Low	4/14 (29%)
Intermediate	1/14 (7%)
High	9/14 (64%)

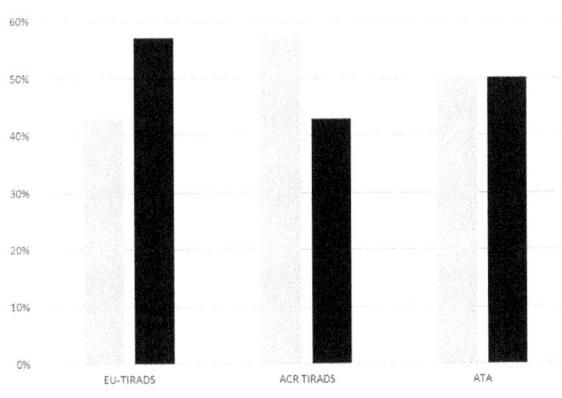

Figure 3. Indication for fine-needle aspiration (FNA) cytology in papillary thyroid cancers according to the criteria set by the 3 US-RSSs.

4. Discussion

The pivotal role of neck ultrasonography in the identification and evaluation of the malignant potential of thyroid nodules, as well as in FNA guiding, has been recognised in the most recent paediatric guidelines [20,21]. Strikingly however, no specific US features to tell apart benign from malignant nodules have been identified, and no dedicated scoring system has been proposed [2]. Some papers have investigated the role of US-RSSs in the paediatric population with conflicting results [22,23]. To our knowledge, this is the first study testing US-RSSs in a selected population of paediatric patients with a history of neck radiation exposure.

In our population, a little less than one third of the radiotherapy-treated patients had developed a DTC; this result is well in line with the data reported in the existing literature [24,25].

Moreover, in this particular setting of patients in which FNA is "a priori" indicated due to the high prevalence of malignancy, we showed that the different US-RSSs can rule out DTCs, having a high NPV ranging from 89 (ATA) up to 91% (ACR TIRADS). Indeed, this finding, similar to that reported in a recent paper comparing the two American systems (i.e., ATA and ACR TIRADS) [23], may have a particular impact on the ability to monitor these subjects at increased risk with reliable, non-invasive procedures. In particular, by contributing to sparing futile and repeated invasive procedures, it can help in reducing stress and anxiety for patients who have been previously heavily pre-treated for non-thyroidal cancer.

We found that, by considering the highest category of each system as positive and the remaining ones as negative, the specificity is very high (from 95 to 97%), with a very low number of false positive US findings. Our data, in this regard, are concordant with a recent meta-analysis by Kim et al. showing that, by using the same interpretation, the pooled specificity of ACR TIRADS in paediatric patients is 97% [26]. On the contrary, the prevalence of DTC within the thyroid nodules classified in the highest categories is even higher than that reported by Kim and colleagues, ranging from 64 for ATA to 71% for ACR TIRADS, without significant differences among the US-RSSs. Generally, we found that all US stratification systems are reliable methods to identify DTCs, and that their diagnostic performances are adequate and higher than those reported by the meta-analysis by Kim et al. [26]. This discrepancy could be related to the higher prevalence of malignancy in the irradiated population and to the histopathology which is exclusively papillary thyroid cancer (PTC). Indeed, a large part of the studies considered in this meta-analysis [22,23,27] excluded patients with a history of radiation exposure and included patients with thyroid cancer other than PTC (10%) for which the US-RSSs are often not reliable enough [17,28].

When we analysed the ability of the three US-RSSs in identifying which thyroid nodule should be investigated by means of FNA, we found that, by rigorously applying the dimensional criteria, all three systems did not provide a proper indication for FNA in more than 40% of DTC patients (from 43 to 57%). Indeed, no significant differences were observed among the three systems. This finding supports the yet unproved indication for FNA in these particular patients with micronodules (i.e., <1 cm) reported in the most recent guidelines [2]. Indeed, there is some evidence that childhood cancer survivors tend to have, on average, smaller thyroid tumours [29]. In addition, it must be underlined that three out of five patients with DTCs smaller than 1 cm already showed loco-regional lymph node involvement (i.e., two with N1a, and one with N1b). This aggressive biological behaviour of small DTCs, which is expected in paediatric patients, should be carefully considered in the drafting of dedicated US paediatric risk stratification systems.

Some limitations should be underlined. First, the retrospective nature of this study may be associated with selection biases that could have affected our results. However, the DTC prevalence and the time from irradiation to DTC onset are in agreement with those estimates by the ATA guidelines [2]. Second, the sample size and the number of DTCs were limited; however, this is the first study evaluating the role of US-RSSs in paediatric patients with a well-known history of irradiation exposure, and overall, the number of patients included in this study is in line with others evaluating non-irradiated patients [23,27,30]. Finally, only for 19 out of 52 patients was a histopathological confirmation available. However, for all patients, cytological results and at least 3 years of clinical and US follow-up were available.

5. Conclusions

We found that the American and European US-RSSs have a high NPV and specificity in detecting DTCs, having the possibility to rule out malignancy even in this particular subgroup of high-risk patients. In addition, the DTC prevalence among the highest system categories was very high, achieving 71%. However, according to all three of the aforementioned US-RSSs, the majority of PTCs would not be selected for FNA. This result is related to the size cut-offs proposed by US-RSSs for indicating FNA rather than US features. Both users of thyroid US-RSSs and panellists of the next TIRADSs should be aware of the present findings.

Author Contributions: Conceptualization, A.P. and P.T.; methodology, G.B. and L.F.; validation, L.F. and U.C.; formal analysis, A.P., M.M. (Monica Muraca) and F.F.; investigation, A.P.; data curation, C.D.L. and M.M. (Michela Massollo); writing—original draft preparation, A.P.; writing—review and editing, P.T. and F.F.; supervision, A.G. All authors have read and agreed to the published version of the manuscript.

Funding: This research received no external funding.

Institutional Review Board Statement: The institutional review board (Comitato Etico Regionale Liguria, Registration Number: 326/2020-DB id 10315 on 23 July 2020) approved this retrospective study, and the requirement to obtain informed consent was waived.

Informed Consent Statement: Patient consent was waived due to a specific review board decision (impossibility to obtain such informed consent retrospectively).

Data Availability Statement: Data regarding the present study are available at the authors' institution and can be obtained upon reasonable request.

Conflicts of Interest: The authors declare no conflict of interest.

References

1. Cimbek, E.A.; Polat, R.; Sonmez, B.; Beyhun, N.E.; Dinc, H.; Saruhan, H.; Karaguzel, G. Clinical, sonographical, and pathological findings of pediatric thyroid nodules. *Eur. J. Pediatr.* **2021**, *180*, 2823–2829. [CrossRef]
2. Francis, G.L.; Waguespack, S.G.; Bauer, A.J.; Angelos, P.; Benvenga, S.; Cerutti, J.M.; Dinauer, C.A.; Hamilton, J.; Hay, I.D.; Luster, M.; et al. Management Guidelines for Children with Thyroid Nodules and Differentiated Thyroid Cancer. *Thyroid* **2015**, *25*, 716–759. [CrossRef]
3. Richman, D.M.; Cherella, C.E.; Smith, J.R.; Modi, B.P.; Zendejas, B.; Frates, M.C.; Wassner, A.J. Clinical utility of sonographic features in indeterminate pediatric thyroid nodules. *Eur. J. Endocrinol.* **2021**, *184*, 657–665. [CrossRef]
4. Elisei, R.; Romei, C.; Vorontsova, T.; Cosci, B.; Veremeychik, V.; Kuchinskaya, E.; Basolo, F.; Demidchik, E.P.; Miccoli, P.; Pinchera, A.; et al. RET/PTC rearrangements in thyroid nodules: Studies in irradiated and not irradiated, malignant and benign thyroid lesions in children and adults. *J. Clin. Endocrinol. Metab.* **2001**, *86*, 3211–3216. [CrossRef] [PubMed]
5. Shulan, J.M.; Vydro, L.; Schneider, A.B.; Mihailescu, D.V. Role of biomarkers in predicting the occurrence of thyroid neoplasms in radiation-exposed children. *Endocr. Relat. Cancer* **2018**, *25*, 481–491. [CrossRef] [PubMed]
6. Jarzab, B.; Handkiewicz-Junak, D. Differentiated thyroid cancer in children and adults: Same or distinct disease? *Hormones* **2007**, *6*, 200–209. [PubMed]
7. Piccardo, A.; Foppiani, L.; Puntoni, M.; Hanau, G.; Calafiore, L.; Garaventa, A.; Arlandini, A.; Villavecchia, G.; Bianchi, P.; Cabria, M. Role of low-cost thyroid follow-up in children treated with radiotherapy for primary tumors at high risk of developing a second thyroid tumor. *Q. J. Nucl. Med. Mol. Imaging* **2012**, *56*, 459–467. [PubMed]
8. Iglesias, M.L.; Schmidt, A.; Ghuzlan, A.A.; Lacroix, L.; Vathaire, F.; Chevillard, S.; Schlumberger, M. Radiation exposure and thyroid cancer: A review. *Arch. Endocrinol. Metab.* **2017**, *61*, 180–187. [CrossRef]
9. Haugen, B.R.; Alexander, E.K.; Bible, K.C.; Doherty, G.M.; Mandel, S.J.; Nikiforov, Y.E.; Pacini, F.; Randolph, G.W.; Sawka, A.M.; Schlumberger, M.; et al. 2015 American Thyroid Association Management Guidelines for Adult Patients with Thyroid Nodules and Differentiated Thyroid Cancer: The American Thyroid Association Guidelines Task Force on Thyroid Nodules and Differentiated Thyroid Cancer. *Thyroid* **2016**, *26*, 1–133. [CrossRef] [PubMed]
10. Mistry, R.; Hillyar, C.; Nibber, A.; Sooriyamoorthy, T.; Kumar, N. Ultrasound Classification of Thyroid Nodules: A Systematic Review. *Cureus* **2020**, *12*, e7239. [CrossRef] [PubMed]
11. Grant, E.G.; Tessler, F.N.; Hoang, J.K.; Langer, J.E.; Beland, M.D.; Berland, L.L.; Cronan, J.J.; Desser, T.S.; Frates, M.C.; Hamper, U.M.; et al. Thyroid Ultrasound Reporting Lexicon: White Paper of the ACR Thyroid Imaging, Reporting and Data System (TIRADS) Committee. *J. Am. Coll. Radiol.* **2015**, *12*, 1272–1279. [CrossRef]
12. Russ, G.; Bonnema, S.J.; Erdogan, M.F.; Durante, C.; Ngu, R.; Leenhardt, L. European Thyroid Association Guidelines for Ultrasound Malignancy Risk Stratification of Thyroid Nodules in Adults: The EU-TIRADS. *Eur. Thyroid J.* **2017**, *6*, 225–237. [CrossRef] [PubMed]
13. Tessler, F.N.; Middleton, W.D.; Grant, E.G.; Hoang, J.K.; Berland, L.L.; Teefey, S.A.; Cronan, J.J.; Beland, M.D.; Desser, T.S.; Frates, M.C.; et al. ACR Thyroid Imaging, Reporting and Data System (TI-RADS): White Paper of the ACR TI-RADS Committee. *J. Am. Coll. Radiol.* **2017**, *14*, 587–595. [CrossRef] [PubMed]

14. Miao, S.; Jing, M.; Sheng, R.; Cui, D.; Lu, S.; Zhang, X.; Jing, S.; Zhang, X.; Shan, T.; Shan, H.; et al. The analysis of differential diagnosis of benign and malignant thyroid nodules based on ultrasound reports. *Gland. Surg.* **2020**, *9*, 653–660. [CrossRef]
15. Sakorafas, G.H.; Mastoraki, A.; Lappas, C.; Safioleas, M. Small (<10 mm) thyroid nodules; how aggressively should they be managed? *Onkologie* **2010**, *33*, 61–64. [CrossRef] [PubMed]
16. Russ, G.; Trimboli, P.; Buffet, C. The New Era of TIRADSs to Stratify the Risk of Malignancy of Thyroid Nodules: Strengths, Weaknesses and Pitfalls. *Cancers* **2021**, *13*, 4316. [CrossRef]
17. Castellana, M.; Castellana, C.; Treglia, G.; Giorgino, F.; Giovanella, L.; Russ, G.; Trimboli, P. Performance of Five Ultrasound Risk Stratification Systems in Selecting Thyroid Nodules for FNA. *J. Clin. Endocrinol. Metab.* **2020**, *105*, dgz170. [CrossRef] [PubMed]
18. Fadda, G.; Basolo, F.; Bondi, A.; Bussolati, G.; Crescenzi, A.; Nappi, O.; Nardi, F.; Papotti, M.; Taddei, G.; Palombini, L.; et al. Cytological classification of thyroid nodules. Proposal of the SIAPEC-IAP Italian Consensus Working Group. *Pathologica* **2010**, *102*, 405–408. [PubMed]
19. Nardi, F.; Basolo, F.; Crescenzi, A.; Fadda, G.; Frasoldati, A.; Orlandi, F.; Palombini, L.; Papini, E.; Zini, M.; Pontecorvi, A.; et al. Italian consensus for the classification and reporting of thyroid cytology. *J. Endocrinol. Investig.* **2014**, *37*, 593–599. [CrossRef] [PubMed]
20. Izquierdo, R.; Shankar, R.; Kort, K.; Khurana, K. Ultrasound-guided fine-needle aspiration in the management of thyroid nodules in children and adolescents. *Thyroid* **2009**, *19*, 703–705. [CrossRef]
21. Buryk, M.A.; Simons, J.P.; Picarsic, J.; Monaco, S.E.; Ozolek, J.A.; Joyce, J.; Gurtunca, N.; Nikiforov, Y.E.; Feldman Witchel, S. Can malignant thyroid nodules be distinguished from benign thyroid nodules in children and adolescents by clinical characteristics? A review of 89 pediatric patients with thyroid nodules. *Thyroid* **2015**, *25*, 392–400. [CrossRef]
22. Creo, A.; Alahdab, F.; Al Nofal, A.; Thomas, K.; Kolbe, A.; Pittock, S.T. Ultrasonography and the American Thyroid Association Ultrasound-Based Risk Stratification Tool: Utility in Pediatric and Adolescent Thyroid Nodules. *Horm. Res. Paediatr.* **2018**, *90*, 93–101. [CrossRef] [PubMed]
23. Martinez-Rios, C.; Daneman, A.; Bajno, L.; van der Kaay, D.C.M.; Moineddin, R.; Wasserman, J.D. Utility of adult-based ultrasound malignancy risk stratifications in pediatric thyroid nodules. *Pediatr. Radiol.* **2018**, *48*, 74–84. [CrossRef]
24. Gupta, A.; Ly, S.; Castroneves, L.A.; Frates, M.C.; Benson, C.B.; Feldman, H.A.; Wassner, A.J.; Smith, J.R.; Marqusee, E.; Alexander, E.K.; et al. A standardized assessment of thyroid nodules in children confirms higher cancer prevalence than in adults. *J. Clin. Endocrinol. Metab.* **2013**, *98*, 3238–3245. [CrossRef] [PubMed]
25. Niedziela, M. Pathogenesis, diagnosis and management of thyroid nodules in children. *Endocr. Relat. Cancer* **2006**, *13*, 427–453. [CrossRef] [PubMed]
26. Kim, P.H.; Yoon, H.M.; Hwang, J.; Lee, J.S.; Jung, A.Y.; Cho, Y.A.; Baek, J.H. Diagnostic performance of adult-based ATA and ACR-TIRADS ultrasound risk stratification systems in pediatric thyroid nodules: A systematic review and meta-analysis. *Eur. Radiol.* **2021**, online ahead of print. [CrossRef]
27. Polat, Y.D.; Ozturk, V.S.; Ersoz, N.; Anik, A.; Karaman, C.Z. Is Thyroid Imaging Reporting and Data System Useful as an Adult Ultrasonographic Malignancy Risk Stratification Method in Pediatric Thyroid Nodules? *J. Med. Ultrasound* **2019**, *27*, 141–145. [CrossRef] [PubMed]
28. Trimboli, P.; Castellana, M.; Piccardo, A.; Romanelli, F.; Grani, G.; Giovanella, L.; Durante, C. The ultrasound risk stratification systems for thyroid nodule have been evaluated against papillary carcinoma. A meta-analysis. *Rev. Endocr. Metab. Disord.* **2021**, *22*, 453–460. [CrossRef]
29. Clement, S.C.; Lebbink, C.A.; Klein Hesselink, M.S.; Teepen, J.C.; Links, T.P.; Ronckers, C.M.; van Santen, H.M. Presentation and outcome of subsequent thyroid cancer among childhood cancer survivors compared to sporadic thyroid cancer: A matched national study. *Eur. J. Endocrinol.* **2020**, *183*, 169–180. [CrossRef]
30. Uner, C.; Aydin, S.; Ucan, B. Thyroid Image Reporting and Data System Categorization: Effectiveness in Pediatric Thyroid Nodule Assessment. *Ultrasound Q.* **2020**, *36*, 15–19. [CrossRef]

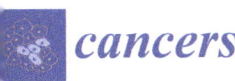

Article

Diagnostic Performance of Kwak, EU, ACR, and Korean TIRADS as Well as ATA Guidelines for the Ultrasound Risk Stratification of Non-Autonomously Functioning Thyroid Nodules in a Region with Long History of Iodine Deficiency: A German Multicenter Trial

Philipp Seifert [1,*], Simone Schenke [2,*], Michael Zimny [3], Alexander Stahl [4], Michael Grunert [5], Burkhard Klemenz [5], Martin Freesmeyer [1], Michael C. Kreissl [2], Ken Herrmann [6] and Rainer Görges [6,7]

[1] Clinic of Nuclear Medicine, Jena University Hospital, 07749 Jena, Germany; martin.freesmeyer@med.uni-jena.de
[2] Division of Nuclear Medicine, Department of Radiology and Nuclear Medicine, Magdeburg University Hospital, 39120 Magdeburg, Germany; michael.kreissl@med.ovgu.de
[3] Institute for Nuclear Medicine Hanau, 63450 Giessen, Germany; zimny@nuklearmedizin-hanau.de
[4] Institute for Radiology and Nuclear Medicine RIZ, 86150 Augsburg, Germany; dr.alexander.stahl@gmx.de
[5] Department of Nuclear Medicine, German Armed Forces Hospital of Ulm, 89081 Ulm, Germany; michael.grunert@uni-ulm.de (M.G.); burkhard.klemenz@uni-ulm.de (B.K.)
[6] Department of Nuclear Medicine, Essen University Hospital, 45147 Essen, Germany; ken.herrmann@uk-essen.de (K.H.); rainer.goerges@uni-due.de (R.G.)
[7] Joint Practice for Nuclear Medicine, Duisburg (Moers), 47441 Duisburg, Germany
* Correspondence: philipp.seifert@med.uni-jena.de (P.S.); simone.schenke@med.ovgu.de (S.S.)

Simple Summary: In Germany, thyroid nodules can be detected by ultrasound examinations in over 30% of the adult population, mainly as a result of prolonged nutritive iodine deficiency. Although only a small proportion of the nodules are malignant, it is important to have a reliable examination method that not only can detect these few thyroid carcinomas with a high degree of certainty, but also not be unnecessarily invasive for the much larger number of benign nodules. Ultrasound is the method of choice, and ultrasound-based risk stratification systems are important tools in clinical care. However, many different systems have been introduced within the last decade. The aim of this study was to evaluate five common ultrasound risk stratification systems for their diagnostic accuracy of thyroid nodules from an area with long history of iodine deficiency.

Abstract: Germany has a long history of insufficient iodine supply and thyroid nodules occur in over 30% of the adult population, the vast majority of which are benign. Non-invasive diagnostics remain challenging, and ultrasound-based risk stratification systems are essential for selecting lesions requiring further clarification. However, no recommendation can yet be made about which system performs the best for iodine deficiency areas. In a German multicenter approach, 1211 thyroid nodules from 849 consecutive patients with cytological or histopathological results were enrolled. Scintigraphically hyperfunctioning lesions were excluded. Ultrasound features were prospectively recorded, and the resulting classifications according to five risk stratification systems were retrospectively determined. Observations determined 1022 benign and 189 malignant lesions. The diagnostic accuracies were 0.79, 0.78, 0.70, 0.82, and 0.79 for Kwak Thyroid Imaging Reporting and Data System (Kwak-TIRADS), American College of Radiology (ACR) TI-RADS, European Thyroid Association (EU)-TIRADS, Korean-TIRADS, and American Thyroid Association (ATA) Guidelines, respectively. Receiver Operating Curves revealed Areas under the Curve of 0.803, 0.795, 0.800, 0.805, and 0.801, respectively. According to the ATA Guidelines, 135 thyroid nodules (11.1%) could not be classified. Kwak-TIRADS, ACR TI-RADS, and Korean-TIRADS outperformed EU-TIRADS and ATA Guidelines and therefore can be primarily recommended for non-autonomously functioning lesions in areas with a history of iodine deficiency.

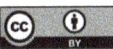

Keywords: thyroid; cancer; nodule; ultrasound; scintigraphy; non-autonomously functioning; thyroid imaging reporting and data systems (TIRADS); risk of malignancy (ROM)

1. Introduction

Iodine deficiency is a well-known risk factor in the development of nodular thyroid disease [1]. Although nutritive iodine supply in the German population has improved in the recent years, Germany has a long history of iodine deficiency and the requirements of the World Health Organization (WHO) have not yet been fully met [2–5]. The prevalence of thyroid nodules (TNs) ranges from 12.5% in young men to over 80% in older women [6–9]. Since the vast majority of the detected TNs are benign, the diagnostic challenge is to reliably detect malignant nodules while avoiding unnecessary interventions for benign lesions [10].

Thyroid ultrasound (US) is a non-invasive, cost-effective, and accurate method for detecting and describing TNs [11]. It is also the method of choice for assessing and selecting TNs for further diagnostic procedures such as fine-needle cytology (FNC) to rule-out malignancy [12–14]. During the last decade, several international societies have published different US-based risk stratification systems (RSSs, Thyroid Imaging Reporting and Data System, TIRADS) based on US features and lesion size. The aim was to improve diagnostic performance of thyroid US, to reduce unnecessary interventions, and to provide a standardized terminology for physicians [12,13,15–18]. In 2011, Kwak et al. published a TIRADS (Kwak-TIRADS) to detect suspicious malignant features: microcalcifications, solid composition, hypoechogenicity, a taller-than-wide shape, and an irregular/microlobulated margin [19]. In 2016, The Korean Thyroid Association/Korean Society of Thyroid Radiology (KTA/KSThR) proposed a pattern-based RSS (Korean-TIRADS) based on solidity and echogenicity with additional suspicious features (microcalcifications, non-parallel orientation, and spiculated/microlobulated margins) [20]. In 2015, The American Thyroid Association (ATA) announced a pattern-based, five-tier RSS with different risks of malignancy [21]. Similar to the Korean-TIRADS, the European Thyroid Association (ETA) in 2017 proposed a pattern-based five-tier RSS (EU-TIRADS) with US features showing a high probability of malignancy (irregular shape and margins, marked hypoechogenicity, solidity, and microcalcifications) [22]. Simultaneously, the American College of Radiology (ACR) published the scoring-based ACR TI-RADS [18].

Recently, several studies were carried out to compare the diagnostic performance of different US-based RSSs [13,14,17,23–30]. Although it is known that hyperfunctioning TNs have a very high probability of being benign and need no further diagnosis [31], none of these studies took the functional status of the TNs into account. Furthermore, in a previous study, our group demonstrated that a relevant proportion of hyperfunctioning TNs were classified as intermediate risk or high risk according to Kwak-TIRADS [32].

The aim of this study was to compare the diagnostic performance of five established US RSSs for non-autonomously functioning TNs in iodine deficiency.

2. Materials and Methods

2.1. Patients and Ethics

Since 2012, an increasing number of physicians specializing in thyroid diagnostics have been in constant communication regarding the diagnostic assessment of TNs, organized in the "German TIRADS Study Group" (GTSG). In recent years, seven institutions set up a continuously growing multicenter database containing the imaging and clinical data of over 2000 consecutive TNs. US features were recorded prospectively in real time immediately after the US examinations (see Section 2.2). Out of this pool, patients recorded between January 2012 and August 2020 were considered for the study. Their cases were consecutively recorded without influencing the treatment course, which was conducted according to guideline-based clinical decisions by the respective sites. Since August 2020, the rating of the RSSs was retrospectively conducted based on prospectively documented US features. Observers were blinded to the clinical results such as cytological and histopathological findings. Communication between the observers regarding difficult cases was, and is, consistently performed to reduce interobserver bias [33].

The inclusion criteria consisted of hypofunctioning or indifferent TNs on thyroid scintigraphy and the availability of cytological (FNC) or histopathological (surgery) diagnoses. Bethesda II lesions were considered benign. Scintigraphically hyperfunctioning TNs and those without scintigraphy as well as FNC findings outside Bethesda category II without histopathological evaluation were excluded. Scintigraphy scans were conducted according to the European guideline using 99 m-technetium-pertechnetate [31].

Recorded data comprised institution site, age, gender, number of TNs per patient, lesion size in three dimensions (crania–caudal, ventral–dorsal, medial–lateral), lesion functionality on scintigram, US features and RSS classifications (see Section 2.2), cytological findings according to the Bethesda System [34], and histopathological results.

The multicentric data collection was conducted according to the guidelines of the Declaration of Helsinki and approved by the Ethics Committee of the Medical Faculty of the University Hospital of Duisburg–Essen, Germany (ID: 16-7022-BO).

2.2. Ultrasound Examinations

US examinations were carried out according to the respective local standards with an emphasis on high-resolution, state-of-the-art image quality, and acquisition in transversal and sagittal orientation. Therefore, examination parameters, such as patient positioning, frequency, focus number and focus positioning, zoom, depth, gain, virtual convex mode, crossbeam mode, harmonic imaging modes, and breath-hold techniques were adapted to individual patient and nodule-specific requirements.

The following US devices were used:

- A Mindray DC-6 (Mindray Medical International Limited, Shenzhen, China) and Esaote MyLab 40 (Esaote SpA, Genova, Italy) equipped with a 10- and 12-MHz small parts probe;
- Hitachi EUB 5000 G (Hitachi Ltd., Chiyoda, Tokyo, Japan) equipped with a 5–10 MHz linear probe;
- Hitachi HI VISION Avius (Hitachi Ltd., Chiyoda, Tokyo, Japan) equipped with a 5–10 MHz linear probe; and
- GE LOGIQ E9 (GE Healthcare, Milwaukee, WI, USA) equipped with a 10–15 MHz linear probe.

The following US features were recorded:

- Composition: solid, <10, 10–50, 50–90, >90% cystic, spongiform;
- Echogenicity: (marked) hypoechoic, isoechoic, hyperechoic, completely cystic;
- Margin: sharp/smooth, macrolobulated, microlobulated, irregular, ill-defined, extrathyroidal extension (ETE);
- Calcifications/spots: none, colloidal-cystic associated spots, macrocalcifications, rim calcifications, rim calcifications with small extrusive soft tissue component (SESTC), microcalcifications; and
- Shape: taller-than-wide (TTW), non-TTW, round.

Of these features, all TNs were classified according to the five RSSs: Kwak-TIRADS [19], ACR TI-RADS [18], EU-TIRADS [22], ATA Guidelines [21], and Korean-TIRADS [20].

2.3. Data Analyses and Statistics

Data were recorded on Excel software (Version 14.7.3, Microsoft Corporation, Redmond, WA, USA) and transferred to SPSS Statistics software (International Business Machines Corporation, Version 26.0, New York, NY, USA) for statistical analyses. Fisher's exact test was conducted to evaluate group differences for ordinal values (e.g., US features). A Student's t test was performed to investigate the differences among groups with normally distributed metric values (e.g., TSH-level, lesion size). For each RSS, calculations were made for positive predictive value (PPV), negative predictive value (NPV), sensitivity, specificity, diagnostic accuracy (ACC), positive likelihood ratio (LHR+), negative likelihood ratio (LHR-), diagnostic odds ratio (DOR), receiver operating curves (ROCs), and area under the curve (AUC). The AUC values were compared using a Hanley and McNeil test on MedCalc software (Version 20.009, Ostend, Belgium). If RSSs classifications were not applicable (N/A), the respective TN was not included in the analyses.

Cutoff values between benign and malignant for performance calculations were defined at 4c, TR5, 5, high, and high for Kwak-TIRADS, ACR TI-RADS, EU-TIRADS, Korean-TIRADS, and ATA Guidelines, respectively. For each test, $p < 0.05$ was considered significant.

3. Results

3.1. Patient Data and Clinical Characteristics of the Thyroid Nodules

A total of 1211 TNs in 849 patients (604 females, 71.1%; 249 males, 28.9%; aged 51 ± 14 years) were included in this study. The majority of the lesions were benign (N = 1022, 84.4%). Malignant lesions were diagnosed in 189 (15.6%) cases, of which 102 (54.0%) were carcinomas: papillary thyroid carcinoma (PTC) containing 19 (10.1%) papillary thyroid microcarcinomas (PTMC) and 43 (22.8%) follicular variants of PTC (FVPTCs), 10 (5.3%) follicular thyroid carcinomas (FTCs), 7 (3.7%) medullary thyroid carcinomas (MTCs), 5 (2.6%) poorly differentiated thyroid carcinomas (PDTCs), 1 (0.5%) anaplastic thyroid carcinoma (ATC), 1 (0.5%) metastasis of a colorectal cancer (CRC), and 1 (0.5%) manifestation of a Non-Hodgkin Lymphoma (NHL).

Histopathological and cytological results were available for 731 (60.4%) and 776 (64.1%) lesions, respectively. In total, 480 (39.6%) TNs were diagnosed as benign by cytology (Bethesda II) only. For 296 (24.4%) lesions, cytological and histopathological results were available. In 142 cases, Bethesda III/IV results were found on cytological examinations. The rate of malignancy in these TNs was 15.5% (Table 1).

Table 1. Histopathological results of thyroid nodules (TNs) with fine-needle cytology (FNC) and surgery.

Bethesda Classifications [34]	All (N = 296) N (%)	Benign (N = 227) N (% of All)	Malignant (N = 69) N (% of All)
I—Nondiagnostic or Unsatisfactory	60 (20.3)	47 (78.3)	13 (21.7)
II—Benign	59 (19.9)	52 (88.1)	7 (11.9)
III/IV—AUS, FLUS, FN, suspicion for a FN	142 (48.0)	120 (84.5)	22 (15.5)
V—Suspicious for Malignancy	17 (5.7)	8 (47.1)	9 (52.9)
VI—Malignant	18 (6.1)	0 (0.0)	18 (100.0)

Abbreviations: AUS—Atypia of Undetermined Significance; FLUS—Follicular Lesion of Undetermined Significance; FN—Follicular Neoplasm.

The mean size (largest diameter) of the TNs was 26 ± 13 mm. Since in Germany thyroid scintigraphy is only regularly performed (irrespective of the TSH level) on TNs ≥ 10 mm, only eight (0.7%) TNs measured < 10 mm and 14 (1.1%) lesions showed a size of 10 mm. These were resected along with other lesions and their RSS classifications as well as scintigraphy findings were retrospectively assessed (with blinded histopathological results). The benign lesions were larger and more frequently hypofunctioning in the present study population (Table 2).

Table 2. Scintigraphy results and lesion sizes.

Scintigraphy and Lesion Size	All (N = 1211) N (%)/Mean ± SD	Benign (N = 1022) N (%)/Mean ± SD	Malignant (N = 189) N (%)/Mean ± SD	p-Value
Scintigraphy	1211 (100.0)	1022 (100.0)	189 (100.0)	
Indifferent	199 (16.4)	152 (14.9)	47 (24.9)	0.001
Hypofunctioning	1012 (83.6)	870 (85.1)	142 (75.1)	
TN Size (mm)	26 ± 13	27 ± 13	19 ± 12	<0.001

Abbreviations: SD—Standard Deviation; TN—Thyroid Nodule.

3.2. Ultrasound Features

US features that were documented for malignant and benign TNs are displayed in Table 3. Over 75% of the included carcinomas showed at least one of the following features: a solid composition, (marked) hypoechogenicity, and micro- or macrocalcifications, respectively. In contrast, over 75% of the benign lesions were characterized by sharp/smooth margins, non-TTW shape, missing calcifications, or demonstrating only colloidal-cystic associated spots. The sensitivity (specificity) of solid composition, hypochogenicity or marked hypoechogenicity, irregular or microlobulated shape, microcalcifications, and TTW for the detection of malignant TNs were 81.5% (47.6%), 84.7% (51.8%), 47.6% (92.2%), 55.0% (81.5%), and 33.3% (85.2%), respectively. The ACC values for solid components, (marked) hypoechogenicity, microlobulated or irregular margins, microcalcifications, and TTW were 52.8%, 56.9%, 85.3%, 77.3%, and 77.1%, respectively.

Table 3. Ultrasound (US) features in relation to cytological and histopathological results.

US Features	All (N = 1211) N (%)	Benign (N = 1022) N (%)	Malignant (N = 189) N (%)	p-Value
Composition				
Solid	696 (57.5)	536 (52.4)	154 (81.5)	<0.001
<10% cystic	296 (24.4)	273 (26.7)	19 (10.1)	<0.001
10–50% cystic	160 (13.2)	148 (14.5)	12 (6.3)	0.002
50–90% cystic	27 (2.2)	24 (2.3)	3 (1.6)	0.788
>90% cystic	16 (1.3)	16 (1.6)	0 (0.0)	0.154
Spongiform	26 (2.1)	25 (2.4)	1 (0.5)	0.106
Echogenicity				
Hypo	530 (43.8)	419 (41.0)	102 (54.0)	<0.001
Marked hypo	132 (10.9)	74 (7.2)	58 (30.7)	<0.001
Iso	534 (44.1)	505 (49.4)	28 (14.8)	<0.001
Hyper	8 (0.7)	7 (0.7)	1 (0.5)	>0.999
Completely cystic	17 (1.4)	17 (1.7)	0 (0.0)	0.092
Margin				
Sharp/smooth	936 (77.3)	858 (84.0)	69 (36.5)	<0.001
Macrolobulated	43 (3.6)	40 (3.9)	2 (1.1)	0.05
Microlobulated	42 (3.4)	27 (2.6)	15 (7.9)	<0.001
Irregular	127 (10.5)	52 (5.1)	75 (39.7)	<0.001
Ill-defined	66 (5.5)	42 (4.1)	24 (12.7)	<0.001
ETE	7 (0.6)	3 (0.3)	4 (2.1)	<0.001
Calcifications				
None	742 (61.3)	660 (64.6)	75 (39.7)	<0.001
Colloidal	157 (13.0)	147 (14.4)	9 (4.8)	<0.001
Macro	155 (12.8)	102 (9.9)	42 (22.2)	<0.001
Rim	17 (1.4)	12 (1.2)	5 (2.6)	<0.001
Rim with SESTC	10 (0.8)	6 (0.6)	4 (2.1)	<0.001
Micro	289 (23.9)	189 (18.5)	104 (55.0)	<0.001
Shape				
TTW	214 (17.7)	151 (14.8)	63 (33.3)	<0.001
Non-TTW	980 (80.9)	857 (83.9)	113 (59.8)	<0.001
Round	27 (2.2)	14 (1.4)	13 (6.9)	<0.001

Abbreviations: US—Ultrasound; ACC—Diagnostic Accuracy; ETE—Extrathyroidal Extension; SESTC—Small Extrusive Soft Tissue Component; TTW—Taller Than Wide.

3.3. Risk Stratification Systems

All TNs were classifiable according to Kwak-TIRADS, ACR TI-RADS, and Korean-TIRADS. A total of 3 (0.2%, 1 malignant) and 135 (11.1%, 16 malignant) TNs could not be classified using EU-TIRADS and ATA Guidelines, respectively (Figure 1). The RSS classification results are displayed in Figure 2.

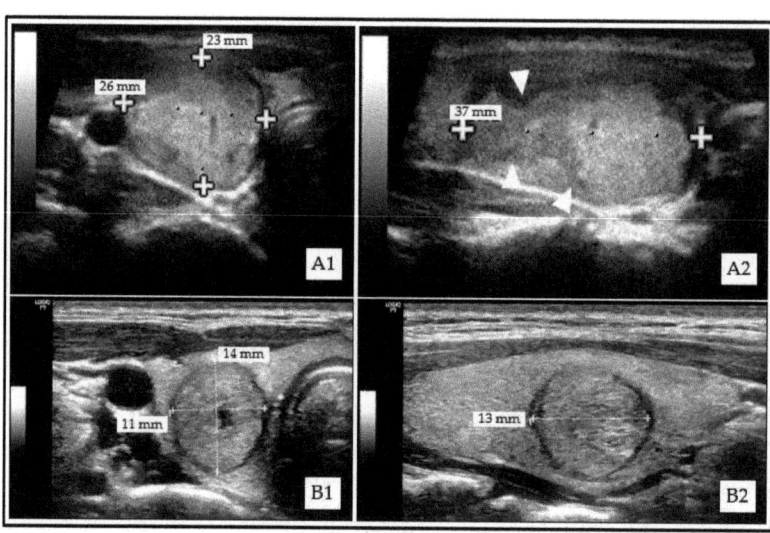

Figure 1. Examples of thyroid nodules (TNs) that could not be classified according to American Thyroid Association (ATA) Guidelines. (**A1**) (transversal)/(**A2**) (sagittal): Solid isoechoic papillary thyroid carcinoma (PTC) with irregular margins (**A2**, white triangle markers). (**B1**) (transversal)/(**B2**) (sagittal): Mainly solid isoechoic benign (Bethesda II) thyroid nodule (TN) with taller-than-wide (TTW) shape.

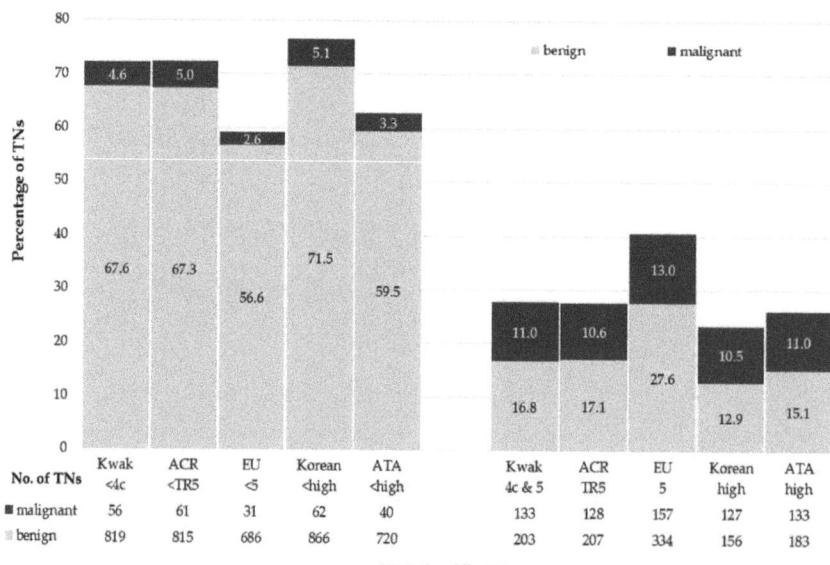

Figure 2. Performance of the risk stratification systems (RSSs). Abbreviations: TNs—Thyroid Nodules; ACR—American College of Radiology; EU—European Union; ATA—American Thyroid Association; RSS—Risk Stratification System.

The PPV, NPV, Sensitivity, Specificity, and diagnostic accuracy ranged between 32.0% (EU-TIRADS) and 44.9% (Korean-TIRADS), 93.0% (ACR TI-RADS) and 95.6% (EU-TIRADS), 67.7% (ACR TI-RADS) and 83.5% (EU-TIRADS), 67.3% (EU-TIRADS) and 84.7% (Korean-TIRADS), and 69.8% (EU-TIRADS) and 82.0% (Korean-TIRADS), respectively (Table 4).

Table 4. Diagnostic performance parameters of the ultrasound risk stratification system (RSSs) for the differentiation between benign and malignant thyroid nodules (TNs).

Diagnostic Parameters	Kwak-TIRADS	ACR TI-RADS	EU-TIRADS	Korean-TIRADS	ATA Guidelines
Cut-off (benign vs. malignant)	4c	TR5	5	high	high
PPV (CI-95)	0.4 (0.36–0.43)	0.38 (0.35–0.42)	0.32 (0.30–0.34)	0.45 (0.41–0.49)	0.42 (0.38–0.46)
NPV (CI-95)	0.94 (0.92–0.95)	0.93 (0.92–0.94)	0.96 (0.94–0.97)	0.93 (0.92–0.94)	0.95 (0.93–0.96)
Sensitivity (CI-95)	0.7 (0.64–0.76)	0.68 (0.61–0.74)	0.84 (0.78–0.88)	0.67 (0.60–0.73)	0.77 (0.70–0.83)
Specificity (CI-95)	0.8 (0.78–0.82)	0.8 (0.77–0.82)	0.67 (0.64–0.70)	0.85 (0.82–0.87)	0.8 (0.77–0.82)
ACC (CI-95)	0.79 (0.76–0.81)	0.78 (0.75–0.80)	0.7 (0.67–0.72)	0.82 (0.79–0.84)	0.79 (0.77–0.82)
LHR+ (CI-95)	3.54 (3.04–4.13)	3.34 (2.86–3.91)	2.55 (2.29–2.84)	4.4 (3.69–5.25)	3.79 (3.23–4.42)
LHR− (CI-95)	0.37 (0.30–0.46)	0.41 (0.33–0.50)	0.25 (0.18–0.34)	0.39 (0.32–0.48)	0.29 (0.22–0.38)
DOR (CI-95)	9.58 (6.78–13.57)	8.26 (5.88–11.62)	10.4 (6.93–15.62)	11.37 (8.03–16.11)	13.08 (8.87–19.30)

Abbreviations: RSS—Risk Stratification Systems; PPV—Positive Predictive Value; CI-95—95% Confidence Intervals; NPV—Negative Predictive Value; ACC—Diagnostic Accuracy; LHR+—Positive Likelihood ratio; LHR—Negative Likelihood ratio; DOR—Diagnostic Odds Ratio; TIRADS/TI-RADS—Thyroid Imaging and Reporting Data System; ATA—American Thyroid Association. Thyroid nodules (TNs) that were not classifiable (N/A) are not included.

The ROCs of the investigated RSSs are shown in Figure 3. The AUC values were 0.803 (95% Confidence Intervals: 0.765–0.840), 0.795 (0.759–0.831), 0.800 (0.765–0.834), 0.805 (0.768–0.842), and 0.801 (0.765–0.837) for Kwak-TIRADS, ACR TI-RADS, EU-TIRADS, Korean-TIRADS, and ATA Guidelines, respectively. There were no differences in the AUC values (Table 5).

Table 5. Comparison of Area under the Curve (AUC) values between the investigated risk stratification systems (RSSs) via Hanley and McNeil Test *.

RSSs	Kwak-TIRADS	ACR TI-RADS	EU-TIRADS	Korean-TIRADS	ATA Guidelines
Kwak-TIRADS	-	$p = 0.760$	$p = 0.909$	$p = 0.941$	$p = 0.939$
ACR TI-RADS	$p = 0.760$	-	$p = 0.844$	$p = 0.702$	$p = 0.814$
EU-TIRADS	$p = 0.909$	$p = 0.844$	-	$p = 0.849$	$p = 0.969$
Korean-TIRADS	$p = 0.941$	$p = 0.702$	$p = 0.849$	-	$p = 0.879$
ATA Guidelines	$p = 0.939$	$p = 0.814$	$p = 0.969$	$p = 0.879$	-

Abbreviations: RSS—Risk Stratification System; TIRADS/TI-RADS—Thyroid Imaging Reporting and Data System; ACR—American College of Radiology; EU—European Union; ATA—American Thyroid Association. * Thyroid nodules (TNs) that were not classifiable (N/A) are not included.

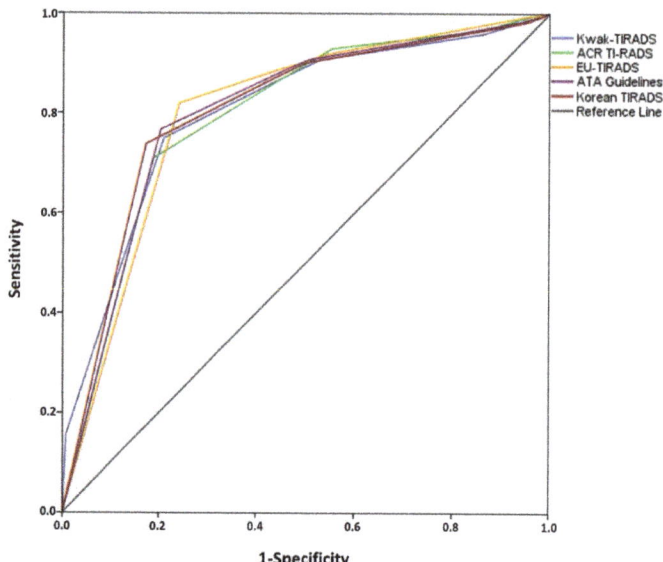

Figure 3. Receiver Operating Curves (ROCs) of the risk stratification systems (RSSs) *. * Thyroid nodules (TNs) that were not classifiable (N/A) are not included.

4. Discussion

One of the most dynamic fields in clinical thyroid research is the sonographic risk stratification of thyroid nodules. US devices are ubiquitous, and the procedure is a patient-friendly, cost-effective, and repeatable approach that has no side effects. Many different RSSs have been published in the recent years, and in the present study the diagnostic performances of five important ultrasound-based risk stratification systems (Kwak-TIRADS, ACR TI-RADS, EU-TIRADS, Korean-TIRADS, and ATA Guidelines) were evaluated in a population that has a high prevalence of TNs due to a long history of iodine deficiency [7,8].

Since 2012, the German TIRADS Study Group has been recording consecutive thyroid nodule cases from seven German institutions where there is a growing number of participating members. In this manner, a large database was built. Constant communication regarding difficult cases and the recent literature was conducted to achieve high performance levels in the application of RSSs and to reduce interobserver variability among the operators [33]. With the present multicenter trial, the group reported the first extensive German dataset regarding the diagnostic performance of five US-based RSSs for non-autonomous TNs.

Because the study focused on TNs that had been invasively diagnosed according to the clinical decision of the treating physicians, the preselected lesions (no hyperfunctioning TN, cytology or histopathology demanded) did not accurately represent the underlying patient population of Germany. Thus, malignant lesions were overrepresented: 15.5% in comparison to their natural incidence of <5% [35]. However, the data also contained TNs that had not been referred to the surgeons primarily for histopathological evaluation but had been resected as part of other surgical indications in multinodular goiters. This mitigates selection bias in favor of a higher classifications of the RSSs.

Meta-analyses are proposing sensitivities (specificities) for the detection of malignancy of 73–87% (53–56%), 63–78% (55–62%), 51–66% (79–83%), 40–54% (80–88%), and 27–53% (77–97%) for solid composition, hypoechogenicity, irregular margins, microcalcifications, and TTW shape, respectively [36–38].The calculated sensitivities and specificities for these US features in the current study were in good concordance with those in the literature.

Diagnostic accuracies ranged between 52.8% (solid composition) and 85.3% (microlobulated or irregular margins).

The diagnostic accuracy of EU-TIRADS (69.8%) was inferior to that of Kwak-TIRADS (78.6%), ACR TI-RADS (77.9%), or Korean-TIRADS (82.0%), because of the relatively high number of EU5 classifications. ATA Guidelines showed a comparably high accuracy of 79.3% but a remarkable number of TNs (11.1%) were N/A. The ATA Guidelines provided an atlas that was primarily pattern-based, which was missing clear definition for isoechoic TNs with suspicious further US features. This problem has already been described in previous studies [33]. However, N/A TNs were excluded from the diagnostic performance calculations. Based on these results, Kwak-TIRADS, ACR TI-RADS, and Korean-TIRADS outperformed EU-TIRADS and ATA Guidelines in the study population, despite the AUC values on ROCs of all five RSSs being very similar (between 0.795 and 0.805) without significant differences (N/A TNs excluded). The diagnostic performance parameters were in concordance with the results of current meta-analyses (Table 6). Wei et al. reported a pooled sensitivity of 79% and a pooled specificity of 71% for mixed TIRADS studies. Pooled sensitivity (specificity) values of 98% (55%), 54–82% (53–90%), 66–74% (64–91%), 55–86% (28–95%), and 74–87% (31–88%) were published for Kwak-TIRADS, EU-TIRADS, ACR TI-RADS, Korean-TIRADS, and ATA guidelines, respectively. However, the cut-off values between benign and malignant lesions were partly different among the respective meta-analyses.

Table 6. Overview of meta-analyses regarding the diagnostic performance of ultrasound risk stratification systems (RSSs) for thyroid nodules (TNs).

Author, Year	No of Studies (TNs)	RSSs	Sensitivity Pooled (CI-95)	Specificity Pooled (CI-95)	LHR+ Pooled (CI-95)	LHR- Pooled (CI-95)	DOR Pooled (CI-95)	AUC on ROC
Wei et al., 2016 [39]	12 (10,437)	mixed TIRADS	0.79 (0.77–0.81)	0.71 (0.70–0.72)	6.62 (4.39–9.99)	0.2 (0.14–0.29)	35.2 (19.5–63.4)	0.918
Migda et al., 2018 [40]	6 (10,926)	Kwak	0.98 (0.98–0.99)	0.55 (0.54–0.56)	2.67 (1.69–4.20)	0.05 (0.04–0.07)	51 (15.2–170.8)	0.938
Kim et al., 2020 [41]	29 (33,748)	ACR	0.66 (0.56–0.75)	0.91 (0.87–0.94)				0.89
		ATA	0.74 (0.62–0.84)	0.88 (0.82–0.93)				0.9
		Korean	0.55 (0.38–0.70)	0.95 (0.90–0.98)				0.88
		EU	0.82 (0.71–0.89)	0.9 (0.77–0.96)				0.91
Kim et al., 2020 [42]	34 (37,585)	ACR	0.7 (0.61–0.79)	0.89 (0.85–0.92)				
		Korean	0.64 (0.58–0.70)	0.93 (0.91–0.95)				
		EU	0.78 (0.64–0.88)	0.89 (0.77–95)				
Castellana et al., 2020 [43]	12 (18,750)	ACR	0.74 (0.61–0.83)	0.64 (0.56–0.70)	1.9 (1.6–2.3)	0.4 (0.3–0.6)	4.9 (3.1–7.7)	
		ATA	0.87 (0.75–0.94)	0.31 (0.24–0.40)	1.2 (1.0–1.4)	0.4 (0.2–0.7)	3.1 (1.3–7.1)	
		EU	0.54 (0.51–0.57)	0.53 (0.51–0.55)	1.4 (1.0–1.8)	0.6 (0.4–1.0)	2.2 (0.9–5.1)	
		Korean	0.86 (0.73–0.94)	0.28 (0.20–0.38)	1.2 (1.0–1.4)	0.5 (0.2–1.0)	2.5 (1.1–5.5)	

Abbreviations: RSSs—Risk Stratification Systems; TNs—Thyroid Nodules; LHR+—Positive Likelihood Ratio; LHR—Negative Likelihood Ratio; DOR—Diagnostic Odds Ratio; AUC—Area Under The Curve; ROC—Receiver Operating Curves; CI-95—95% Confidence Intervals; TIRADS—Thyroid Imaging Reporting and Data System; ACR—American College of Radiology; EU—European Union; ATA—American Thyroid Association.

Considering the data from former iodine deficiency areas specifically, Dobruch-Sobczak et al. observed a sensitivity of 93.4% and a specificity of 54.6% for EU-TIRADS with a cut-off for EU5 in a Polish multicenter study containing 842 TNs (229 malignant) [44]. In a smaller study population from Austria ($N = 195$), EU-TIRADS, Kwak-TIRADS, ATA Guidelines, and French-TIRADS were assessed suitable for the differentiation between benign and malignant TNs. The authors found a sensitivity of 85% and a specificity of 45% with a cut-off of two or more positive US criteria. However, this was only true for the 45 included PTCs, but not for the eight FTCs [29]. In the present study, a large variety of different malignant lesions were observed, containing 54.0% PTC, 5.3% FTC, 3.7% MTC, 2.6% PDTC, 0.5% ATC, and 1% other cancer types. Therefore, to the best of our knowledge, the current data provide the most comprehensive results from an area with history of iodine deficiency. In a recently published Italian real-life setting study (single-center, retrospective, observational) that included 6474 cytologically investigated TNs and comprised five different RSSs, inferior sensitivities (50.1–94.5%), PPV (7.7–11.5%), and AUC values in ROC analyses (0.606–0.632) were reported [45]. Among other reasons, such as a different history of iodine supply between Germany and Italy [46], the superior performance of the RSSs in the current study may be due to the exclusion of non-autonomously functioning lesions. In a previous study, the GTSG revealed that a relevant number of hyperfunctioning TNs showed high-risk US patterns [32]. Scintigraphically guided preselection can therefore be recommended to improve the US-based risk stratification of TNs.

Further clinical examination data revealed larger sizes and a higher frequency of scintigraphically hypofunctioning lesions for benign compared to malignant TNs. However, since the decision for or against cytological or histopathological clarification of a TN was carried out as a comprehensive clinical decision, the data were affected by a selection bias after considering several additional findings such as laboratory results and disease-related symptoms. Therefore, over 80% of the lesions were hypofunctioning in the study population. The data showed a high sensitivity (75.1%) but a very low specificity (14.9%) for the hypofunctional feature for detecting malignant lesions. Due to this selection bias (especially the exclusion of hyperfunctioning lesions) these diagnostic parameters did not display the findings in a clinical routine. However, the majority of the malignant TNs showed up as hypofunctioning on scintigraphy scans, which was in accordance with the literature [47].

The multicentric study design allowed a patient enrolled in the study to be managed by different approaches during clinical practice. It needs to be underlined that this could have affected the results. Since only TNs that were characterized by scintigraphy were included, less than 1% of the TNs measured were < 10 mm. However, it is known that lesions < 10 mm can be detected as hyperfunctioning on scintigraphy and can be reliably assessed by I-124 positron emission tomography (PET)/US fusion imaging even in unfavorable localizations [47–49]. Furthermore, TIRADS have been proven to perform well in TNs < 10 mm [50].

So far, no uniform RSS has been established worldwide, although work has recently begun on a new international US-based RSS for TN. With the participation of several scientific societies, the so-called I-TIRADS will be proposed and established internationally as a uniform evidence-based system. Currently, different working groups are investigating individual ultrasound criteria [51]. In addition, promising data already exist regarding the use of artificial intelligence (AI) to identify ultrasound patterns. This technique could significantly reduce interobserver variability and account for regional differences such as site-typical normal findings via variable databases [52]. Another important pillar in the evaluation of TNs is related to the aforementioned topics: the establishment of (automated) structured reporting (SR). It is already well advanced in other diagnostic examination procedures such as mammography or prostate MRI as well as in professional study protocols [53,54]. Concepts for the implementation of AI pattern detection and SR in the field of thyroid US have already been proposed. In particular, the generation of automated findings from manually acquired ultrasound image data has the potential to provide considerable time savings for medical staff and may thus also have health and economic relevance for regions with a high prevalence of thyroid disease [55–57].

5. Conclusions

Kwak-TIRADS, ACR TI-RADS, Korean-TIRADS, and ATA Guidelines revealed high performance levels with diagnostic accuracies of about 80% and AUC values of approximately 0.8 without significant differences. However, over 10% of the TNs were not classifiable according to ATA Guidelines. The diagnostic performance of EU-TIRADS was slightly inferior in comparison with the aforementioned ultrasound risk stratification systems for thyroid nodules. Therefore, Kwak-TIRADS, ACR TI-RADS, and Korean-TIRADS can be preferentially recommended in areas with a history of iodine deficiency. Scintigraphic preselection to exclude hyperfunctioning nodules may improve the performance of ultrasound-based risk stratification systems.

Author Contributions: Conceptualization, P.S., S.S., M.Z. and R.G.; methodology, P.S., S.S., M.Z. and R.G.; software, P.S.; validation, M.F., M.C.K. and R.G.; formal analysis, P.S.; investigation, P.S., S.S., M.Z., A.S., B.K., M.G. and R.G.; resources, M.Z., A.S., M.F., M.C.K., K.H. and R.G.; data curation, P.S.; writing—original draft preparation, P.S. and S.S.; writing—review and editing, M.Z., A.S., B.K., M.F., M.C.K., K.H. and R.G.; visualization, P.S.; supervision, M.C.K., K.H. and R.G.; project administration, S.S.; funding acquisition, N/A. All authors have read and agreed to the published version of the manuscript.

Funding: This research received no external funding.

Institutional Review Board Statement: The study was conducted according to the guidelines of the Declaration of Helsinki and approved by the Institutional Ethics Committee of the Medical Faculty of the University Hospital of Duisburg–Essen, Germany (protocol code: 16-7022-BO, 04-AUG-2016, date of approval at 4 August 2016).

Informed Consent Statement: Informed consent for clinical investigations was obtained from all subjects involved in the study.

Data Availability Statement: The data presented in this study are openly available in FigShare at 10.6084/m9.figshare.14988171, reference number [58].

Acknowledgments: The authors thank Elena Gilman for her support with statistical analyses.

Conflicts of Interest: The authors declare no conflict of interest.

References

1. Carle, A.; Krejbjerg, A.; Laurberg, P. Epidemiology of nodular goitre. Influence of iodine intake. *Best Pract. Res. Clin. Endocrinol. Metab.* **2014**, *28*, 465–479. [CrossRef]
2. Johner, S.A.; Thamm, M.; Nothlings, U.; Remer, T. Iodine status in preschool children and evaluation of major dietary iodine sources: A german experience. *Eur. J. Nutr.* **2013**, *52*, 1711–1719. [CrossRef]
3. Johner, S.A.; Thamm, M.; Schmitz, R.; Remer, T. Examination of iodine status in the german population: An example for methodological pitfalls of the current approach of iodine status assessment. *Eur. J. Nutr.* **2016**, *55*, 1275–1282. [CrossRef] [PubMed]
4. World Health Organization. *Assessment of Iodine Deficiency Disorders and Monitoring Their Elimination: A Guide for Programme Managers*, 3rd ed.; World Health Organization: Geneva, Switzerland, 2007; ISBN 978-92-4-159582-7.
5. World Health Organization. *Iodine Status Worldwide: Who Global Database on Iodine Deficiency*; World Health Organization: Geneva, Switzerland, 2004.
6. Volzke, H. Study of health in pomerania (ship). Concept, design and selected results. *Bundesgesundheitsblatt Gesundh. Gesundh.* **2012**, *55*, 790–794.
7. Reiners, C.; Wegscheider, K.; Schicha, H.; Theissen, P.; Vaupel, R.; Wrbitzky, R.; Schumm-Draeger, P.M. Prevalence of thyroid disorders in the working population of germany: Ultrasonography screening in 96,278 unselected employees. *Thyroid* **2004**, *14*, 926–932. [CrossRef]
8. Verburg, F.A.; Grelle, I.; Tatschner, K.; Reiners, C.; Luster, M. Prevalence of thyroid disorders in elderly people in germany. A screening study in a country with endemic goitre. *Nuklearmedizin* **2017**, *56*, 9–13. [CrossRef] [PubMed]
9. Russ, G.; Leboulleux, S.; Leenhardt, L.; Hegedus, L. Thyroid incidentalomas: Epidemiology, risk stratification with ultrasound and workup. *Eur. Thyroid J.* **2014**, *3*, 154–163. [CrossRef]

10. Paschke, R.; Schmid, K.W.; Gartner, R.; Mann, K.; Dralle, H.; Reiners, C. Epidemiology, pathophysiology, guideline-adjusted diagnostics, and treatment of thyroid nodules. *Med. Klin.* **2010**, *105*, 80–87. [CrossRef] [PubMed]
11. Chaudhary, V.; Bano, S. Thyroid ultrasound. *Indian J. Endocrinol. Metab.* **2013**, *17*, 219–227. [CrossRef] [PubMed]
12. Floridi, C.; Cellina, M.; Buccimazza, G.; Arrichiello, A.; Sacrini, A.; Arrigoni, F.; Pompili, G.; Barile, A.; Carrafiello, G. Ultrasound imaging classifications of thyroid nodules for malignancy risk stratification and clinical management: State of the art. *Gland. Surg.* **2019**, *8*, S233–S244. [CrossRef]
13. Kim, P.H.; Suh, C.H.; Baek, J.H.; Chung, S.R.; Choi, Y.J.; Lee, J.H. Unnecessary thyroid nodule biopsy rates under four ultrasound risk stratification systems: A systematic review and meta-analysis. *Eur. Radiol.* **2021**, *31*, 2877–2885. [CrossRef]
14. Xu, T.; Wu, Y.; Wu, R.X.; Zhang, Y.Z.; Gu, J.Y.; Ye, X.H.; Tang, W.; Xu, S.H.; Liu, C.; Wu, X.H. Validation and comparison of three newly-released thyroid imaging reporting and data systems for cancer risk determination. *Endocrine* **2018**, *64*, 299–307. [CrossRef] [PubMed]
15. Wei, X.; Li, Y.; Zhang, S.; Gao, M. Thyroid imaging reporting and data system (ti-rads) in the diagnostic value of thyroid nodules: A systematic review. *Tumour. Biol.* **2014**, *35*, 6769–6776. [CrossRef]
16. Wang, Y.; Lei, K.R.; He, Y.P.; Li, X.L.; Ren, W.W.; Zhao, C.K.; Bo, X.W.; Wang, D.; Sun, C.Y.; Xu, H.X. Malignancy risk stratification of thyroid nodules: Comparisons of four thyroid imaging reporting and data systems in surgically resected nodules. *Sci. Rep.* **2017**, *7*, 11560. [CrossRef] [PubMed]
17. Grani, G.; Lamartina, L.; Ascoli, V.; Bosco, D.; Biffoni, M.; Giacomelli, L.; Maranghi, M.; Falcone, R.; Ramundo, V.; Cantisani, V.; et al. Reducing the number of unnecessary thyroid biopsies while improving diagnostic accuracy: Toward the "right" tirads. *J. Clin. Endocrinol. Metab.* **2019**, *104*, 95–102. [CrossRef]
18. Tessler, F.N.; Middleton, W.D.; Grant, E.G.; Hoang, J.K.; Berland, L.L.; Teefey, S.A.; Cronan, J.J.; Beland, M.D.; Desser, T.S.; Frates, M.C.; et al. Acr thyroid imaging, reporting and data system (ti-rads): White paper of the acr ti-rads committee. *J. Am. Coll. Radiol.* **2017**, *14*, 587–595. [CrossRef] [PubMed]
19. Kwak, J.Y.; Han, K.H.; Yoon, J.H.; Moon, H.J.; Son, E.J.; Park, S.H.; Jung, H.K.; Choi, J.S.; Kim, B.M.; Kim, E.K. Thyroid imaging reporting and data system for us features of nodules: A step in establishing better stratification of cancer risk. *Radiology* **2011**, *260*, 892–899. [CrossRef] [PubMed]
20. Shin, J.H.; Baek, J.H.; Chung, J.; Ha, E.J.; Kim, J.H.; Lee, Y.H.; Lim, H.K.; Moon, W.J.; Na, D.G.; Park, J.S.; et al. Ultrasonography diagnosis and imaging-based management of thyroid nodules: Revised korean society of thyroid radiology consensus statement and recommendations. *Korean J. Radiol.* **2016**, *17*, 370–395. [CrossRef]
21. Haugen, B.R.; Alexander, E.K.; Bible, K.C.; Doherty, G.M.; Mandel, S.J.; Nikiforov, Y.E.; Pacini, F.; Randolph, G.W.; Sawka, A.M.; Schlumberger, M.; et al. 2015 american thyroid association management guidelines for adult patients with thyroid nodules and differentiated thyroid cancer: The american thyroid association guidelines task force on thyroid nodules and differentiated thyroid cancer. *Thyroid* **2016**, *26*, 1–133. [CrossRef] [PubMed]
22. Russ, G.; Bonnema, S.J.; Erdogan, M.F.; Durante, C.; Ngu, R.; Leenhardt, L. European thyroid association guidelines for ultrasound malignancy risk stratification of thyroid nodules in adults: The eu-tirads. *Eur. Thyroid J.* **2017**, *6*, 225–237. [CrossRef]
23. Chng, C.L.; Tan, H.C.; Too, C.W.; Lim, W.Y.; Chiam, P.P.S.; Zhu, L.; Nadkarni, N.V.; Lim, A.Y.Y. Diagnostic performance of ata, bta and tirads sonographic patterns in the prediction of malignancy in histologically proven thyroid nodules. *Singap. Med. J.* **2018**, *59*, 578–583. [CrossRef] [PubMed]
24. Ha, S.M.; Baek, J.H.; Choi, Y.J.; Chung, S.R.; Sung, T.Y.; Kim, T.Y.; Lee, J.H. Malignancy risk of initially benign thyroid nodules: Validation with various thyroid imaging reporting and data system guidelines. *Eur. Radiol.* **2019**, *29*, 133–140. [CrossRef] [PubMed]
25. Koh, J.; Kim, S.Y.; Lee, H.S.; Kim, E.K.; Kwak, J.Y.; Moon, H.J.; Yoon, J.H. Diagnostic performances and interobserver agreement according to observer experience: A comparison study using three guidelines for management of thyroid nodules. *Acta Radiol.* **2018**, *59*, 917–923. [CrossRef] [PubMed]
26. Middleton, W.D.; Teefey, S.A.; Reading, C.C.; Langer, J.E.; Beland, M.D.; Szabunio, M.M.; Desser, T.S. Comparison of performance characteristics of american college of radiology ti-rads, korean society of thyroid radiology tirads, and american thyroid association guidelines. *AJR Am. J. Roentgenol.* **2018**, *210*, 1148–1154. [CrossRef]
27. Migda, B.; Migda, M.; Migda, A.M.; Bierca, J.; Slowniska-Srzednicka, J.; Jakubowski, W.; Slapa, R.Z. Evaluation of four variants of the thyroid imaging reporting and data system (tirads) classification in patients with multinodular goitre-initial study. *Endokrynol. Pol.* **2018**, *69*, 156–162.
28. Shen, Y.; Liu, M.; He, J.; Wu, S.; Chen, M.; Wan, Y.; Gao, L.; Cai, X.; Ding, J.; Fu, X. Comparison of different risk-stratification systems for the diagnosis of benign and malignant thyroid nodules. *Front. Oncol.* **2019**, *9*, 378. [CrossRef] [PubMed]
29. Tugendsam, C.; Petz, V.; Buchinger, W.; Schmoll-Hauer, B.; Schenk, I.P.; Rudolph, K.; Krebs, M.; Zettinig, G. Ultrasound criteria for risk stratification of thyroid nodules in the previously iodine deficient area of austria—A single centre, retrospective analysis. *Thyroid Res.* **2018**, *11*, 3. [CrossRef]
30. Yoon, S.J.; Na, D.G.; Gwon, H.Y.; Paik, W.; Kim, W.J.; Song, J.S.; Shim, M.S. Similarities and differences between thyroid imaging reporting and data systems. *AJR Am. J. Roentgenol.* **2019**, *213*, W76–W84. [CrossRef]
31. Giovanella, L.; Avram, A.M.; Iakovou, I.; Kwak, J.; Lawson, S.A.; Lulaj, E.; Luster, M.; Piccardo, A.; Schmidt, M.; Tulchinsky, M.; et al. Eanm practice guideline/snmmi procedure standard for raiu and thyroid scintigraphy. *Eur. J. Nucl. Med. Mol. Imaging* **2019**, *46*, 2514–2525. [CrossRef]

32. Schenke, S.; Seifert, P.; Zimny, M.; Winkens, T.; Binse, I.; Goerges, R. Risk stratification of thyroid nodules using thyroid imaging reporting and data system (tirads): The omission of thyroid scintigraphy increases the rate of falsely suspected lesions. *J. Nucl. Med.* **2019**, *60*, 342–347. [CrossRef]
33. Seifert, P.; Gorges, R.; Zimny, M.; Kreissl, M.C.; Schenke, S. Interobserver agreement and efficacy of consensus reading in kwak-, eu-, and acr-thyroid imaging recording and data systems and ata guidelines for the ultrasound risk stratification of thyroid nodules. *Endocrine* **2020**, *67*, 143–154. [CrossRef] [PubMed]
34. Cibas, E.S.; Ali, S.Z. The bethesda system for reporting thyroid cytopathology. *Am. J. Clin. Pathol.* **2009**, *132*, 658–665. [CrossRef] [PubMed]
35. Farahati, J.; Mader, U.; Gilman, E.; Gorges, R.; Maric, I.; Binse, I.; Hanscheid, H.; Herrmann, K.; Buck, A.; Bockisch, A. Changing trends of incidence and prognosis of thyroid carcinoma. *Nuklearmedizin* **2019**, *58*, 86–92. [CrossRef] [PubMed]
36. Remonti, L.R.; Kramer, C.K.; Leitao, C.B.; Pinto, L.C.; Gross, J.L. Thyroid ultrasound features and risk of carcinoma: A systematic review and meta-analysis of observational studies. *Thyroid* **2015**, *25*, 538–550. [CrossRef]
37. Brito, J.P.; Gionfriddo, M.R.; Al Nofal, A.; Boehmer, K.R.; Leppin, A.L.; Reading, C.; Callstrom, M.; Elraiyah, T.A.; Prokop, L.J.; Stan, M.N.; et al. The accuracy of thyroid nodule ultrasound to predict thyroid cancer: Systematic review and meta-analysis. *J. Clin. Endocrinol. Metab.* **2014**, *99*, 1253–1263. [CrossRef] [PubMed]
38. Razavi, S.A.; Hadduck, T.A.; Sadigh, G.; Dwamena, B.A. Comparative effectiveness of elastographic and b-mode ultrasound criteria for diagnostic discrimination of thyroid nodules: A meta-analysis. *AJR Am. J. Roentgenol.* **2013**, *200*, 1317–1326. [CrossRef]
39. Wei, X.; Li, Y.; Zhang, S.; Gao, M. Meta-analysis of thyroid imaging reporting and data system in the ultrasonographic diagnosis of 10,437 thyroid nodules. *Head Neck* **2016**, *38*, 309–315. [CrossRef]
40. Migda, B.; Migda, M.; Migda, M.S.; Slapa, R.Z. Use of the kwak thyroid image reporting and data system (k-tirads) in differential diagnosis of thyroid nodules: Systematic review and meta-analysis. *Eur. Radiol.* **2018**, *28*, 2380–2388. [CrossRef]
41. Kim, P.H.; Suh, C.H.; Baek, J.H.; Chung, S.R.; Choi, Y.J.; Lee, J.H. Diagnostic performance of four ultrasound risk stratification systems: A systematic review and meta-analysis. *Thyroid* **2020**, *30*, 1159–1168. [CrossRef] [PubMed]
42. Kim, D.H.; Chung, S.R.; Choi, S.H.; Kim, K.W. Accuracy of thyroid imaging reporting and data system category 4 or 5 for diagnosing malignancy: A systematic review and meta-analysis. *Eur. Radiol.* **2020**, *30*, 5611–5624. [CrossRef]
43. Castellana, M.; Castellana, C.; Treglia, G.; Giorgino, F.; Giovanella, L.; Russ, G.; Trimboli, P. Performance of five ultrasound risk stratification systems in selecting thyroid nodules for fna. *J. Clin. Endocrinol. Metab.* **2020**, *105*, 1659–1669. [CrossRef]
44. Dobruch-Sobczak, K.; Adamczewski, Z.; Szczepanek-Parulska, E.; Migda, B.; Wolinski, K.; Krauze, A.; Prostko, P.; Ruchala, M.; Lewinski, A.; Jakubowski, W.; et al. Histopathological verification of the diagnostic performance of the eu-tirads classification of thyroid nodules-results of a multicenter study performed in a previously iodine-deficient region. *J. Clin. Med.* **2019**, *8*, 1781. [CrossRef]
45. Sparano, C.; Verdiani, V.; Pupilli, C.; Perigli, G.; Badii, B.; Vezzosi, V.; Mannucci, E.; Maggi, M.; Petrone, L. Choosing the best algorithm among five thyroid nodule ultrasound scores: From performance to cytology sparing-a single-center retrospective study in a large cohort. *Eur. Radiol.* **2021**, *31*, 5689–5698. [CrossRef]
46. Gartner, R. Recent data on iodine intake in germany and europe. *J. Trace Elem. Med. Biol.* **2016**, *37*, 85–89. [CrossRef]
47. Seifert, P.; Freesmeyer, M. Preoperative diagnostics in differentiated thyroid carcinoma. *Nuklearmedizin* **2017**, *56*, 201–210. [CrossRef] [PubMed]
48. Seifert, P.; Winkens, T.; Kuhnel, C.; Guhne, F.; Freesmeyer, M. I-124-pet/us fusion imaging in comparison to conventional diagnostics and tc-99m pertechnetate spect/us fusion imaging for the function assessment of thyroid nodules. *Ultrasound Med. Biol.* **2019**, *45*, 2298–2308. [CrossRef] [PubMed]
49. Winkens, T.; Seifert, P.; Hollenbach, C.; Kuhnel, C.; Guhne, F.; Freesmeyer, M. The fusion iena study: Comparison of i-124-pet/us fusion imaging with conventional diagnostics for the functional assessment of thyroid nodules by multiple observers. *Nuklearmedizin* **2019**, *58*, 434–442. [CrossRef] [PubMed]
50. Schenke, S.; Klett, R.; Seifert, P.; Kreissl, M.C.; Gorges, R.; Zimny, M. Diagnostic performance of different thyroid imaging reporting and data systems (kwak-tirads, eu-tirads and acr ti-rads) for risk stratification of small thyroid nodules (</=10 mm). *J. Clin. Med.* **2020**, *9*, 236. [CrossRef]
51. Trimboli, P.; Durante, C. Ultrasound risk stratification systems for thyroid nodule: Between lights and shadows, we are moving towards a new era. *Endocrine* **2020**, *69*, 1–4. [CrossRef]
52. Moon, J.H.; Steinhubl, S.R. Digital medicine in thyroidology: A new era of managing thyroid disease. *Endocrinol. Metab.* **2019**, *34*, 124–131. [CrossRef]
53. Ganeshan, D.; Duong, P.T.; Probyn, L.; Lenchik, L.; McArthur, T.A.; Retrouvey, M.; Ghobadi, E.H.; Desouches, S.L.; Pastel, D.; Francis, I.R. Structured reporting in radiology. *Acad. Radiol.* **2018**, *25*, 66–73. [CrossRef] [PubMed]
54. Scher, H.I.; Morris, M.J.; Stadler, W.M.; Higano, C.; Basch, E.; Fizazi, K.; Antonarakis, E.S.; Beer, T.M.; Carducci, M.A.; Chi, K.N.; et al. Trial design and objectives for castration-resistant prostate cancer: Updated recommendations from the prostate cancer clinical trials working group 3. *J. Clin. Oncol.* **2016**, *34*, 1402–1418. [CrossRef] [PubMed]
55. Ernst, B.P.; Strieth, S.; Katzer, F.; Hodeib, M.; Eckrich, J.; Bahr, K.; Rader, T.; Kunzel, J.; Froelich, M.F.; Matthias, C.; et al. The use of structured reporting of head and neck ultrasound ensures time-efficiency and report quality during residency. *Eur. Arch. Otorhinolaryngol.* **2020**, *277*, 269–276. [CrossRef] [PubMed]

56. Ernst, B.P.; Strieth, S.; Kunzel, J.; Hodeib, M.; Katzer, F.; Eckrich, J.; Bahr, K.; Matthias, C.; Sommer, W.H.; Froelich, M.F.; et al. Evaluation of optimal education level to implement structured reporting into ultrasound training. *Med. Ultrason* **2020**, *22*, 445–450. [CrossRef] [PubMed]
57. Wildman-Tobriner, B.; Ngo, L.; Jaffe, T.A.; Ehieli, W.L.; Ho, L.M.; Lerebours, R.; Luo, S.; Allen, B.C. Automated structured reporting for thyroid ultrasound: Effect on reporting errors and efficiency. *J. Am. Coll. Radiol.* **2021**, *18*, 265–273. [CrossRef]
58. SPSS Data. Available online: https://figshare.com/s/8f070a42e1e59919d84e (accessed on 15 July 2021).

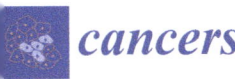

Review

The New Era of TIRADSs to Stratify the Risk of Malignancy of Thyroid Nodules: Strengths, Weaknesses and Pitfalls

Gilles Russ [1,*], Pierpaolo Trimboli [2,3] and Camille Buffet [1]

1. Groupe de Recherche Clinique n°16 Tumeurs Thyroïdiennes, Thyroid and Endocrine Tumors Unit, Institute of Endocrinology, Pitié-Salpêtrière Hospital, Sorbonne University, F-75013 Paris, France; camille.buffet@aphp.fr
2. Clinic for Endocrinology and Diabetology, Lugano Regional Hospital, Ente Ospedaliero Cantonale, 6900 Lugano, Switzerland; Pierpaolo.Trimboli@eoc.ch
3. Faculty of Biomedical Sciences, Università della Svizzera Italiana (USI), 6900 Lugano, Switzerland
* Correspondence: gilles.russ@orange.fr

Simple Summary: The aim of this review is to provide the reader with a comprehensive overview of thyroid imaging and reporting data systems used for thyroid nodules, so as to understand how nodules are scored with all existing systems. Both ultrasound based risk stratification systems and indications for fine-needle aspirations are described. Systems are compared by analyzing their strengths and weaknesses. Studies show satisfactory sensitivities and specificities for the diagnosis of malignancy for all systems, and none of them have shown a real significant advantage over the others in terms of raw diagnostic value. Interobserver agreement is also very similar for all systems, fairly adequate to robust. Dimensional cut-offs for fine-needle aspiration are quite similar and all RSSs seem to reduce effectively the number of unnecessary FNAs. Merging all existing systems in a common international one is desirable.

Abstract: Since 2009, thyroid imaging reporting and data systems (TI-RADS) have been playing an increasing role in the field of thyroid nodules (TN) imaging. Their common aims are to provide sonologists of varied medical specialties and clinicians with an ultrasound (US) based malignancy risk stratification score and to guide decision making of fine-needle aspiration (FNA). Schematically, all TI-RADSs scores can be classified as either pattern-based or point-based approaches. The main strengths of these systems are their ability (i) to homogenize US TN descriptions among operators, (ii) to facilitate and shorten communication on the malignancy risk of TN between sonologists and clinicians, (iii) to provide quantitative ranges of malignancy risk assessment with high sensitivity and negative predictive values, and (iv) to reduce the number of unnecessary FNAs. Their weaknesses are (i) the remaining inter-observer discrepancies and (ii) their insufficient sensitivity for the diagnosis of follicular cancers and follicular variant of papillary cancers. Most common pitfalls are degenerating shrinking nodules and confusion between individual and coalescent nodules. The benefits of all TI-RADSs far outweigh their shortcomings, explaining their rising use, but the necessity to improve and merge the different existing systems remains.

Keywords: thyroid; nodule; risk stratification; TI-RADS; fine-needle aspiration

1. Introduction

Risk stratification systems (RSSs) have two main aims. The first one is to homogenize the results of thyroid ultrasound (US) reports, by using a quantitative cancer risk estimation approach, in order to facilitate communication between practitioners and with the patients. Ambiguities of qualitative descriptions such as "multinodular goiter to be confronted with biological tests" are reduced and allow for a quick understanding of the risk level of a thyroid nodule. The second one is to provide guidelines regarding the indications for fine-needle aspiration biopsy (FNA). There again, the limitation of subjectivity for this decision is crucial for patients to hope to get homogenized care.

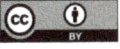

Some of these systems, but not all, have incorporated a lexicon and even more rarely a standardized report. At least the former seems mandatory to increase inter-observer description agreement.

However, all RSSs tend to base the whole stratification and decision making process solely on US criteria and nodular size, whereas obviously many other factors should, and are, integrated when accomplishing these tasks. Among these are patient's age and sex; age of the disease; family history of thyroid cancer; personal history of cervical irradiation; clinical symptoms such as dysphonia, dysphagia, or dyspnea; nodular location; number of nodules; and presence of suspicious cervical lymph nodes. Thus, a more thorough algorithm, also including laboratory tests such as TSH and calcitonin and thyroid scintigraphy when deemed adapted, may be sought in the future. This review will describe present RSSs, their strengths, weaknesses, and pitfalls via a comprehensive analysis of the literature and make some suggestions for the future.

1.1. Description of Present RSSs

Several national and international professional organizations have developed US-based risk-stratification systems. They are often referred to as thyroid imaging reporting and data systems, or TIRADS, terms derived from those used for breast cancer imaging. Some societies have chosen to stay with their own name to refer to their system (e.g., the American Thyroid Association). RSSs assign thyroid nodules to categories characterized by increasing risk ranges for cancer, based on the presence or not of specific US features. Two of the eight RSSs described below, ACR- and C-TIRADS, are point-based systems and the six others are pattern-based. Pattern-based scoring consists of recognizing a grouping of US features in a single figure, whereas point-based scoring systems consist of summing points that have been formerly attributed to US features.

1.1.1. Chilean TIRADS (2009)

Historically, it was the first TIRADS to be published [1]. Ten US patterns were defined, called colloid 1 to 3 (TIRADS 2), pseudo-nodule (TIRADS 3), simple neoplastic, De Quervain and suspicious neoplastic patterns (TIRADS 4A), malignant A (TIRADS 4B), B, and C patterns (TIRADS 5). TIRADS 2 corresponded to anechoic with hyperechoic spots, nonvascularized lesions, or to nonencapsulated, mixed isoechoic with hyperechoic spots lesions and to spongiform nodules. TIRADS 3 nodules referred to hyper, iso, or hypoechoic, partially encapsulated nodules with peripheral vascularization, in Hashimoto's thyroiditis. TIRADS 4A nodules were solid or mixed hyper, iso, or hypoechoic nodules, with a thin capsule, or hypoechoic lesion with ill-defined borders but without calcifications or hyper, iso, or hypoechoic, hypervascularized, encapsulated nodules with a thick capsule, containing calcifications (coarse or microcalcifications). TIRADS 4B corresponded to hypoechoic, nonencapsulated nodules, with irregular shape and margins, penetrating vessels, and with or without calcifications, and TIRADS 5 referred to iso or hypoechoic, nonencapsulated nodules with multiple peripheral microcalcifications and hypervascularization or nonencapsulated, isoechoic mixed hypervascularized nodules with or without calcifications, without hyperechoic spots. The TIRADS classification was evaluated in a sample of 1097 nodules (benign: 703; follicular lesions: 238; and carcinoma: 156), among which all nodules with a malignant FNAB result were submitted to surgery, benign ones by FNAB were followed, and in the group of patients with indeterminate or follicular lesions, 31% were operated on, and the rest followed. Sensitivity, specificity, positive predictive value (PPV), negative predictive value (NPV), and accuracy were 88, 49, 49, 88, and 94%, respectively.

In 2016, in a study on 210 patients with 502 nodules, the same team found a 99.6% sensitivity, a 74.35% specificity, an 82.1% PPV, and a 99.4% NPV [2].

1.1.2. BTA Classification (British Thyroid Association) (2014)

In 2014 the British Thyroid Association guidelines for the management of thyroid cancer were introduced [3]. The BTA system classifies the thyroid US features in 5 categories at increasing risk of malignancy, from U1 (normal thyroid gland) to U5 (very suspicious lesion). The U2 (benign) category is characterized by isoechoic or mildly hyperechoic nodules with halo, cystic change with or without "ring down sign," microcystic or spongiform appearance, peripheral eggshell calcification, or peripheral vascularity. The U3 (indeterminate/equivocal) category comprises homogeneous, hyperechoic (markedly), solid nodules with halo (follicular lesion); hypoechoic nodules with equivocal echogenic foci cystic change; or mixed/central vascularity. The U4 (suspicious) category is characterized by solid hypoechoic or very hypoechoic nodules with disrupted peripheral calcification and hypoechoic lobulated outline. The U5 (malignant) category comprises solid hypoechoic nodules with lobulated or irregular outline and with or without microcalcification or globular calcification. Other U5 malignant features are intranodular vascularity, taller-than-wide shape, and characteristic associated lymphadenopathy.

In 2020, a retrospective observational study was carried out among 1465 patients. Thyroid surgery was performed in 129 patients, of which malignancy was seen in 35 (27.1%). The proportions of patients with cancer in U1–U5 categories were 0%, 13.6%, 30.4%, 40%, and 100%, respectively [4]. In another study of 73 consecutive patients with 17 histological confirmed malignant nodules, it was found that the sensitivity and NPV of BTA-U score in detecting and predicting malignancy were 100%, whereas the specificity and PPV were 34% and 32%, respectively [5].

1.1.3. AACE (American Association of Clinical Endocrinologists) Grading System (2016)

In 2016 the American Association of Clinical Endocrinologists (AACE), American College of Endocrinology (ACE) and Associazione Medici Endocrinologi (AME) Medical Guidelines for Clinical Practice for the Diagnosis and Management of Thyroid Nodules [6] were released. These included recommendations on reporting, an illustrated atlas, and an assessment of the malignancy risk of all US features, including Doppler and elastography and suggested a 3-tier RSS subdivided into low, intermediate, and high risks. Low risk nodules corresponded to cystic and spongiform ones and intermediate risk nodules to mildly hypoechoic and isoechoic ones with no features of high suspicion. The latter included marked hypoechogenicity, spiculated or lobulated margins, microcalcifications, taller-than-wide shape, extrathyroidal growth, and/or a pathologic lymph node.

In 2017, a study on 859 FNAs from 598 patients showed that 88.5% and 74.9% of low and intermediate risk nodules, respectively, were cytologically benign, whereas 84.6% of high risk nodules had a moderate-to-elevated risk of malignancy or were malignant [7].

1.1.4. ATA (American Thyroid Association) Grading System (2016)

In 2016, the American Thyroid Association Management Guidelines for Adult Patients with Thyroid Nodules and Differentiated Thyroid Cancer were published [8]. The RSS was composed of 5 categories ranging from benign to high suspicion. Irregular margins (infiltrative, microlobulated), microcalcifications, taller than wide shape, rim calcifications with small extrusive soft tissue component, and evidence of extra-thyroidal extension were considered highly suspicious in hypoechoic nodules, and, on the contrary, cystic nodules were classified as benign and spongiform nodules as very low suspicion. Low suspicion and intermediate suspicion nodules depended on their echogenicity and composition (hypoechoic solid-intermediate suspicion and isoechoic solid or partially cystic-low suspicion). The ATA risk assessment was validated in a prospective study on 206 nodules [9]. Malignancy rates determined by cytology/surgical pathology were 100%, 11%, 8%, and 2% in high, intermediate, low, and very low classes, respectively, which were closely aligned with ATA malignancy risk estimates (high 70–90%, intermediate 10–20%, low 5–10%, and very low 3%).

1.1.5. K-TIRADS (Korean-TIRADS) (2016)

The last published version of the Korean Society of Thyroid Radiology was issued in 2016 [10], including a detailed lexicon, an RSS, and management recommendations. The main specificities of the lexicon were to detail definitions of composition and of hyperechoic foci. Composition can be solid, predominantly solid, or cystic (with a 50% cut-off) or (entirely) cystic (meaning no solid portion). Hyperechoic foci can correspond either to microcalcifications when measuring 1 mm or less and located in the solid portion, or to colloid when located in the cystic portion and generating comet-tail artifacts. The RSS ranges from 1 to 5, 1 corresponding to the absence of nodule. It is based on both composition and echogenicity. Pure cysts and spongiform nodules are scored as K-TIRADS 2 (benign). Iso/hyperechoic nodules and partially cystic nodules are classified as K-TIRADS 3 (low suspicion) in the absence of features of high suspicion and as K-TIRADS 4 (intermediate suspicion) if there is any suspect feature, likewise solid hypoechoic nodules without features of high suspicion. Solid hypoechoic nodules with any suspicious features (microcalcification, nonparallel orientation, spiculated/microlobulated margins) are K-TIRADS 5 (high suspicion).

Its diagnostic value has been evaluated in a prospective multicenter study on 902 nodules [11]. The calculated malignancy risk in K-TIRADS categories 5, 4, 3, and 2 nodules was 73.4, 19.0, 3.5, and 0.0%, respectively. The sensitivity, specificity, PPV, NPV, and accuracy for malignancy were 95.5, 58.6, 44.5, 96.9, and 69.5%, respectively.

1.1.6. EU-TIRADS (European-TIRADS) (2017)

Published in 2017, the European Thyroid Association (ETA) guidelines include a lexicon, a standardized report, an RSS, and management recommendations [12]. The lexicon incorporates illustrations and the report a drawing example used to locate nodules simply and precisely. The RSS ranges from 1 to 5, with 1 corresponding to no nodule. EU-TIRADS 2 correspond to purely cystic and spongiform nodules. EU-TIRADS 3 are isoechoic nodules with no features of high suspicion and EU-TIRADS 4 mildly hypoechoic nodules also with no such features, knowing that here the presence of a mildly hypoechoic zone, even in minority, is sufficient to classify the nodule as intermediate risk. Features of high suspicion are marked hypoechogenicity, microcalcifications, taller-than-wide shape, spiculated/microlobulated margins, and the presence of at least one of these categorizes the nodule as EU-TIRADS 5.

A multicenter retrospective validation study on 1058 nodules using final histology as a gold standard found a cancer rate within or close to the given range described in the EU-TIRADS guidelines and a satisfactory diagnostic value with 93% sensitivity and 97% NPV [13]. A meta-analysis published in 2020 including seven studies and evaluating 5672 nodules showed that the prevalence of malignancy in each EU-TIRADS class was 0.5%, 5.9%, 21.4%, and 76.1%, from class 2 to 5 respectively. The sensitivity, specificity, PPV, and NPV of EU-TIRADS class 5 for the detection of malignancy were 83.5%, 84.3%, 76.1%, and 85.4%, respectively [14].

1.1.7. ACR-TIRADS (American College of Radiology-TIRADS) (2017)

The lexicon was issued in 2015 [15] and the RSS and management recommendations in 2017 [16]. In contrast to most other RSSs, the ACR-TIRADS is point-based, considering five US categories, which are composition, echogenicity, shape, margin, and echogenic foci. In each category, US features are attributed a certain number of points ranging from 0 to 3. Summing the points allows one to obtain the final classification of the nodule, which goes from 1 to 5, with 1 corresponding to benign, 2 to not suspicious, 3 to mildly suspicious, 4 to moderately suspicious, and 5 to highly suspicious. Features attributing 1 point are mixed composition, isoechogenicity, and macrocalcifications. Solid composition, hypoechogenicity, irregular margins, and peripheral calcifications correspond to 2 points. Marked hypoechogenicity, a taller-than-wide shape, extra-thyroidal extension, and all punctate echogenic foci give 3 points.

In a retrospective study on 100 nodules, sensitivity, specificity, and accuracy were 92% (95% CI: 68%, 98%), 44% (95% CI: 33%, 56%), and 52% (95% CI: 40%, 63%), respectively [17]. In a multi-institutional study aiming to analyze thyroid nodule risk stratification on 3422 nodules including 352 carcinomas, 2948 (86.1%) had risk levels that were within 1% of the TIRADS risk thresholds defined in the guidelines. Of the 474 nodules that were more than 1% outside these thresholds, 88.0% (417/474) had a risk level that was below the TIRADS threshold [18]. In a systematic review and meta-analysis on 31,552 nodules, the pooled sensitivity and specificity were 89% (95% CI 81–93%) and 70% (95% CI 60–78%), respectively. The calculated area under summary ROC was 0.86 (95% CI 0.83–0.89) [19].

1.1.8. C-TIRADS (Chinese-TIRADS) (2020)

Realizing that in China, as many as ten versions of TIRADS had been used in different hospitals nationwide, causing a lot of confusion, the Chinese-TIRADS, in line with China's national conditions and medical status, was established based on literature review, expert consensus, and multicenter data provided by the Chinese Artificial Intelligence Alliance for Thyroid and Breast Ultrasound [20]. It includes a terminology section and a score. The score ranges from 1 to 5, 1 corresponding to the absence of nodule. Each US feature is attributed a number of points ranging from -1 to 1 and the points are summed. Vertical orientation, solid composition, markedly hypoechoic, microcalcifications, ill-defined and irregular margins, and extra-thyroidal extension each are attributed 1 point, whereas comet-tail artifacts correspond to -1. The sum corresponds to the C-TIRADS score: 1, no nodule; 2, benign (-1 point); 3, probably benign (0 point); 4A, low suspicion (1 point); 4B, moderate suspicion (2 points); 4C, high suspicion (3–4 points); 5, highly suggestive of malignancy (5 points). The corresponding expected malignancy risks are 0, 0, ≤ 2, 2–10, 10–50, 50–90, and ≥ 90%, respectively. C-TIRADS 6 corresponds to a proven malignancy.

A multicentric retrospective validation study on 2141 thyroid nodules that were neither cystic nor spongiform was simultaneously published [21]. It was designed to determine which of three methods, namely regression equation, weighting, and counting would be the most suitable to determine the malignant risk of thyroid nodules. The counting value of positive and negative ultrasound features was retained to define the C-TIRADS. The malignancy risk of each TIRADS score was in agreement with what was predicted in the guidelines.

1.2. Pattern-Based and Point Based Systems

Two of the eight RSSs described above, ACR- and C-TIRADS, are point-based systems and the six others are pattern-based. Of note, however, another point-based system was published in 2011, sometimes referred as "Kwak-TIRADS", and has gained acceptance in some parts of South Korea, in China, and other countries or regions [22]. The TI-RADS scores ranged from 1 to 5, with 1 corresponding to no nodule, 2 and 3 to benign and probably benign with no suspicious US features, and then 4a, 4b, 4c, and 5 to 1, 2, 3, or 4 and 5 suspicious US features, respectively. In a retrospective study on 1000 patients [23], a significant association was found between the TI-RADS score and Bethesda classification ($p < 0.001$). Most individuals with TI-RADS 2 or 3 had Bethesda 2 result (95.5% and 92.5%, respectively). Among those classified as TI-RADS 4C and 5, most presented Bethesda 6 (68.2% and 91.3%, respectively; $p < 0.001$). The proportion of malignancies among TI-RADS 2 was 0.8%, and TI-RADS 3 was 1.7%. Among those classified as TI-RADS 4A, proportion of malignancies was 16.0%, 43.2% in 4B, 72.7% in 4C, and 91.3% among TI-RADS 5 ($p < 0.001$), showing clear association between TI-RADS and FNA results.

Pattern-based scoring consists of recognizing a grouping of US features. It is the basis of most RSSs. Pattern-based systems have the advantage of quickness and pedagogy, in the way that they easily show and transmit patterns which are frequently encountered in daily practice. For instance, the pattern of an EU-TIRADS 3 [12] is a nodule with oval shape, regular margins, and isoechoic solid component. It describes common aspects of thyroid nodules and simplifies reality as it groups various patterns into a single recognizable one.

However, here also lies its disadvantage as it may sometimes go too far in simplifying. For example, a nodule with taller-than-wide shape is considered as high risk by the EU-TIRADS, regardless of its echogenicity and composition, although its malignancy risk would rather be intermediate. The K-TIRADS tries to overcome this problem by dividing the intermediate category into two, depending on echogenicity and composition [10].

Point-based scoring systems consist of summing points that have been formerly attributed to US features. It is the core of the ACR-TIRADS and of the C-TIRADS. The advantages are that all existing US features can be included and that the system can easily be modified with experience and virtually tested. A disadvantage is the necessity of learning by heart the number of points of each feature and having to sum them for every nodule, which can be quite time consuming if these are numerous and or if the workload is very intense. Another disadvantage is that the point assignment to each US feature is basically arbitrary. Interestingly, the ACR-TIRADS has been the attempt of a revision using artificial intelligence (AI) [24]. A genetic AI algorithm was applied to a training set of 1325 nodules and to create an optimized scoring system. This AI TI-RADS assigned new point values for eight features, including a simplified scheme for some categories. For example, only assigning points to solid nodules and eliminating point assignments to other composition features represented one such modification.

Direct implementation of the calculation algorithm in US machines could significantly simplify the use of both point-based and pattern-based RSSs.

1.3. Other Similarities and Differences

The aims of RSSs are identical: provide the highest possible diagnostic accuracy and reduce the number of unnecessary FNAs. All RSSs stratify the risk of malignancy with a qualitative approach ranging from normal to high risk linked to quantitative risk ranges appreciated by clinical studies. However, they differ by the number of classes used, the features defined as highly suspicious and the use of composition and ETE for risk stratification (Table 1).

Table 1. Comparison of some specificities of existent risk stratification systems (RSSs). Note: ETE = extra-thyroidal extension; RSS = risk stratification system.

RSS	Number of Classes	Meaning of TIRADS 1	Pattern or Point-Based RSS	Features of High Suspicion	Composition Included in the RSS	ETE Included in the RSS
Chilean TIRADS	6 TIRADS 4 divided into 2 subclasses	Normal examination	Pattern	Irregular margins Irregular shape Multiple peripheral microcalcifications Penetrating vessels	Yes	No
Kwak-TIRADS	5 TIRADS 4 divided into 3 subclasses	No nodule	Point	Marked hypoechogenicity Irregular margins Microcalcifications Taller than wide	No	No
BTA	5	Normal	Pattern	In a solid hypoechoic nodule: Irregular margins Microcalcifications Globular calcifications Intranodular vascularity Taller than wide Lymphadenopathy	Yes	No

Table 1. Cont.

RSS	Number of Classes	Meaning of TIRADS 1	Pattern or Point-Based RSS	Features of High Suspicion	Composition Included in the RSS	ETE Included in the RSS
AACE	3	Low risk	Pattern	Marked hypoechogenicity Irregular margins Microcalcifications Taller-than-wide Extrathyroidal growth Pathologic lymph node.	No	Yes
ATA	5	Benign	Pattern	In a solid hypoechoic nodule: Irregular margins Microcalcifications Taller than wide Rim calcifications with small extrusive soft tissue component Extra-thyroidal extension	Yes	Yes
K-TIRADS	5	Absence of nodule	Pattern	In a solid hypoechoic nodule: Irregular margins Microcalcification Nonparallel orientation	Yes	No
EU-TIRADS	5	Absence of significant nodule	Pattern	Marked hypoechogenicity Irregular margins Microcalcifications Taller than wide	No	No
ACR-TIRADS	5	Benign	Point	Marked hypoechogenicity All punctate echogenic foci Taller-than-wide Extra-thyroidal extension	Yes	Yes
C-TIRADS	5 TIRADS 4 divided into 3 subclasses	No nodule	Point	Markedly hypoechogenicity Ill-defined and irregular margins Vertical orientation Solid composition Microcalcifications Extra-thyroidal extension	Yes	Yes

For abbreviations of the names of the RSSs, please refer to Section 1.1. Note: ETE = extra-thyroidal extension; RSS = risk stratification system.

1.3.1. Lexicon

Lexicons have many similarities, in particular regarding the categories (composition, echogenicity, shape, margins) and terms that have been chosen to describe nodules. In particular, the taller-than-wide shape has a common definition. However, significant differences exist:

Echogenicity: the EU-TIRADS considers that even a small hypoechoic part is sufficient to classify the nodule as hypoechoic, whereas K-TIRADS and ACR-TIRADS define the echogenicity of the nodule by its predominant one in heterogeneous nodules. The correctness of the definition of the K-TIRADSs seems to have been confirmed in a report on 2255 nodules, with a retrospective design [25]. Finally, the term markedly hypoechoic applies in the K-TIRADS as more or of equivalent hypoechogenicity to the strap muscles and in the other systems only as more hypoechoic than strap muscles.

Composition: this not taken into account in the EU-TIRADS. The 2016 Korean Society of Thyroid Radiology–Korean Thyroid Association guidelines recommend the use of solid composition for nodules with no obvious cystic change even considering that nodules with minimal cystic changes (<10%) do not have a high malignancy risk. By the ACR-TIRADS, cystic changes are considered as significant if they represent at least 50% in volume.

Hyperechoic foci: the EU- and K-TIRADS differentiate the ones which are located in the cystic part of the nodule (with a comet-tail artifact in the K-TIRADS), in favor of benignity, opposite to the one in the solid part, whereas the ACR-TIRADS does not discriminate between the two.

1.3.2. Classification

The lowest grade has different definitions from one RSS to another: in K- and EU-TIRADS, class 1 corresponds to a normal examination whereas it means benign for the ACR-TIRADS, very low suspicion for the ATA, and low risk for the AACE system. The number of classes varies from 3 in the AACE to 4 for the ATA and 5 for most other systems.

1.3.3. Patterns

Spongiform and purely cystic nodules are universally recognized as benign or at very low risk. Microcalcifications, taller-than-wide shape, marked hypoechogenicity, and irregular margins are also widely considered as weighing a high risk of malignancy. However, the K-TIRADS and the ATA system consider that these features as high risk only in solid hypoechoic nodules, whereas they are considered to be so in all nodules for the EU-TIRADS and AACE/ACE/AME system. In the ACR-TIRADS, a taller-than-wide shape, very hypoechoic and punctate echogenic foci are attributed 3 points but irregular margins only 2. Risk stratification differences are illustrated on Figure 1.

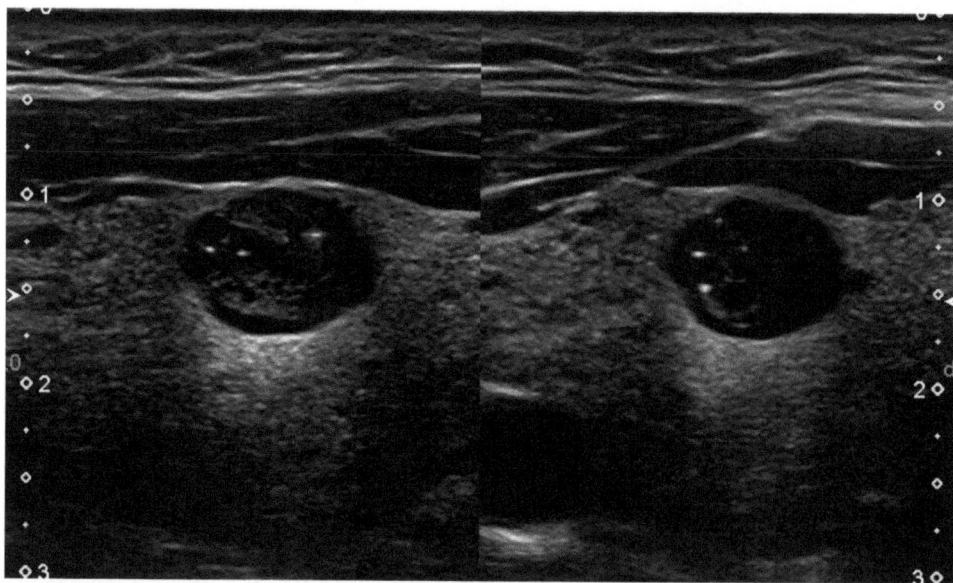

Figure 1. Longitudinal (**left** picture) and transverse (**right** picture) of an oval shaped, isoechoic nodule of mixed composition with hyperechoic spots located at the bottom of microcystic cavities. The nodule measures $11 \times 9 \times 7$ mm. Classification: Chilean-TIRADS 2, Kwak-TIRADS 4a, BTA U3, AACE Class 2, ATA not classifiable as being of mixed composition with hyperechoic spots, K-TIRADS 4, EU-TIRADS 3, ACR-TIRADS 4, C-TIRADS 4A. Note: magnification $\times$ 3; scale bar: 1 cm/unit; TIRADS = Thyroid Imaging and Reporting Data System.

1.4. Raw Diagnostic Values in Comparative Studies (before Applying Size Cut-Offs for the Decision to Perform FNA)

Many studies have attempted to compare the systems with each other. In particular, a comparison was performed between the BTA, AACE, and ATA RSSs [26]. The conclusions were that classification systems had elevated positive predictive value of malignancy in high-risk classes. ATA and AACE/ACE/AME systems were effective for ruling-out indication to FNA in low US risk nodules. A similar diagnostic accuracy and a substantial inter-observer agreement was provided by the 3- and the 5-category classifications.

Systematic reviews and meta-analyses are available. In a study including 10,437 thyroid nodules and 12 studies on different TIRADS, a pooled sensitivity of 0.79 and a pooled specificity of 0.71 were found [27]. Subgroup analyses showed that the most important factor of heterogeneity in studies was the final diagnostic references (histological and cytological standards or only histological results). In the report by Kim et al. [28], a total of 29 articles including 33,748 thyroid nodules met the eligibility criteria and were included in the analysis. The report concluded that the overall diagnostic performance of the four US-based risk stratification systems (ACR, ATA, K, and EU-TIRADS) was comparable. However, most of these studies used cytology as a gold standard and eliminated indeterminate ones of the assessment, thus introducing a significant recruitment bias. An interesting report used histology as a gold standard while comparing the ACR- and EU-TIRADS [29]. It was found that ACR-TIRADS and EU-TIRADS score had similar and satisfactory accuracy values for predicting thyroid malignancy (AUC: 0.835 for ACR-TIRADS vs. 0.827 for EU-TIRADS).

Thus, up to now, no RSS has shown a real significant advantage over the others in terms of raw diagnostic value.

1.5. Inter-Observer Agreement

One of the main aims of the TIRADS was to improve interobserver discrepancies in the description of US features. Yime et al. reported that the concordance rate of nodules classified as high- or intermediate-suspicion was high (84.1–100%), but low or mildly-suspicious nodules exhibited relatively low concordance (63.8–83.8%) between the K-TIRADS, ATA, and ACR-TIRADS [30].

In a blinded multicenter study [31], thyroid nodules were classified according to AACE/ACE/AME, EU-TIRADS, ATA, and ACR-TIRADS US classifications. Intra- and interobserver agreement was calculated using cross-tabulation expressed as mean Cohen's Kappa (K-coefficient). It was judged that intraobserver reproducibility for thyroid nodule US reporting and US classification systems appears fairly adequate, while the interobserver agreement between different centers is lower than in single-center trials. Reporting and rating ability of thyroid US examiners still appeared inconsistent.

The impact of radiologist experience was evaluated for the ACR-TIRADS [32]. Three experienced and three less experienced radiologists assessed 150 thyroid nodules using the TI-RADS lexicon. Concordance was significantly higher for less experienced readers in identifying margins (84.3% vs. 67.4%), echogenic foci (76.9% vs. 69.3%), comet tail artifact (89.6% vs. 79.2%), and punctate echogenic foci (85.3% vs. 75.5%), and lower for peripheral rim calcifications (95.0% vs. 97.8 %), but was not different for the remaining categories and features. However, the overall TI-RADS level and recommendation for FNA were unaffected, supporting the robustness of the TI-RADS lexicon and its continued use in practice.

In a study comparing Kwak, ACR, and EU-TIRADS and ATA system [33], it was found that after a first session and a consensus reading, interobserver agreement (IA) significantly increased but did not affect the diagnostic accuracy. Interobserver agreement and diagnostic accuracy were very similar for the four investigated risk stratification systems.

Finally, in a study comparing Kwak- and EU-TIRADS [34], it was found that the interobserver agreement (Cohen's κ) was 0.52 and 0.67 for Kwak-TIRADS and EU-TIRADS, respectively, and rated as substantial.

The synthesis of all these reports leads to believe that interobserver agreement is very similar for all systems: fairly adequate to robust. However, it may be better for high- or intermediate-suspicion nodules than for lower mildly-suspicious ones. Moreover, while intraobserver reproducibility for thyroid nodule US reporting and US classification systems appears fairly adequate, the interobserver agreement between different centers may be lower than previously assessed in single-center trials. Thus, and unfortunately, it seems that despite what was expected, reporting and rating ability of thyroid US examiners is not much better for classification systems than it is for individual US features. Dedicated training is necessary and proven to be able to achieve this goal.

2. Indications for FNA and Diagnostic Values of RSSs after Applying Size Cut-Offs for FNA

2.1. Dimensional Cut-Offs

Each US risk-stratification system has set its own cut-offs for guiding fine needle aspiration cytology indications (Table 2).

Table 2. Size cut-offs for performing FNA recommended by each RSS.

RSS	TIRADS 2 or Very Low Risk	TIRADS 3 or Low Risk	TIRADS 4 or Intermediate Risk	TIRADS 5 or High Risk	Small Nodules < 10 mm
Chilean TIRADS	No FNA or follow-up	FNA (no cut-off) or follow-up	FNA (no cut-off)	FNA (no cut-off)	FNA if >3–4 mm and feasible
Kwak-TIRADS	No FNA	No FNA	TIRADS 4a: $\geq$25 mm TIRADS 4B: 15 mm	TIRADS 4 C and 5: $\geq$10 mm	No FNA
BTA	No FNA	All nodules	All nodules	All nodules	-
AACE	No FNA	$\geq$20 mm and growing lesion or risk factors	$\geq$20 mm	$\geq$10 mm	<5 mm no FNA 5–10 mm FNA if clinical or US risk factors or PP
ATA	$\geq$20 mm or observation	$\geq$15 mm	$\geq$10 mm	$\geq$10 mm	5–10 mm FNA if clinical or US risk factors or PP
K-TIRADS	$\geq$20 mm	$\geq$15 mm	$\geq$10 mm	$\geq$10 mm	$\geq$5 mm selective cases
EU-TIRADS	No FNA	>20 mm	>15 mm	>10 mm	FNA or active surveillance, PP
ACR-TIRADS	No FNA	$\geq$25 mm	$\geq$15 mm	$\geq$10 mm	No FNA
C-TIRADS	No FNA	No FNA	$\geq$15 mm	$\geq$10 mm	US risk factors

Note: PP = patient's preference.

For BTA guidelines [3], US appearances that are indicative of a benign nodule (U1–U2) should be regarded as reassuring not requiring FNA, unless the patient has a statistically high risk of malignancy (i.e., age less than 20 or older than 60 years; firmness of the nodule on palpation; rapid growth; fixation to adjacent structures; vocal cord paralysis; regional lymphadenopathy; history of neck irradiation; family history of thyroid cancer). US guided FNA is indicated for all U3–5 nodules (i.e., equivocal, indeterminate or suspicious of malignancy nodules), independent of their size. Cytologically benign nodules with indeterminate or suspicious US features should undergo repeat FNA for confirmation, due to the significant rate of malignancy. Nodules with FDG uptake should be investigated with FNA unless the patient has limited life-expectancy.

AACE guidelines [6] recommend FNA for high US risk thyroid lesions $\geq$10 mm and intermediate US risk thyroid lesions >20 mm. For low US risk thyroid lesions, FNA is recommended only when size is >20 mm and increasing or associated with a risk history and before thyroid surgery or minimally invasive ablation therapy. These guidelines highlight that nodules <5 mm should be monitored with US, rather than biopsied, irrespective of their sonographic appearance, in light of the low clinical risk. For nodules measuring 5–10 mm, FNA sampling or watchful waiting can either be considered according to the clinical setting and patient preference. US-guided FNA is recommended for subcapsular or paratracheal nodules, suspicious lymph nodes or suspicion of extrathyroidal spread, positive personal or family history of thyroid cancer, or coexistent suspicious clinical findings (e.g., dysphonia). A retrospective series on 859 FNA from 598 patients showed that moderate-to-elevated risk of malignancy (i.e., Bethesda III to VI categories) [35] lesions would have been missed for 13 out of 17 nodules, if intermediate risk nodules <20 mm had been excluded from FNAC, of which 11 were malignant at definitive histology [7]. Cytological confirmation of diagnosis would have been missed in 8 out of 26 cases of high-risk lesion <10 mm if a watchful waiting attitude has been chose over FNA sampling.

ATA guidelines [8] recommend FNA for nodules ≥10 mm in greatest dimension with high and intermediate suspicion US pattern, ≥15 mm in case of low suspicion US pattern, and ≥20 mm in greatest dimension with very low suspicion US pattern (e.g., spongiform). Alternatively, observation without FNAC is also stated as a reasonable option. FNA is not required for purely cystic nodules.

The 2016 revised Korean Society of Thyroid Radiology Consensus Statement and Recommendations [10] stated that FNA should be restricted to K-TIRADS 2 spongiform nodules ≥ 20 mm, K-TIRADS 3 ≥ 15 mm, K-TIRADS 4 or 5 ≥ 10 mm, and in selective cases of K-TIRADS 5 > 5 mm. Applying cut-off of ≥10 mm for K-TIRADS categories 4 or 5 and ≥15 mm for K-TIRADS 3, the negative predictive value was 94.3% according to a study where 85.5% of the malignant tumors were papillary thyroid cancer (PTC) [36], meaning less than 6% of missed carcinomas.

Because the false negative rate of an initial benign findings of FNA could be relatively high (11.3–56.6%) for thyroid nodules with suspicious US features [10], FNA should be repeated in these cases within 6–12 months after the initial FNAC.

The European Thyroid Association Guidelines [12] stated that FNA should usually be performed only for nodules EU-TIRADS 3 > 20 mm, EU-TIRADS 4 > 15 mm, and Eu-TIRADS 5 > 10 mm. Patients with highly suspicious EU-TIRADS 5 nodule < 10 mm can have the choice between active surveillance or immediate FNAC if surgery is decided.

Regarding EU-TIRADS 3 nodule, it should be pointed out that entirely solid isoechoic nodules can correspond to follicular cancer or a follicular variant of PTC [36] in <4% of cases. As a consequence, few carcinomas will be missed after applying FNA cut-off for EU-TIRADS 3 nodules.

The ACR committee [16] recommends FNA for TI-RADS 5 nodules (7 points or more) ≥ 10 mm, for TI-RADS 4 nodules (4 to 6 points) ≥ 15 mm, for TI-RADS 3 nodules (3 points) ≥ 25 mm. FNA is not indicated for TI-RADS 1 (0 point) and TI-RADS 2 (2 points) nodules regardless of their size. The 10 mm size-threshold to indicate FNA for highly suspicious nodules is consistent with most other guidelines. However the ACR thresholds for mildly and moderately suspicious nodules (25 mm and 15 mm respectively) are higher than the cut-offs advocated by the ATA and the Korean Society of Thyroid Radiology. Rational for the ACR cut-offs relies on the one hand, on the discrepancy regarding the size of PTC at definitive histology (26.5 ± 10.7 mm) and the size on ultrasound (19.7 ± 11.7 mm) on a retrospective series including 205 PTC [36]. However, all series reporting outcome of thyroid cancers are based on the size of resected specimen. On the other hand the ACR cut-offs rely on a slight decrease in 10-year thyroid cancer-specific survival for nodules ≥30 mm [37].

The Chinese Guidelines for US Malignancy Risk Stratification of Thyroid [20] does not recommend FNA for TIRADS 2 and 3 nodules but recommend FNA for TIRADS 4A nodules > 15 mm. FNA is recommended for TIRADS 4B or 4C or 5 nodules > 10 mm. In case of parameters predictors of poor prognosis of PTC such as multifocality, or nodule(s) immediately adjacent to the trachea or recurrent laryngeal nerve, then US-guided FNA can be considered if the nodule is TIRADS 4A > 10 mm or TIRADS 4B or 4C or 5 > 5 mm. If

TIRADS 4B or 4C nodules <5 mm are multiple, or are immediately adjacent to the capsule, trachea, or the recurrent laryngeal nerve, then biopsy is required by comprehensively considering the skills of the doctor and the anxiety level of the patient. For patients with familial thyroid carcinoma or history of radiation exposure during childhood, the size threshold for FNA can be appropriately reduced. These guidelines recommend taking into account the patient's personal preference and anxiety level to determine if FNA is appropriate in each specific case.

Apart from the BTA classification system, which had not defined size cut-offs for the selection of nodules that should be submitted to FNA, most US RSS agree on the threshold of 10 mm for indicating FNA in highly suspicious nodule, although some RSS (AACE, KThRS) recommend FNA for nodules between 5 and 10 mm in selected cases and systematically for Chinese TIRADS. The threshold for indicating FNA for intermediate-risk nodule varies from 10 mm for the ATA classification system and the K-TIRADS, to 15 mm for the ACR classification system and the EU-TIRADS and even 20 mm for the AACE classification system. A low threshold of 5 mm for intermediate risk nodules is only recommended by the Chinese TIRADS. The threshold for indicating FNA for low suspicion nodule varies from 15 mm for ATA classification system, K-TIRADS and Chinese TIRADS, to 20 mm for EU-TIRADS and even 25 mm for ACR TIRADS. Most RSS do not recommend FNAC for very low suspicion nodules, i.e., AACE (FNAC can be performed in selective cases), ATA, ACR classification systems, EU-TIRADS, and Chinese TIRADS. Only K-TIRADS and ATA guidelines retain FNA indication for spongiform or partially cystic nodules $\geq$ 20 mm.

2.2. Diagnostic Value after Applying Cut-Offs: Decision Guidance, Avoided FNAs, and Missed Carcinomas

Different retrospective series demonstrated that a very small proportion of thyroid cancers are missed after applying size cut-offs for FNA of the ACR committee. This would decrease with lower cut-offs, but create a substantial increase in the number of benign nodules that would be explored. A series showed that 13 cancers (11 PTC, one follicular and one medullary thyroid cancer) among nodules measuring 15–25 mm, would have been missed if FNA would have not been performed for the 874 nodules measuring less than 25 mm included in this series [38]. Middleton et al. showed, in a series of 3822 nodules Bethesda II or VI, that among 352 malignant nodules (303 were histologically confirmed), 40 nodules would have received a recommendation for no further evaluation, among which were 16 malignant nodules $\geq$10 mm [38].

A recent meta-analysis [39], including 12 studies [7,13,26,40–48] representing 18,750 nodules, evaluated the ability of 5 US RSSs (AACE, ACR, ATA, EU-TIRADS, K-TIRADS) for the appropriate selection of thyroid nodules for FNA. Diagnostic odds ratio, representing the test performance and corresponding to the odds of the FNA being indicated in a malignant nodule compared to the odds of the FNA being indicated in a benign one, were calculated for each US RSS. Keeping in mind that data on AACE and EU-TIRADS were sparse, diagnostic odd ratio was higher for ACR-TIRADS in comparison with the other systems. The higher discriminative power was related to a higher ability of ACR-TIRADS to select malignant nodules for FNA, while no difference was found for benign nodules. This cannot be explained by the size cut-offs for FNA in intermediate- and high-risk-nodules, given that it is similar to that of the other US RSSs. However, fewer nodules will probably be classified as intermediate- or high suspicious than in other systems, because of the point-based pattern of this RSS. As intermediate risk nodules are frequent, this could explain the advantage of the ACR-TIRADS over the other systems.

For example, in the series of Xu et al. [43], comparing the diagnostic value of three RSS (i.e., ACR-, EU- and K-TIRADS) in 2465 thyroid nodules, the rate of unnecessary FNA was lowest with the ACR-TIRADS (17.3%), followed by ETA-TIRADS (25.2%), and K-TIRADS (32.1%). Among nodules not submitted to FNA, 33.1%, 37.7%, and 38.2% thyroid cancers would be missed by the same TI-RADS, respectively. Finally, after applying adequate FNA cut-offs of each of these TI-RADS, 62.6%, 54.6%, and 43.9% FNAC were avoided, respectively.

In the work by Grani et al. [44] that prospectively compared the performances of five internationally endorsed sonographic classification systems (those of the ATA, the AACE, the ACR, the ETA, and the KSThR) in 477 patients, application of the systems' FNA criteria would have reduced the number of biopsies performed by 17.1% to 53.4% (17.1% for K-TIRADS, 30.7% for EU-TIRADS, 34.9% for AACE, 43.8% for ATA, and 53.4% for ACR TIRADS). The percentage of missed carcinomas was low comprised between 2.2% for ACR TIRADS and 4.1% for ATA.

In the work of Yoon et al. [49] comparing the diagnostic performance of US-guided FNAC criteria for detecting malignant thyroid nodules in ACR TI-RADS and EU-TIRADS, the percentage of unnecessary FNAC was estimated at 53% for the EU-TIRADS and 28% for the ACR-TIRADS.

As a conclusion, all RSSs seem to reduce effectively the number of unnecessary FNAs. However, this is at the cost of temporarily missing a significant proportion of carcinomas. Their diagnosis will be postponed until they eventually grow and are then diagnosed after they reach the cut-off threshold defined for FNA according to their US risk category. Most of the time, this strategy implies no significant loss of chance for the patient. This is due to the statistical predominance of papillary carcinomas of low and intermediate risks among all thyroid cancers. However, looking for lymph node or extra-thyroidal extension, including clinical factors such as age, sex, personal and family history with risk factors of thyroid cancer, tumor growth rate, and also serum calcitonin whenever judged relevant is critical for making the right decision to prevent missing more aggressive carcinomas. Thus, the recommendation for no further evaluation, as specifically formulated in the ACR-TIRADS, should be considered with caution and put into perspective including clinical and biological data.

3. Weaknesses of TIRADSs

3.1. Insufficient Sensitivity for the Diagnosis of Follicular Thyroid Carcinoma and Follicular Variant of PTC

While historically the follicular variant of PTC (FVPTC) was considered a diagnostic pitfall of US, this notion was not confirmed in a report published in 2018 on 34 cases [50]. The K-TIRADS score was 3, 4, and 5 in 5.9%, 2.9%, and 91.2%, respectively. Thus, the false negative rate does not seem to exceed 6%.

In a study on 45 follicular thyroid carcinomas (FTCs) from 45 consecutive patients, with a median tumor diameter of 32 mm, an ovoid isoechoic nodule with or without lobulated margins was the most frequent presentation [51]. When FTCs were classified according to RSSs, the most common categories were intermediate and high risk, though 1 out of 3 cases was not classifiable. FTCs were classified as high risk/high suspicion/malignant in 11% to 74% of cases, with a statistically significant difference among the systems. More specifically, 26.7% were classified as EU-TIRADS 3 but all submitted to FNA due to their size and 2.2% and 26.7% were classified as ACR-TIRADS 2 and 3, respectively and among these 25% were not submitted to FNA, also due to size cut-offs. To conclude, in FTCs cases, the RSSs false negative rate seems persistently higher than for FVPTCs, around 25%. Clinicians should be aware of this, especially in the era of thermal ablation, to try to avoid treating such nodules by alternatives to surgery. More specifically, exclusively solid isoechoic and mildly hypoechoic nodules should always be considered with caution.

3.2. Insufficient Specificity to Rule-Out Autonomously Functioning/Hot Thyroid Nodules from FNA

Autonomously functioning thyroid nodules (AFTN) account for 5–10% of palpable lesions and are very rarely malignant. In a study on 87 AFTNs from 85 consecutive patients who had undergone US, scintigraphy, and thyroid function evaluation, AFTNs were reclassified according to AACE/ACE/AME, ACR-TIRADS, ATA, BTA, EU-TIRADS, K-TIRADS, and TIRADS [52]. An ovoid isoechoic nodule with median diameter of 22 mm (range 10–59) was the most frequent US presentation. When AFTNs were reclassified according to US RSSs, the most common categories were low and intermediate risk. AFTNs were assessed as being at high risk/high suspicion/malignant in 1–9%, with good agreement among AACE/ACE/AME, ATA, EU-TIRADS, K-TIRADS, and TIRADS. Remarkably, FNA was indicated in 27–90% of AFTNs. It was concluded that ultrasound RSSs prompt inappropriate FNA in a significant number of patients with AFTN. The management strategy of thyroid nodules being essentially based on US risk stratification and size cut-offs, it could be considered that, depending on the RSS used, 2.7% to 9% of all nodules should have been excluded from FNA.

However, the reverse strategy of submitting all TNs to scintigraphy to exclude an AFTN before US exploration would drastically augment the costs with no diagnostic gain in, at least, 90% of all nodules.

3.3. High Rates of Nodules Classified at Intermediate Risk (Usually TI-RADS 4)

Based on the high negative predictive value of all RSSs, it could be considered that FNA could be avoided for most nodules classified as low risk, especially for those of mixed composition. At the opposite end, the high positive predictive value of high-risk categories prompt the indication for FNA in most cases if the size is over 10 mm, knowing these represent a minority of all nodules.

Conversely, the indication for FNA in intermediate risk nodules is still a matter of concern. Indeed, these nodules represent a substantial part of all nodules discovered during US thyroid imaging and even a more substantial part of those referred for FNA. Using the ATA US pattern risk assessment, nodules were classified as intermediate risk in 31% of cases [9]. Regarding the AACE, 56.9% were considered at intermediate risk in another report [7]. In a study on 305 nodules with final histology as gold standard, it was shown that ACR-TIRADS 4 nodules represented 28.8% of all nodules and EU-TIRADS 4 category 22% [29]. Finally, in a study with a prospective design with cytological examination as a gold standard on 4550 nodules [53], the rate of TIRADS 4A nodules (equivalent to EU-TIRADS 4) was 44.5%.

Thus, the main difficulty in significantly and appropriately reducing the indications for FNA is the high rate of intermediate risk nodules. Research has been performed to improve the low specificity of the category for the diagnostic of malignancy by using either Doppler or elastography. In a report on 80 nodules, no significant differences were observed in elasticity score or strain ratio between benign and malignant nodules [54]. 18F-FDG PET/CT could be a more useful tool to discriminate intermediate risk nodules [55]. 18F-FDG PET/CT showed 85.7% sensitivity and 41.4% specificity. Thus, 18F-FDG PET/CT may have a role in stratifying the cancer risk of thyroid nodules with an intermediate ultrasound assessment. More specifically, thyroid lesions classified as EU-TIRADS 4 without 18F-FDG uptake could be ruled out from further examination. Further prospective and cost-effectiveness studies are however needed.

3.4. Thyroid Diffuse Masses

All RSSs have been studied and developed for nodules. However, it is unclear whether diffuse thyroid masses have been taken into account in those systems. These are most of the time responsible for pressure symptoms with a rapid development. The most common US presentation is a hypoechoic mass invading one lobe or all the thyroid gland. It is usually hypoechoic, with poorly defined margins. Vascularity and stiffness are variable and they can be accompanied or not by suspect cervical lymph nodes. The following main aspects should be considered:

- First, several etiological hypotheses should always be mentioned in the US report, including anaplastic carcinoma, lymphoma, metastases from non-thyroidal origin, and large differentiated papillary and follicular carcinomas. Riedel's thyroiditis could be added to this list. In this case, marked hypoechogenicity and absorption of the US beam, absence of vascularity, and high stiffness are relatively characteristic features.

- The context helps refining the hypotheses. Knowledge of a prior renal cell carcinoma is for instance in favor of a metastasis and rapid development in an elderly subject with severe pressure symptoms in favor of an anaplastic carcinoma.
- Core-needle biopsy or surgical biopsy, depending on the center's habits, should systematically be added to FNA, due to its low diagnostic power in this situation.
- Quick referral to a tertiary care center is advised.

3.5. Absence of Validation in Large Non-Specialized Medical Communities

One of the main issues in adopting RSSs in daily life is the limited evidence regarding their diagnostic value when applied by non-specialized teams, most of the available literature on the subject being produced by expert centers. Studies carried out outside the specialized world of thyroid imaging without dedicated US machines are necessary to confirm the real world efficiency of all RSSs.

4. Pitfalls

4.1. Shrinking Nodules

Nodules with a cystic or hemorrhagic component can evolve by shrinking. Risk factors for such evolution include abundant blood supply, non-smooth margin of the internal solid portion, and a spongiform internal content [56]. The process can be of variable length, sometimes lasting for years, but frequently leads to ambiguous US features mimicking malignancy. Such nodules often harbor a taller-than-wide shape, marked hypoechogenicity or some hyperechoic spots and can easily be classified at high risk of malignancy, whatever the RSS used. Some sonographic imaging features, such as regular eggshell calcifications, peripheral hypoechoic or hypoechoic rim, posterior shadowing, and absence of intranodular vascularization have been described [57] to help diagnosing this pattern, named "mummified thyroid syndrome" and later on "degenerating thyroid nodules" [58]. Knowledge, if available, of previous images showing the thyroid nodule shrinkage over time is useful for reaching the correct final diagnosis. In case of doubt, FNA of such suspicious thyroid nodules and sonographic follow-up contribute to establishing the final diagnosis of benign thyroid findings. The cytology is mainly composed of thick colloid and macrophages and the cytopathologist should be informed of the hypothesis. Otherwise, the result could be considered as non-diagnostic instead of representative of the lesion [59].

4.2. Subacute Thyroiditis

Subacute thyroiditis can also mimic malignancy by US, because frequently displaying a taller-than-wide shape and marked hypoechogenicity. However, the existence of spontaneous thyroid pain, low TSH, and elevated serum inflammatory markers frequently allows the diagnosis. On the US point of view, it has been shown that the lesions have poorly defined margins that can help differentiating from a carcinoma [60]. In case of persistent doubt, it is advised to proceed to FNA if TSH is normal, or to scintigraphy if TSH is low, which will show an absence of tracer uptake. US follow-up is also advised, showing progressive regression of the hypoechoic zone and absence of a true nodule that could also have been hidden initially by the marked hypoechogenicity of the lesions.

4.3. Confusion or Absence of Clear Distinction between Nodular Disease and Hyperplasia

Hyperplasia of the follicular epithelium is the most common morphological change in the thyroid seen by the pathologist [61]. The manifestation of this process is the goiter (diffuse or nodular hyperplasia). The US features range from a simple isoechoic enlargement of the thyroid gland to multiple coalescent isoechoic nodules, usually of small size individually with no or poor definite margins. This pattern is very frequent in regions of endemic goiter. Solely did the EU-TIRADS address this issue, but it should be included in the future in RSSs, because of its very low risk of malignancy and of the feeble interest of FNA, that may even lead to false positive results [62].

5. Suggestions for the Future

5.1. Absence of Classification for TNs Treated with Thermal Ablation

Thermal ablation, especially laser and radiofrequency (RFA), is of increasing use in the treatment of benign thyroid nodules and is considered as a possible alternative to surgery [63]. In a systematic review, it has been shown that RFA induces a volume reduction ratio ranging between 66.9% and 97.9% three years after the procedure [59]. These treatments induce important changes in the US features of nodules that can mimic malignancy. Nodules turn solid and hypoechoic, even markedly hypoechoic, sometimes with irregular margins and calcifications [64]. As radiofrequency is of frequent use for liver tumors, the LI-RADS Treatment Response (LR-TR) algorithm was introduced in 2017 to assist radiologists in assessing hepatocellular carcinoma (HCC) response following locoregional therapy [65]. A comparable addendum should be part of future thyroid RSSs.

5.2. Incorporating in the Algorithm the Number of Nodules Especially If They Belong to the Same Category

Different studies demonstrated that a single nodule increases the risk of malignancy compared to multiple nodules [29,66]. Moreover, this parameter has high inter-observer agreement and is easy to implement. Taking into account in the algorithm of future US RSSs the number of nodules to decrease the estimated risk of malignancy, especially if all are low to intermediate risk nodules, could be valuable.

5.3. Taking into Account Age, Sex, Time Since Discovery, Results of Previous FNAs

Many risk factors for thyroid nodules malignancy have been suggested, such as patient age, sex, nodule size, and composition, but our understanding of the specific risk attributable to these is not precisely known. An interesting study [66] demonstrated in 20 001 thyroid nodules evaluated by FNA from 1995 to 2017 a significant increased risk of malignancy for patient age >52, male sex, nodule size with growing risk from 20 mm until more than 40 mm in comparison with nodules less than 20 mm. On the opposite side, cystic content (at least 25% of the nodule) was associated with a decreased risk of malignancy compared with predominantly solid nodule, as well as the presence of additional nodules with lowest risk for greater than 4 nodules. Interestingly, a free online calculator was constructed to provide malignancy-risk estimates based on these variables.

5.4. Taking into Account the Serum Value of TSH (to Exclude a AFTN) and Calcitonin (to Detect a Medullary Cancer), When Available

Serum TSH should be measured during the initial evaluation of a patient with one or more thyroid nodule(s). If the serum TSH is low, a radionuclide (preferably 123I) thyroid scan should be performed to exclude AFTN from FNAC and to explore the etiology of hyperthyroidism, provided that there is no evidence of Graves' disease. In case of normal serum TSH value, there are no US features correlated with autonomous nodules [67,68]. The cost-effectiveness of submitting all nodules to a thyroid scan to avoid unnecessary FNA for AFTN is questioned.

Calcitonin may detect C-cell hyperplasia and medullary thyroid cancer (MTC). However, most guidelines cannot recommend for or against routine calcitonin measurement in patients with thyroid nodules. A recent review [69] demonstrated that calcitonin has good sensitivity and specificity to diagnose MTC and could be useful when available in the evaluation of thyroid nodules. The literature and the experience show that for a calcitonin level over 100 pg/mL nodule larger than 1 cm are MTC. For levels below 100 ng/L and that in nodules larger than 1 cm the systematic calcitonin measurement does not bring a clear advantage for the diagnosis, especially if at low or intermediate US risk. However, the value of routine testing in patients with thyroid nodules remains questionable, due to the low prevalence of MTC, and whether routine calcitonin testing improves prognosis in MTC patients remains unclear. In clinical practice, situations associated with false positivity of calcitonin tests (e.g., renal insufficiency, treatment with proton pump inhibitor, obesity) and the correlation of calcitonin value with the nodule volume should be taken into account for the interpretation of the result. Calcitonin measurement remains mandatory in case active surveillance of EU-TIRADS 5 nodules or proven microcarcinomas is considered and before surgery or thermal ablation. Regardless, the heterogeneous US presentation of MTC [70] and the low sensitivity of FNA in detecting MTC [71] has to be taken into account during the clinical practice.

5.5. D Vascularity

Advanced ultrasound techniques may improve the risk estimation and could be used more extensively. For example, Borlea et al. [72] demonstrated that adding 4D vascularity to the French TIRADS score proved beneficial for predicting the malignancy risk and may add important knowledge in uncertain situations.

An international team has been set up and is currently working on a global new TIRADS, to be called I-TIRADS for International TIRADS. It will include a lexicon, an RSS, and recommendations for FNA and follow-up. Maybe some of these suggestions could be taken into account to create this new version. The pitfalls they imply are detailed in Table 3.

Table 3. Current pitfalls of most known risk stratification systems (RSSs) of thyroid nodules and recommendations to improve these.

Current Pitfalls of Existent RSSs Variables Not Taken into Account for Risk Stratification	Suggested Correction
Modifications of nodules treated by thermal ablation are classified as highly suspect	Incorporate a treatment response (TR) algorithm
The number of nodules is an independent predictor of the malignancy risk	Add the number of nodules in the risk stratification algorithm, especially if they look all alike and are of low or intermediate risk
Some clinical variables and previous results of FNA(s) are predictors of the malignancy risk	Incorporate age, sex, time since discovery, results of previous FNAs in the risk stratification algorithm
TSH and serum calcitonin are predictors of the malignancy risk	Incorporate TSH and serum calcitonin in the risk stratification algorithm
Complementary tools not used in most RSSs, such as vascularity and elastography	At least, incorporate these in the lexicon, to allow comparative studies on the subject

6. Conclusions

The different US RSSs introduced since the late 2000s have facilitated the effective interpretation and communication of thyroid US findings among physicians and cytopathologists and with the patient. On the whole, there are similarities among the different RSS regarding the lexicons used and the categorization of nodules, although differences and specificities remain. Diagnostic performance and efficacy of FNA performed according to the different RSS vary, mainly influenced by different size cut-offs and partially by different risk categorizations of nodules. Understanding the strengths and weakness of the different RSSs will help to improve each system and may provide the basis for an ultimate international standardization. Efforts should be made to merge the different systems utilized around the world with the ultimate aim of eliminating unnecessary thyroid biopsies without jeopardizing the detection of clinically significant malignancies.

Author Contributions: All the authors participated in the preparation, writing and revision of the manuscript. All authors have read and agreed to the published version of the manuscript.

Funding: This research received no external funding.

Institutional Review Board Statement: Not applicable.

Informed Consent Statement: Not applicable.

Data Availability Statement: Not applicable.

Conflicts of Interest: The authors declare no conflict of interest.

References

1. Horvath, E.; Majlis, S.; Rossi, R.; Franco, C.; Niedmann, J.P.; Castro, A.; Dominguez, M. An ultrasonogram reporting system for thyroid nodules stratifying cancer risk for clinical management. *J. Clin. Endocrinol. Metab.* **2009**, *94*, 1748–1751. [CrossRef]
2. Horvath, E.; Silva, C.F.; Majlis, S.; Rodriguez, I.; Skoknic, V.; Castro, A.; Rojas, H.; Niedmann, J.P.; Madrid, A.; Capdeville, F.; et al. Prospective validation of the ultrasound based TIRADS (Thyroid Imaging Reporting And Data System) classification: Results in surgically resected thyroid nodules. *Eur. Radiol.* **2017**, *27*, 2619–2628. [CrossRef]
3. Perros, P.; Boelaert, K.; Colley, S.; Evans, C.; Evans, R.M.; Gerrard Ba, G.; Gilbert, J.; Harrison, B.; Johnson, S.J.; Giles, T.E.; et al. Guidelines for the management of thyroid cancer. *Clin. Endocrinol.* **2014**, *81* (Suppl. 1), 1–122. [CrossRef]
4. Arambewela, M.H.; Wijesinghe, A.M.; Randhawa, K.; Bull, M.; Wadsley, J.; Balasubramanian, S.P. A pragmatic assessment of the British Thyroid Association "U classification" of thyroid nodules with a focus on their follow-up. *Clin. Radiol.* **2020**, *75*, 466–473. [CrossRef]
5. Weller, A.; Sharif, B.; Qarib, M.H.; St Leger, D.; De Silva, H.S.; Lingam, R.K. British Thyroid Association 2014 classification ultrasound scoring of thyroid nodules in predicting malignancy: Diagnostic performance and inter-observer agreement. *Ultrasound* **2020**, *28*, 4–13. [CrossRef]
6. Gharib, H.; Papini, E.; Garber, J.R.; Duick, D.S.; Harrell, R.M.; Hegedus, L.; Paschke, R.; Valcavi, R.; Vitti, P. American Association of Clinical Endocrinologists, American College of Endocrinology, and Associazione Medici Endocrinologi Medical Guidelines for Clinical Practice for the Diagnosis and Management of Thyroid Nodules—2016 Update. *Endocr. Pract.* **2016**, *22*, 622–639. [CrossRef]
7. Negro, R.; Greco, G.; Colosimo, E. Ultrasound Risk Categories for Thyroid Nodules and Cytology Results: A Single Institution's Experience after the Adoption of the 2016 Update of Medical Guidelines by the American Association of Clinical Endocrinologists and Associazione Medici Endocrinologi. *J. Thyroid Res.* **2017**, *2017*, 8135415. [CrossRef]
8. Haugen, B.R.; Alexander, E.K.; Bible, K.C.; Doherty, G.M.; Mandel, S.J.; Nikiforov, Y.E.; Pacini, F.; Randolph, G.W.; Sawka, A.M.; Schlumberger, M.; et al. 2015 American Thyroid Association Management Guidelines for Adult Patients with Thyroid Nodules and Differentiated Thyroid Cancer: The American Thyroid Association Guidelines Task Force on Thyroid Nodules and Differentiated Thyroid Cancer. *Thyroid* **2016**, *26*, 1–133. [CrossRef]
9. Tang, A.L.; Falciglia, M.; Yang, H.; Mark, J.R.; Steward, D.L. Validation of American Thyroid Association Ultrasound Risk Assessment of Thyroid Nodules Selected for Ultrasound Fine-Needle Aspiration. *Thyroid* **2017**, *27*, 1077–1082. [CrossRef]
10. Shin, J.H.; Baek, J.H.; Chung, J.; Ha, E.J.; Kim, J.H.; Lee, Y.H.; Lim, H.K.; Moon, W.J.; Na, D.G.; Park, J.S.; et al. Ultrasonography Diagnosis and Imaging-Based Management of Thyroid Nodules: Revised Korean Society of Thyroid Radiology Consensus Statement and Recommendations. *Korean J. Radiol.* **2016**, *17*, 370–395. [CrossRef]
11. Ha, E.J.; Moon, W.J.; Na, D.G.; Lee, Y.H.; Choi, N.; Kim, S.J.; Kim, J.K. A Multicenter Prospective Validation Study for the Korean Thyroid Imaging Reporting and Data System in Patients with Thyroid Nodules. *Korean J. Radiol.* **2016**, *17*, 811–821. [CrossRef]
12. Russ, G.; Bonnema, S.J.; Erdogan, M.F.; Durante, C.; Ngu, R.; Leenhardt, L. European Thyroid Association Guidelines for Ultrasound Malignancy Risk Stratification of Thyroid Nodules in Adults: The EU-TIRADS. *Eur. Thyroid J.* **2017**, *6*, 225–237. [CrossRef]
13. Trimboli, P.; Ngu, R.; Royer, B.; Giovanella, L.; Bigorgne, C.; Simo, R.; Carroll, P.; Russ, G. A multicentre validation study for the EU-TIRADS using histological diagnosis as a gold standard. *Clin. Endocrinol.* **2019**, *91*, 340–347. [CrossRef]
14. Castellana, M.; Grani, G.; Radzina, M.; Guerra, V.; Giovanella, L.; Deandrea, M.; Ngu, R.; Durante, C.; Trimboli, P. Performance of EU-TIRADS in malignancy risk stratification of thyroid nodules: A meta-analysis. *Eur. J. Endocrinol.* **2020**, *183*, 255–264. [CrossRef]
15. Grant, E.G.; Tessler, F.N.; Hoang, J.K.; Langer, J.E.; Beland, M.D.; Berland, L.L.; Cronan, J.J.; Desser, T.S.; Frates, M.C.; Hamper, U.M.; et al. Thyroid Ultrasound Reporting Lexicon: White Paper of the ACR Thyroid Imaging, Reporting and Data System (TIRADS) Committee. *J. Am. Coll. Radiol.* **2015**, *12*, 1272–1279. [CrossRef] [PubMed]
16. Tessler, F.N.; Middleton, W.D.; Grant, E.G.; Hoang, J.K.; Berland, L.L.; Teefey, S.A.; Cronan, J.J.; Beland, M.D.; Desser, T.S.; Frates, M.C.; et al. ACR Thyroid Imaging, Reporting and Data System (TI-RADS): White Paper of the ACR TI-RADS Committee. *J. Am. Coll. Radiol.* **2017**, *14*, 587–595. [CrossRef]
17. Hoang, J.K.; Middleton, W.D.; Farjat, A.E.; Langer, J.E.; Reading, C.C.; Teefey, S.A.; Abinanti, N.; Boschini, F.J.; Bronner, A.J.; Dahiya, N.; et al. Reduction in Thyroid Nodule Biopsies and Improved Accuracy with American College of Radiology Thyroid Imaging Reporting and Data System. *Radiology* **2018**, *287*, 185–193. [CrossRef] [PubMed]
18. Middleton, W.D.; Teefey, S.A.; Reading, C.C.; Langer, J.E.; Beland, M.D.; Szabunio, M.M.; Desser, T.S. Multiinstitutional Analysis of Thyroid Nodule Risk Stratification Using the American College of Radiology Thyroid Imaging Reporting and Data System. *Am. J. Roentgenol.* **2017**, *208*, 1331–1341. [CrossRef]
19. Li, W.; Wang, Y.; Wen, J.; Zhang, L.; Sun, Y. Diagnostic Performance of American College of Radiology TI-RADS: A Systematic Review and Meta-Analysis. *Am. J. Roentgenol.* **2021**, *216*, 38–47. [CrossRef] [PubMed]

20. Zhou, J.; Yin, L.; Wei, X.; Zhang, S.; Song, Y.; Luo, B.; Li, J.; Qian, L.; Cui, L.; Chen, W.; et al. 2020 Chinese guidelines for ultrasound malignancy risk stratification of thyroid nodules: The C-TIRADS. *Endocrine* **2020**, *70*, 256–279. [CrossRef]
21. Zhou, J.; Song, Y.; Zhan, W.; Wei, X.; Zhang, S.; Zhang, R.; Gu, Y.; Chen, X.; Shi, L.; Luo, X.; et al. Thyroid imaging reporting and data system (TIRADS) for ultrasound features of nodules: Multicentric retrospective study in China. *Endocrine* **2021**, *72*, 157–170. [CrossRef] [PubMed]
22. Kwak, J.Y.; Han, K.H.; Yoon, J.H.; Moon, H.J.; Son, E.J.; Park, S.H.; Jung, H.K.; Choi, J.S.; Kim, B.M.; Kim, E.K. Thyroid imaging reporting and data system for US features of nodules: A step in establishing better stratification of cancer risk. *Radiology* **2011**, *260*, 892–899. [CrossRef]
23. Rahal, A.J.; Falsarella, P.M.; Rocha, R.D.; Lima, J.P.; Iani, M.J.; Vieira, F.A.; Queiroz, M.R.; Hidal, J.T.; Francisco, M.J.N.; Garcia, R.G.; et al. Correlation of Thyroid Imaging Reporting and Data System [TI-RADS] and fine needle aspiration: Experience in 1000 nodules. *Einstein* **2016**, *14*, 119–123. [CrossRef] [PubMed]
24. Wildman-Tobriner, B.; Buda, M.; Hoang, J.K.; Middleton, W.D.; Thayer, D.; Short, R.G.; Tessler, F.N.; Mazurowski, M.A. Using Artificial Intelligence to Revise ACR TI-RADS Risk Stratification of Thyroid Nodules: Diagnostic Accuracy and Utility. *Radiology* **2019**, *292*, 112–119. [CrossRef] [PubMed]
25. Lee, J.Y.; Na, D.G.; Yoon, S.J.; Gwon, H.Y.; Paik, W.; Kim, T.; Kim, J.Y. Ultrasound malignancy risk stratification of thyroid nodules based on the degree of hypoechogenicity and echotexture. *Eur. Radiol.* **2020**, *30*, 1653–1663. [CrossRef]
26. Persichetti, A.; Di Stasio, E.; Guglielmi, R.; Bizzarri, G.; Taccogna, S.; Misischi, I.; Graziano, F.; Petrucci, L.; Bianchini, A.; Papini, E. Predictive Value of Malignancy of Thyroid Nodule Ultrasound Classification Systems: A Prospective Study. *J. Clin. Endocrinol. Metab.* **2018**, *103*, 1359–1368. [CrossRef]
27. Wei, X.; Li, Y.; Zhang, S.; Gao, M. Meta-analysis of thyroid imaging reporting and data system in the ultrasonographic diagnosis of 10,437 thyroid nodules. *Head Neck* **2016**, *38*, 309–315. [CrossRef] [PubMed]
28. Kim, P.H.; Suh, C.H.; Baek, J.H.; Chung, S.R.; Choi, Y.J.; Lee, J.H. Diagnostic Performance of Four Ultrasound Risk Stratification Systems: A Systematic Review and Meta-Analysis. *Thyroid* **2020**, *30*, 1159–1168. [CrossRef]
29. Magri, F.; Chytiris, S.; Croce, L.; Molteni, M.; Bendotti, G.; Gruosso, G.; Tata Ngnitejeu, S.; Agozzino, M.; Rotondi, M.; Chiovato, L. Performance of the ACR TI-RADS and EU TI-RADS scoring systems in the diagnostic work-up of thyroid nodules in a real-life series using histology as reference standard. *Eur. J. Endocrinol.* **2020**, *183*, 521–528. [CrossRef]
30. Yim, Y.; Na, D.G.; Ha, E.J.; Baek, J.H.; Sung, J.Y.; Kim, J.H.; Moon, W.J. Concordance of Three International Guidelines for Thyroid Nodules Classified by Ultrasonography and Diagnostic Performance of Biopsy Criteria. *Korean J. Radiol.* **2020**, *21*, 108–116. [CrossRef]
31. Persichetti, A.; Di Stasio, E.; Coccaro, C.; Graziano, F.; Bianchini, A.; Di Donna, V.; Corsello, S.; Valle, D.; Bizzarri, G.; Frasoldati, A.; et al. Inter- and Intraobserver Agreement in the Assessment of Thyroid Nodule Ultrasound Features and Classification Systems: A Blinded Multicenter Study. *Thyroid* **2020**, *30*, 237–242. [CrossRef] [PubMed]
32. Chung, R.; Rosenkrantz, A.B.; Bennett, G.L.; Dane, B.; Jacobs, J.E.; Slywotzky, C.; Smereka, P.N.; Tong, A.; Sheth, S. Interreader Concordance of the TI-RADS: Impact of Radiologist Experience. *Am. J. Roentgenol.* **2020**, *214*, 1152–1157. [CrossRef]
33. Seifert, P.; Gorges, R.; Zimny, M.; Kreissl, M.C.; Schenke, S. Interobserver agreement and efficacy of consensus reading in Kwak-, EU-, and ACR-thyroid imaging recording and data systems and ATA guidelines for the ultrasound risk stratification of thyroid nodules. *Endocrine* **2020**, *67*, 143–154. [CrossRef]
34. Sych, Y.P.; Fadeev, V.V.; Fisenko, E.P.; Kalashnikova, M. Reproducibility and Interobserver Agreement of Different Thyroid Imaging and Reporting Data Systems (TIRADS). *Eur. Thyroid J.* **2021**, *10*, 161–167. [CrossRef]
35. Cibas, E.S.; Ali, S.Z. The 2017 Bethesda System for Reporting Thyroid Cytopathology. *Thyroid* **2017**, *27*, 1341–1346. [CrossRef] [PubMed]
36. Na, D.G.; Kim, J.H.; Kim, D.S.; Kim, S.J. Thyroid nodules with minimal cystic changes have a low risk of malignancy. *Ultrasonography* **2016**, *35*, 153–158. [CrossRef] [PubMed]
37. Nguyen, X.V.; Choudhury, K.R.; Eastwood, J.D.; Lyman, G.H.; Esclamado, R.M.; Werner, J.D.; Hoang, J.K. Incidental thyroid nodules on CT: Evaluation of 2 risk-categorization methods for work-up of nodules. *AJNR Am. J. Neuroradiol.* **2013**, *34*, 1812–1817. [CrossRef] [PubMed]
38. Koseoglu Atilla, F.D.; Ozgen Saydam, B.; Erarslan, N.A.; Diniz Unlu, A.G.; Yilmaz Yasar, H.; Ozer, M.; Akinci, B. Does the ACR TI-RADS scoring allow us to safely avoid unnecessary thyroid biopsy? single center analysis in a large cohort. *Endocrine* **2018**, *61*, 398–402. [CrossRef]
39. Castellana, M.; Castellana, C.; Treglia, G.; Giorgino, F.; Giovanella, L.; Russ, G.; Trimboli, P. Performance of Five Ultrasound Risk Stratification Systems in Selecting Thyroid Nodules for FNA. *J. Clin. Endocrinol. Metab.* **2020**, *105*, 1659–1669. [CrossRef]
40. Yoon, J.H.; Han, K.; Kim, E.K.; Moon, H.J.; Kwak, J.Y. Diagnosis and Management of Small Thyroid Nodules: A Comparative Study with Six Guidelines for Thyroid Nodules. *Radiology* **2017**, *283*, 560–569. [CrossRef]
41. Ha, E.J.; Na, D.G.; Moon, W.J.; Lee, Y.H.; Choi, N. Diagnostic Performance of Ultrasound-Based Risk-Stratification Systems for Thyroid Nodules: Comparison of the 2015 American Thyroid Association Guidelines with the 2016 Korean Thyroid Association/Korean Society of Thyroid Radiology and 2017 American College of Radiology Guidelines. *Thyroid* **2018**, *28*, 1532–1537. [CrossRef] [PubMed]

42. Middleton, W.D.; Teefey, S.A.; Reading, C.C.; Langer, J.E.; Beland, M.D.; Szabunio, M.M.; Desser, T.S. Comparison of Performance Characteristics of American College of Radiology TI-RADS, Korean Society of Thyroid Radiology TIRADS, and American Thyroid Association Guidelines. *Am. J. Roentgenol.* **2018**, *210*, 1148–1154. [CrossRef]
43. Xu, T.; Wu, Y.; Wu, R.X.; Zhang, Y.Z.; Gu, J.Y.; Ye, X.H.; Tang, W.; Xu, S.H.; Liu, C.; Wu, X.H. Validation and comparison of three newly-released Thyroid Imaging Reporting and Data Systems for cancer risk determination. *Endocrine* **2019**, *64*, 299–307. [CrossRef]
44. Grani, G.; Lamartina, L.; Ascoli, V.; Bosco, D.; Biffoni, M.; Giacomelli, L.; Maranghi, M.; Falcone, R.; Ramundo, V.; Cantisani, V.; et al. Reducing the Number of Unnecessary Thyroid Biopsies While Improving Diagnostic Accuracy: Toward the "Right" TIRADS. *J. Clin. Endocrinol. Metab.* **2019**, *104*, 95–102. [CrossRef]
45. Mohammadi, M.; Betel, C.; Burton, K.R.; Higgins, K.M.; Ghorab, Z.; Halperin, I.J. Retrospective Application of the 2015 American Thyroid Association Guidelines for Ultrasound Classification, Biopsy Indications, and Follow-up Imaging of Thyroid Nodules: Can Improved Reporting Decrease Testing? *Can. Assoc. Radiol. J.* **2019**, *70*, 68–73. [CrossRef]
46. Ruan, J.L.; Yang, H.Y.; Liu, R.B.; Liang, M.; Han, P.; Xu, X.L.; Luo, B.M. Fine needle aspiration biopsy indications for thyroid nodules: Compare a point-based risk stratification system with a pattern-based risk stratification system. *Eur. Radiol.* **2019**, *29*, 4871–4878. [CrossRef] [PubMed]
47. Wu, X.L.; Du, J.R.; Wang, H.; Jin, C.X.; Sui, G.Q.; Yang, D.Y.; Lin, Y.Q.; Luo, Q.; Fu, P.; Li, H.Q.; et al. Comparison and preliminary discussion of the reasons for the differences in diagnostic performance and unnecessary FNA biopsies between the ACR TIRADS and 2015 ATA guidelines. *Endocrine* **2019**, *65*, 121–131. [CrossRef] [PubMed]
48. Ha, E.J.; Na, D.G.; Baek, J.H.; Sung, J.Y.; Kim, J.H.; Kang, S.Y. US Fine-Needle Aspiration Biopsy for Thyroid Malignancy: Diagnostic Performance of Seven Society Guidelines Applied to 2000 Thyroid Nodules. *Radiology* **2018**, *287*, 893–900. [CrossRef]
49. Yoon, S.J.; Na, D.G.; Gwon, H.Y.; Paik, W.; Kim, W.J.; Song, J.S.; Shim, M.S. Similarities and Differences Between Thyroid Imaging Reporting and Data Systems. *Am. J. Roentgenol.* **2019**, *213*, W76–W84. [CrossRef]
50. Baek, H.J.; Kim, D.W.; Shin, G.W.; Heo, Y.J.; Baek, J.W.; Lee, Y.J.; Cho, Y.J.; Park, H.K.; Ha, T.K.; Kim, D.H.; et al. Ultrasonographic Features of Papillary Thyroid Carcinomas According to Their Subtypes. *Front. Endocrinol.* **2018**, *9*, 223. [CrossRef] [PubMed]
51. Castellana, M.; Piccardo, A.; Virili, C.; Scappaticcio, L.; Grani, G.; Durante, C.; Giovanella, L.; Trimboli, P. Can ultrasound systems for risk stratification of thyroid nodules identify follicular carcinoma? *Cancer Cytopathol.* **2020**, *128*, 250–259. [CrossRef]
52. Castellana, M.; Virili, C.; Paone, G.; Scappaticcio, L.; Piccardo, A.; Giovanella, L.; Trimboli, P. Ultrasound systems for risk stratification of thyroid nodules prompt inappropriate biopsy in autonomously functioning thyroid nodules. *Clin. Endocrinol.* **2020**, *93*, 67–75. [CrossRef]
53. Russ, G.; Royer, B.; Bigorgne, C.; Rouxel, A.; Bienvenu-Perrard, M.; Leenhardt, L. Prospective evaluation of thyroid imaging reporting and data system on 4550 nodules with and without elastography. *Eur. J. Endocrinol.* **2013**, *168*, 649–655. [CrossRef]
54. Yang, B.R.; Kim, E.K.; Moon, H.J.; Yoon, J.H.; Park, V.Y.; Kwak, J.Y. Qualitative and Semiquantitative Elastography for the Diagnosis of Intermediate Suspicious Thyroid Nodules Based on the 2015 American Thyroid Association Guidelines. *J. Ultrasound Med.* **2018**, *37*, 1007–1014. [CrossRef] [PubMed]
55. Trimboli, P.; Piccardo, A.; Alevizaki, M.; Virili, C.; Naseri, M.; Sola, S.; Paone, G.; Russ, G.; Giovanella, L. Dedicated neck (18) F-FDG PET/CT: An additional tool for risk assessment in thyroid nodules at ultrasound intermediate risk. *Clin. Endocrinol.* **2019**, *90*, 737–743. [CrossRef] [PubMed]
56. Yang, H.; Zhao, S.; Zhang, Z.; Chen, Y.; Wang, K.; Shang, M.; Chen, B. The associated factors for spontaneous intranodular hemorrhage of partially cystic thyroid nodules: A retrospective study of 101 thyroid nodules. *Medicine* **2020**, *99*, e23846. [CrossRef] [PubMed]
57. Lacout, A.; Chevenet, C.; Marcy, P.Y. Mummified Thyroid Syndrome. *Am. J. Roentgenol.* **2016**, *206*, 837–845. [CrossRef] [PubMed]
58. Ren, J.; Baek, J.H.; Chung, S.R.; Choi, Y.J.; Jung, C.K.; Lee, J.H. Degenerating Thyroid Nodules: Ultrasound Diagnosis, Clinical Significance, and Management. *Korean J. Radiol.* **2019**, *20*, 947–955. [CrossRef]
59. Bernardi, S.; Palermo, A.; Grasso, R.F.; Fabris, B.; Stacul, F.; Cesareo, R. Current Status and Challenges of US-Guided Radiofrequency Ablation of Thyroid Nodules in the Long Term: A Systematic Review. *Cancers* **2021**, *13*, 2746. [CrossRef]
60. Pan, F.S.; Wang, W.; Wang, Y.; Xu, M.; Liang, J.Y.; Zheng, Y.L.; Xie, X.Y.; Li, X.X. Sonographic features of thyroid nodules that may help distinguish clinically atypical subacute thyroiditis from thyroid malignancy. *J. Ultrasound Med.* **2015**, *34*, 689–696. [CrossRef] [PubMed]
61. Sheu, S.Y.; Gorges, R.; Schmid, K.W. Hyperplasia of the thyroid gland. *Pathologe* **2003**, *24*, 348–356. [CrossRef] [PubMed]
62. Zhu, Y.; Song, Y.; Xu, G.; Fan, Z.; Ren, W. Causes of misdiagnoses by thyroid fine-needle aspiration cytology (FNAC): Our experience and a systematic review. *Diagn Pathol* **2020**, *15*, 1. [CrossRef] [PubMed]
63. Papini, E.; Monpeyssen, H.; Frasoldati, A.; Hegedus, L. 2020 European Thyroid Association Clinical Practice Guideline for the Use of Image-Guided Ablation in Benign Thyroid Nodules. *Eur. Thyroid J.* **2020**, *9*, 172–185. [CrossRef] [PubMed]
64. Deandrea, M.; Trimboli, P.; Mormile, A.; Cont, A.T.; Milan, L.; Buffet, C.; Giovanella, L.; Limone, P.P.; Poiree, S.; Leenhardt, L.; et al. Determining an energy threshold for optimal volume reduction of benign thyroid nodules treated by radiofrequency ablation. *Eur. Radiol.* **2021**, *31*, 5189–5197. [CrossRef] [PubMed]
65. Elsayes, K.M.; Hooker, J.C.; Agrons, M.M.; Kielar, A.Z.; Tang, A.; Fowler, K.J.; Chernyak, V.; Bashir, M.R.; Kono, Y.; Do, R.K.; et al. 2017 Version of LI-RADS for CT and MR Imaging: An Update. *Radiographics* **2017**, *37*, 1994–2017. [CrossRef]

66. Angell, T.E.; Maurer, R.; Wang, Z.; Kim, M.I.; Alexander, C.A.; Barletta, J.A.; Benson, C.B.; Cibas, E.S.; Cho, N.L.; Doherty, G.M.; et al. A Cohort Analysis of Clinical and Ultrasound Variables Predicting Cancer Risk in 20,001 Consecutive Thyroid Nodules. *J. Clin. Endocrinol. Metab.* **2019**, *104*, 5665–5672. [CrossRef]
67. Noto, B.; Eveslage, M.; Pixberg, M.; Gonzalez Carvalho, J.M.; Schafers, M.; Riemann, B.; Kies, P. Prevalence of hyperfunctioning thyroid nodules among those in need of fine needle aspiration cytology according to ATA 2015, EU-TIRADS, and ACR-TIRADS. *Eur. J. Nucl. Med. Mol. Imaging* **2020**, *47*, 1518–1526. [CrossRef]
68. Schenke, S.; Seifert, P.; Zimny, M.; Winkens, T.; Binse, I.; Gorges, R. Risk Stratification of Thyroid Nodules Using the Thyroid Imaging Reporting and Data System (TIRADS): The Omission of Thyroid Scintigraphy Increases the Rate of Falsely Suspected Lesions. *J. Nucl. Med.* **2019**, *60*, 342–347. [CrossRef]
69. Verbeek, H.H.; de Groot, J.W.B.; Sluiter, W.J.; Muller Kobold, A.C.; van den Heuvel, E.R.; Plukker, J.T.; Links, T.P. Calcitonin testing for detection of medullary thyroid cancer in people with thyroid nodules. *Cochrane Database Syst. Rev.* **2020**, *3*, CD010159. [CrossRef]
70. Trimboli, P.; Giovanella, L.; Valabrega, S.; Andrioli, M.; Baldelli, R.; Cremonini, N.; Rossi, F.; Guidobaldi, L.; Barnabei, A.; Rota, F.; et al. Ultrasound features of medullary thyroid carcinoma correlate with cancer aggressiveness: A retrospective multicenter study. *J. Exp. Clin. Cancer Res.* **2014**, *33*, 87. [CrossRef]
71. Trimboli, P.; Treglia, G.; Guidobaldi, L.; Romanelli, F.; Nigri, G.; Valabrega, S.; Sadeghi, R.; Crescenzi, A.; Faquin, W.C.; Bongiovanni, M.; et al. Detection rate of FNA cytology in medullary thyroid carcinoma: A meta-analysis. *Clin. Endocrinol.* **2015**, *82*, 280–285. [CrossRef] [PubMed]
72. Borlea, A.; Borcan, F.; Sporea, I.; Dehelean, C.A.; Negrea, R.; Cotoi, L.; Stoian, D. TI-RADS Diagnostic Performance: Which Algorithm is Superior and How Elastography and 4D Vascularity Improve the Malignancy Risk Assessment. *Diagnostics* **2020**, *10*, 180. [CrossRef] [PubMed]

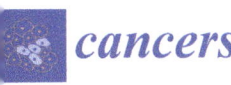

Review

Overview of the Ultrasound Classification Systems in the Field of Thyroid Cytology

Esther Diana Rossi [1,*], Liron Pantanowitz [2], Marco Raffaelli [3] and Guido Fadda [1,4]

1. Division of Anatomic Pathology and Histology, Fondazione Policlinico Universitario Agpstino Gemelli, 00168 Rome, Italy; guido.fadda@unime.it
2. Department of Pathology & Clinical Labs, University of Michigan, Ann Arbor, MI 48103, USA; lironp@med.umich.edu
3. Division of Endocrine-Surgery, Fondazione Policlinico Universitario Agpstino Gemelli, 00168 Rome, Italy; marco.raffaelli@policlinicogemelli.it
4. D.A.I. Diagnostic Department of Anatomic Pathology, University of Messina, 98100 Messina, Italy
* Correspondence: esther.rossi@policlinicogemelli.it

Simple Summary: Ultrasound (US) is the preferred imaging modality for thyroid nodule evaluation. Accurate US assessment of thyroid lesions can help decrease unwarranted FNA procedures of benign nodules. Several thyroid nodule risk classification systems that focus on US features have been published. Some of them highlight simple US patterns, while others rely on the presence of multiple US features to categorize thyroid nodules. The current review offers an evaluation of different US system, combining them with the use of fine needle aspiration and the cytological classification systems.

Abstract: The increasing application of ultrasound (US) in recent years has led to a greater number of thyroid nodule diagnoses. Consequently, the number of fine needle aspirations performed to evaluate these lesions has increased. Although the majority of thyroid nodules are benign, identifying methods to define specific lesions and tailor risk of malignancy has become vital. Some of the tools employed to stratify thyroid nodule risk include clinical factors, thyroid US findings, and reporting systems for thyroid cytopathology. Establishing high concordance between US features and cytologic diagnoses might help reduce healthcare costs by diminishing unnecessary thyroid procedures and treatment. This review aims to review radiology US classification systems that influence the practice of thyroid cytology.

Keywords: thyroid; classification system; follicular neoplasm; ultrasound classification system; TIRAD

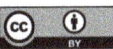

1. Introduction

Thyroid nodules are common in adults. In recent years, the incidence rate of thyroid cancer has increased, as has the rate of thyroidectomy [1,2]. However, the overall mortality for thyroid malignancy during this time period showed no significant changes. The increase in diagnosing thyroid lesions is partly attributed to improvements in imaging technology and increased use of imaging, which leads to higher rates of thyroid nodule detection [3–5]. As a result, finer needle aspiration (FNA) biopsies and, accordingly, a higher incidence of subclinical thyroid cancer has risen. FNA is the first and perhaps most important minimally invasive diagnostic tool employed in the evaluation of thyroid nodules [6–11]. Around 70% of thyroid nodules are benign, with only 5–10% reported to be malignant [1,2]. The remaining 20–25% of thyroid lesions comprise grey zone indeterminate proliferations that include either benign or malignant lesions, for which morphological discrimination alone is not always possible. These aspects raised concerns over the costs and morbidity linked with the management of patients with thyroid nodules. On the whole, it often leads to unnecessary surgical resections and drives up healthcare cost. It stands to reason that a more refined and accurate approach to the management of thyroid lesions needs to start from an accurate initial workup including US evaluation, avoiding the over-diagnosis of low-risk lesions [2–6].

According to the American Thyroid Association (ATA), ultrasound (US) is the main and preferred imaging modality for thyroid nodule evaluation [7]. Accurate US assessment of thyroid lesions can help decrease unwarranted FNA procedures of benign nodules. Several thyroid nodule risk classification systems that focus on US features have already been published. Some of them highlight only simple US patterns, while others rely on the presence of multiple US features to categorize thyroid nodules. In 2009, Horvath et al. proposed a Thyroid Imaging, Reporting and Data System (TIRADS) [12] (Table 1) accepted and then proposed by the American College of Radiology (ACR) and based upon the distribution of US features in five categories (composition, echogenicity, shape, margin, and echogenic foci) [13,14]. The TIRADS reporting system has notably been modeled after the 2009 Breast Imaging Reporting and Data System (BIRADS) [15].

Table 1. Summary of the main features of ultrasound-based thyroid nodule systems.

ACR-TIRADS	Korean System	UK BTA System
TR 1 0 points Benign	K-TIRADS 1: no nodule	U1: No nodule
TR 2 2 points no suspicious	K-TIRADS 2: Benign	U2: Benign hyperechoic or isoechoic with a halo cystic change with ring-down artifact (colloid) • microcystic or spongiform appearance • peripheral egg-shell calcification • peripheral vascularity
TR 3 3 points Mildly suspicious	K-TIRADS 3: Low partially cystic/isohyperechoic with no suspicious features	U3: Indeterminate solid homogenous markedly hyperechoic nodule with halo (follicular lesions) • hypoechoic with equivocal echogenic foci or cystic change • mixed or central vascularity
TR 4 TR4a = 4 TR4b = 5 TR4c = 6 from 4 to 6 points Moderately suspicious	K-TIRADS 4: Intermediate as for K-TIRADS 3 but with any suspicious features or as for K-TIRADS 5 without suspicious features	U4: Suspicious solid hypoechoic (compared with thyroid) • solid very hypoechoic (compared with strap muscles) • hypoechoic with disrupted peripheral calcification • lobulated outline
TR 5 > 7 points Highly suspicious	K-TIRADS 5: High solid hypoechoic nodule with any suspicious feature	U5 Malignant solid hypoechoic with a lobulated or irregular outline and microcalcification • papillary carcinoma • solid hypoechoic with a lobulated or irregular outline and globular calcification • medullary carcinoma • intranodular vascularity • taller than wide axially (AP > ML) • characteristic associated lymphadenopathy

American College of Radiology Thyroid Imaging, Reporting and Data System (ACR-TIRADS); K-TIRADS: Korean Tirads; UK BTA TIRADS: United Kingdom British Thyroid Association TIRADS. TR = TI-RADS; AP = anteroposterio; ML = mediolateral.

In 2015, Grant et al. published a thyroid ultrasound reporting lexicon in which all thyroid nodules were classified on the basis of TIRADS categories which, in turn, not only defined their risk of malignancy but offered evidence-based recommendations to manage thyroid nodules based on their size and sonographic features [5]. After the first Korean version of the TIRADS system by Kwak et al. [14], Shin et al. (2016) subsequently proposed a revised Korean Society of Thyroid Radiology (KSThR) consensus statement with recommendations in which specific sonographic features were used to stratify the risk of thyroid nodules into four categories [8]. According to the published literature, the Korean-TIRADS has been successfully used for US evaluation of thyroid nodules in order to stratify the need for these nodules to undergo FNA (Table 1).

The 2015 ATA guideline includes a detailed description of sonographic features, categorizing thyroid nodules that utilize one of the described patterns [7]. The most suspicious US features include margins, microcalcifications, "taller-than-wide" shape", rim calcifications, and evidence of extrathyroidal extension. Specifically, the ATA defined and identified five categories: (1) Benign (ROM < 1%); (2) very low suspicion (ROM < 3% in lesions $\geq$ 20 mm); (3) low suspicion (ROM 5–10% in lesions $\geq$ 15 mm); (4) Intermediate suspicion (ROM 10–20% in lesions $\geq$10 mm); and (5) high suspicion (ROM 70–90% in lesions $\geq$ 10 mm).

Furthermore, the European Thyroid Association (ETA) TIRADS, which includes five categories, was published in 2017 by Russ et al., with the main purpose of identifying thyroid malignancies while maintaining both high negative predictive value and sensitivity [16]. Since then, several similar systems have been promoted including the recommendations from the American Association of Clinical Endocrinology (AACE), American College of Endocrinology (ACE), Associazione Medici Endocrinologi (AME), as well as comprehensive cancer network guidelines [17–19].

The current article reviews these different US classification systems and the influence they have on the practice of thyroid cytology.

2. Overview of ACR-TIRADS

In an attempt to stratify the risk of thyroid cancer utilizing US features, the TIRADS imaging risk stratification system was proposed by Horvath et al. from Chile in 2009 and further modified by Kwak et al. from Seoul in 2011 [12,14]. TIRADS is now accepted by the ACR and has been described in a paper published by the ACR TIRADS Committee [5].

The ACR-TIRADS is designed to reduce the number of unnecessary FNA procedures performed for benign thyroid nodules with an objective to increase the diagnostic efficacy of evaluating thyroid nodules. The idea behind this system is to codify all thyroid lesions into diagnostic US categories. Specifically, five different US characteristics of a thyroid nodule are evaluated, including: (a) composition, (b) echogenicity, (c) shape, (d) margin, and (e) echogenic foci (Table 2). Points are assigned to each of these US features. For composition, the values are as follows: cystic or spongiform = 0, mixed solid-cystic = 1, and solid = 2. For echogenicity, they are anechoic = 0, isoechoic or hyperechoic = 1, hypoechoic = 2, and very hypoechoic = 3. For shape, wider-than-tall = 0, whilst taller-than-wide = 3. Margins are classified as follows: smooth or ill-defined = 0, irregular or lobulated = 2, and extrathyroidal extension = 3. The echogenic foci are classified as: none or comet-tail = 0, macrocalcifications = 1, peripheral or rim calcifications = 2, and punctate = 3. Points are totaled by adding single selections from the five nodular characteristics and they are then used to classify thyroid nodules into TIRADS categories as follow: TR1 = Benign (requires no FNA), TR2 = not suspicious for malignancy (requires no FNA-Figure 1), TR3 = mildly suspicious (FNA if $\geq$2.5 cm and follow if $\geq$1.5 cm), TR4 = moderately suspicious (FNA if $\geq$1.5 cm and follow if $\geq$1.0 cm-Figure 2), and TR5 = highly suspicious (FNA if $\geq$1.0 cm and follow if $\geq$0.5 cm-Figure 3). Concerning TR4, there was a further subclassification including TR4a with one malignant sign and possibly benign; TR4b with two malignant signs and possible malignant; TR4c with three or four malignant signs and highly possible malignant. Furthermore, the TIRAD Committee underlined the risk of malignancy (ROM) for each category as follows: 2% or less for TR1 and TR2, 2.1–5% for TR3, 5.1–20% for TR4, and greater than 20% for TR5. As indicated, the categories along with thyroid nodule size help determine recommendations for FNA and follow-up management.

Table 2. Criteria adopted for the definition of the TIRADS system score categories.

Criteria	Definitions
Composition	Cystic = 0 Spongiform = 0 Mixed solid and cystic = 1 Solid = 2
Echogenecity	Anechoic = 0 Hyperechoic or isoechoic = 1 Hypoechoic = 2 Very hypoechoic = 3
Shape	Wider-than-tall = 0 Taller-than-wide = 3
Margins	Smooth = 0 Ill-defined = 0 Lobulated or irregular = 2 Extrathyroid extension = 3
Echogenic foci	None or large comet-tail artifacts = 0 Macrocalcifications = 1 Peripheral calcifications = 2 Punctate echogenic foci = 3

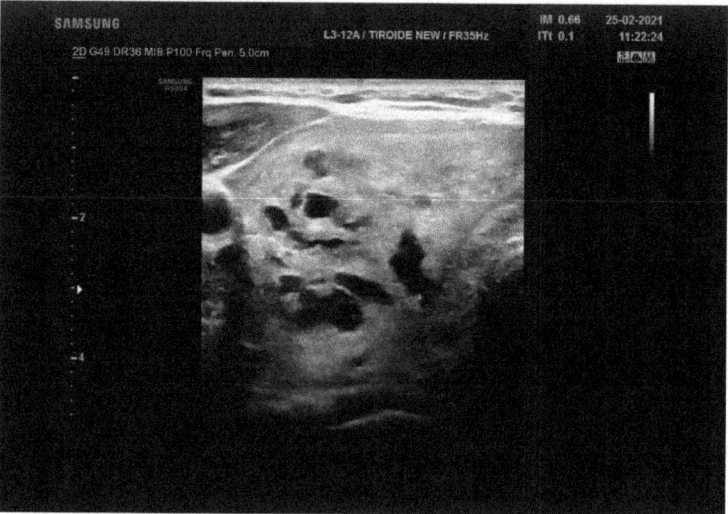

Figure 1. Ultrasound features from a thyroid nodule (50 mm size) resulting into a score 2 (solid and cystic plus hyperechoic-isoechoic) belonging to TR 2. The lesion was diagnosed as adenomatous goiter.

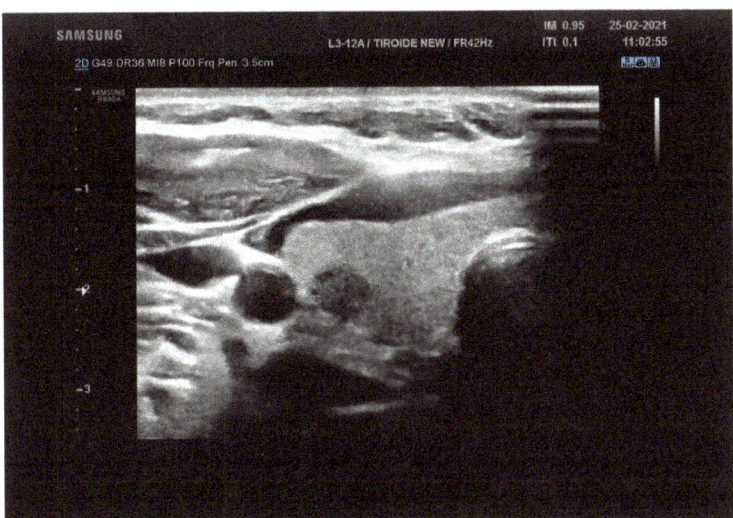

Figure 2. Ultrasound features from a thyroid nodule (15 mm size) resulting into a score 5 (solid, hypoechoic with a calcification) belonging to TR 4. The lesion was diagnosed as Follicular nodule.

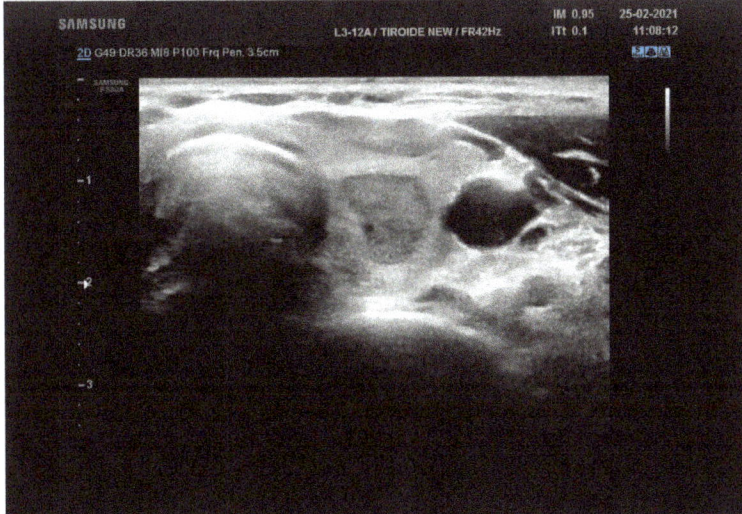

Figure 3. Ultrasound features from a thyroid nodule (15 mm size) resulting into a score 7 belonging to TR 5 (solid, very hypoechoic, lobulated). The lesion was diagnosed as Follicular nodule.

The novelty of ACR-TIRADS is the method of scoring both echogenic foci and calcifications, which are additive features given more weight than in other systems. Some authors have suggested modifying TIRADS [13,20–24]. Park et al. established a new system with 12 characteristics even though its application proved to be difficult, [13] and Kwak et al. proposed a more practical classification system including only five US features [14]. Several studies have evaluated the efficacy of ACR-TIRADS [20–24]. Among the others, Koseoglu et al. documented that in a series of 2847 patients who underwent FNA of their thyroid lesions ACR-TIRADS was able to classify 98.8% as benign nodules with only a minimal number of malignant lesions classified as TR2 and TR3 [20]. Ha et al. compared seven society guidelines, of which ACR-TIRADS resulted in the lowest rate (25.3%) of unnecessary thyroid FNA procedures [21].

3. TIRADS Challenges and Pitfalls

The implementation and adoption of any new classification system are likely to present some challenges [2–6]. For ACR-TIRADS, such issues were mostly due to education, workflow, and interpretation of this reporting system. An initial step in the global adoption of a unique classification such as TIRADS is the education and training of sonographers to recognize the relevant US features. In general, a report of a thyroid nodule that received US examination should be structured and written in order to avoid colorful descriptive terms. Tappouni et al. suggested an algorithmic approach to stratify thyroid nodules, further aiding radiologists to discriminate benign from suspicious nodules [4].

As documented by Eze et al., FNA-induced reactive changes in thyroid nodules can appear worrisome and may include features such as atypical nuclei, hemorrhage, infarction, fibrinoid necrosis, fibrosis, cystic degeneration, pseudocapsular invasion, and squamous metaplasia that may resemble suspicious imaging findings, resulting in incorrectly classifying a previously aspirated thyroid nodule as TIRADS 4a [22]. Such FNA-induced changes may explain a subset of false-positive TIRADS cases, in which subsequent surgical resection of these surgeries is negative (so-called vanishing tumors).

4. Results from Applying TIRADS

Various studies have evaluated the prediction of thyroid malignancy using TIRADS [25–39] (Table 3). Shayganfar et al. studied 239 thyroid nodules combining TIRADS and FNA outcome using the Bethesda System for Reporting Thyroid Cytopathology (TBSRTC) [25]. The BSRTC includes six diagnostic categories including: bon-diagnostic (I); benign and bon-beoplastic (II); atypia of undetermined significance or follicular lesion of undetermined significance (AUS/FLUS) (III); follicular neoplasm or suspicious for follicular neoplasm (FN/SFN) (IV); suspicious for malignancy (SM) (V); and malignant (VI) [9]. In their study, the Bethesda system documented that thyroid nodules with TIRADS > 4 and a diameter lower than 12 mm were highly suspicious for malignancy, with a sensitivity of 91.7% and specificity of 52.8%. They found an inverse relationship between nodular size and malignancy risk [25].

Table 3. prediction of thyroid malignancy using TIRADS in some of the proposed studies.

Series	N° Cases	Sensitivity	Specificity	PPV	NPV	Diagnostic Accuracy	ROM (Ranged According to the Cytologic Categories)
Shayganfar [25]	239	91.7%	52.8%	/	/	/	0–25%
Barbosa [26]	140	95.3%	84.6%	87%	94%	90.2%	20–92.9%
Zhang [27]	319	86.7%	91.4%	75.6%	95.3%	96%	0–90.5%
Maia [28]	242	80%	84%	71%	90%	66.7%	8.7%–77%
Rocha [29]	143	80.4%	94%	52.4%	95%	/	0–72%
Chaigeau [30]	602	95%%	/	77.6%	55%	/	20–100%
Rahal [32]	1000	/	/	/	/	/	16–92%
Grani [33]	502	83.3%	56.2%	12.8%	97.8%	/	2–20%
Wu [39]	346	96%	53%	76%	89%	79%	

PPV: positive predictive value, NPV = negative predictive value; ROM = risk of malignancy

Barbosa et al. analyzed the correlation of ACR-TIRADS and ATA guidelines in the evaluation of 140 indeterminate thyroid lesions [26]. According to their study, the combination of US classification, ACR-TIRADS, and ATA along with TBSRTC is useful for detecting benign lesions in Bethesda III nodules and malignant lesions in Bethesda IV/V nodules. The ROM increased according to US suspicion categories ($p < 0.001$) for both US classifications (i.e.,

TIRADS and ATA). Whilst thyroid nodules with the lowest TIRADS categories had 95.3% sensitivity and 94% negative predictive value (NPV), the highest TIRADS categories were significantly associated with cancer.

Several other studies have also evaluated the use of US patterns to stratify the risk of malignancy for indeterminate thyroid lesions. Grani et al. studied 49 indeterminate lesions combined with TIRADS and ATA systems. They concluded that nodules classified as TIRADS 3 or as having a very low suspicion could be followed-up with FNA, whilst TIRADS 4c nodules had a high positive predictive value (PPV) of 71% with a suggestion for surgical procedure [33]. Moreover, Maia et al. studied 136 indeterminate thyroid lesions combining TIRADS with TBSRTC [28]. They found that Bethesda III nodules with a TIRADS 3 and 4a had high sensitivity (80%) and NPV (90%), implying that conservative management was adequate. On the other hand, thyroid nodules scored as TIRAD 4c and 5 with Bethesda IV and V had a high ROM at 75% and 76.9%, respectively. Rocha et al. investigated 143 indeterminate thyroid lesions, classified as Bethesda III and IV, who were referred to surgery and they hey found a ROM ranging from 0% to 72% [29]. Chaigneau et al. studied 602 indeterminate thyroid nodules classified as TIRADS score 3, 4a, 4b, and 5 with different ROM as 20.5%, 29%, 63.4%, and 100%, respectively [30].

Friedrich-Rust et al. demonstrated promising results in a study including three observers for 114 thyroid nodules [34]. They found that the interobserver agreement was only fair for TIRADS categories 2–5 (Cohen kappa-ck = 0.27, p = 0.000001) and TIRADS categories 2/3 versus 4/5 (ck = 0.25, p = 0.0020). The NPV was 92–100% for TIRADS categories 4 and 5 in the same study. Valderrabano et al. [31] and Barbosa et al. [26] concluded that there were no differences in the prevalence of malignancy between indeterminate nodules with low or intermediate ATA suspicious patterns, confirming that hypoechogenicity alone did not seem to improve the risk stratification of indeterminate lesions. In contrast, any additional suspicious US feature significantly increases the risk of malignancy of the indeterminate nodules. Rahal et al. assessed a significant association between TIRADS outcome and TBSRTC (p < 0.001) in the evaluation of 1000 retrospective thyroid nodules [32]. Benign Bethesda results (95.5%) had been classified as TIRADS 2 or 3, whilst among those classified as TIRADS 4c and 5, the majority belonged to Bethesda VI (68.2% and 91.3%, respectively). Furthermore, among TIRADS 4a–c and 5, the proportion of malignancy was 16%, 43.2%, 72.7%, and 91.3%, respectively. Hence, this study supports the role of TIRADS for the correct assessment and management of thyroid nodules [32]. Zhang et al. studied 319 thyroid nodules combining TIRADS classification and the contrast-enhanced ultrasound (CEUS) enhancement pattern of thyroid nodules concluding that the accuracy in the diagnosis was 96% especially for TIRADS class-4 thyroid nodules [27].

Grani et al. assessed the performance of five internationally endorsed sonographic classification systems [33]. They included 502 cases classified with both the Italian classification system and TBSRTC. The application of the FNA criteria systems reduced the number of biopsies performed by 17.1% to 53.4% for the Italian and TBSRTC, respectively. Among the sonographic risk stratification systems, ACR-TIRADS allowed the largest reduction of biopsies (more than 50%) and the lowest false negative rate (2.2%). Middleton et al., in a multi-institutional reevaluation of thyroid nodules, found that TIRADS was favorably comparable with the ATA and the Korean society of thyroid radiology classifications in reducing the number of biopsies [35].

Other controversial areas for TIRADS include microcarcinoma, growth of nodules, number of nodules to be aspirated and the evaluation of cervical nodes [6]. A paper by Tessler et al. also discussed these issues [6]. Concerning the performance of FNAs for subcentimeter nodules, the ACR-TIRADS agree with other guidelines in limiting FNA of nodules smaller than 1 cm, even if they are highly suspicious. Nevertheless, due to the possibility of active surveillance, ablation, or lobectomy for microcarcinoma, an FNA may be performed.

The committee defined the number of nodules to be biopsied [6]. They recommended one targets no more than two nodules defined by the most worrisome TIRADS. Among the criteria, size should be one of the primary criteria for FNA. Furthermore, the evaluation of cervical lymph nodes is a vital part of every thyroid sonographic examination, and it should be recommended for suspicious nodes.

Another point of discussion is represented by the growth of nodules [6]. The ACR-TIRADS defines a significant enlargement when there is a 20% increase in at least two nodular dimensions and a minimal increase of 2 mm, or a 50% or greater increase in volume, compared with the immediately previous US evaluation [6].

Yang et al. discussed the role of ARC-TIRADS in triaging thyroid follicular cells with papillary-like nuclear features obtained by FNA in order to evaluate the extent of surgery [37]. They found that ACR TI-RADS can be combined with morphology, including NIFTP among cytological diagnoses.

In another paper, Yang et al. studied 179 cases including 72 (40.2%) noninvasive follicular thyroid neoplasm with papillary-like nuclear features (NIFTP), 37 (20.7%) encapsulated FVPTC with invasion (EFVPTC), and 70 (39.1%) infiltrative FVPTC (IFVPTC) without a capsule [38]. They underlined that either NIFTPs or minimally invasive EFVPTC have a circumscribed oval/round border and a hypoechoic rim, and hypervascularity with Doppler. On the other hand, the ultrasound findings for IFVPTCs found at least one of the malignant gray-scale features: markedly hypoechoic, taller-than-wide, microcalcifications, or blurred margins.

Wu studied the same correlation with TIRAD, including 346 thyroid FNAC. They found an overall 0.465 r-value between TI-RADS scores and TBSRTC categories. Furthermore, the comparative analysis between TBSRTC and TIRADS showed that sensitivity, specificity, PPV, NPV, and accuracy are 96%, 53%, 76%, 89%, 79% for TI-RADS vs. 100%, 93%, 96%, 100%, 97% for TBSRTC, respectively ($p = 0.038$) [39].

5. Other Thyroid Nodule Ultrasound Scoring Systems

Lee et al. assessed the accuracy of rendering a US diagnosis for benign and malignant solid thyroid nodules using a different classification system comprised of five categories [36] (Table 2). These categories included: malignant, suspicious for malignancy, borderline, probably benign, and benign. The criteria, used for fitting the nodules into the different categories, focused on their hypoechogenicity, nodular margins, microcalcifications, a "taller-than-wider" shape, and associated regional lymphadenopathy. In their series of 103 thyroid lesions, Lee et al. demonstrated that this novel thyroid US system had 86% sensitivity, 95% specificity, 91% positive, and 92% negative predictive values, as well as 92% diagnostic accuracy in discriminating benign from malignant lesions [36]. Nonetheless, the suspicious for malignancy US category had a low diagnostic accuracy value, whilst all malignant US nodules were confirmed to be correctly categorized.

The British Thyroid Association (BTA) in 2014 provided guidelines for US scoring of thyroid nodules (BTA-U score) to assist in the management of thyroid cancer [40]. Briefly, it allows for stratifying thyroid nodules as benign, suspicious, or malignant based on ultrasound appearances termed U1-U5. They include five categories as U1 (normal parenchyma; U2 (benign); U3 (indeterminate); U4 (suspicious); and U5 (malignant). The categories are linked with different management. In fact, U2 nodules do not require FNA or follow-up imaging in the absence of concerning clinical features. The assignation of U3-U5 to nodules require FNA with further management based on resultant cytology, radiology and clinical findings. The US features should be combined with the cytological evaluation and the diagnostic categories. The Royal College of Pathologists in 2009 recommended the subdivision of the Thy-3 (indeterminate) category into Thy-3a (atypia) and Thy-3f (follicular neoplasm) [41,42].

Weller et al. studied 73 consecutive cases evaluated by five sonographers [40]. Their results suggested that there was substantial inter-observer agreement, culminating in 100% sensitivity and negative predictive value, with low specificity (32%) and specificity (34%). On the other hand, a study by Brophy et al. using the BTA system on 151 indeterminate thyroid lesions (Thy3) found no statistically significant differences in the ROM between Thy3a and Thy3f [42].

Ulisse et al. combined the Italian system for classifying thyroid nodules with the TIRADS scoring system in a series of 70 thyroid lesions classified as indeterminate lesions (TIR3A or TIR3B) [43]. The authors reported a different rate of malignancy between TIR3A (13%) and TIR3B (44.5%). They also subclassified their patients into three subgroups showing low (8.3%), indeterminate (21.4%), and high (80%) risk of malignancy. Adoption of the second edition of the Italian cytologic classification system has offered better stratification of malignant risk for indeterminate thyroid lesions [11]. This finding was corroborated by Chng et al. using the BTA system and TIRADS, confirming that the risk of malignancy increased from TIRADS 4A (14.3%), TIRADS 4B (23.1%), TIRADS 4C (87.5%), and TIRADS 5 (100%) [44].

The KSThR published their first recommendation in 2011 for utilizing an US-based diagnosis to assist with the management of thyroid nodules [14]. Subsequently in 2016, a taskforce revised these Korean recommendations [8]. Of note, their changes included revising the US malignancy risk stratification system for thyroid nodules now known as the Korean Thyroid Imaging Reporting and Data System (K-TIRADS), adding a risk stratification system of cervical lymph nodes on the basis of US and computed tomography (CT) features, and recommendations for image-guided ablation of benign thyroid nodules. Their data included a detailed analysis of thyroid nodules encompassing: (1) internal composition (solid, predominantly solid, cystic, predominantly cystic); (2) echogenicity (marked hypoechogenicity, mild hypoechogenicity, isoechogenicity, hyperechogenicity); (3) shape (round to oval, irregular); (4) orientation (parallel, non-parallel); (5) margin (smooth, spiculated, ill-defined); (6) calcification (microcalcification, macrocalcification, rim calcification); (7) halo (present or absent); (8) spongiform (present or not); (9) colloid (present or not); and (10) vascularity (from type 1 to 4). Using this score, the system defines five categories including no nodule, benign category with a <3% ROM, low suspicious category with a 3–15% ROM, intermediate suspicion with a 15–50% ROM, and high suspicion category with >60% ROM [45].

6. Conclusions

The adoption of an ultrasound (US) system for classifying thyroid nodules is useful for tailoring the diagnostic approach when evaluating these lesions and combining their workup with FNA biopsy [45–48]. Accurate categorization of thyroid nodules based on an US classification system, irrespective of whether it is the ACR-TIRADS or an alternative system, may help physicians in predicting their ROM and thus rationalize adequate management. Furthermore, combined analysis including TIRADS in concert with the patient's age, gender, clinical findings, and thyroid nodule size is essential in determining the pre-FNA ROM. Even if TIRADS or another related US-based system demonstrates satisfactory sensitivity in detecting malignant thyroid nodules, it is unlikely going to replace FNA, as the latter remains the gold standard to define the nature of these nodules, especially when cytomorphology is combined with ancillary molecular testing for indeterminate lesions. However, when TIRADS is combined with US-guided FNA this has been shown to greatly improve the accuracy of diagnosing malignant thyroid nodules.

Author Contributions: Conceptualization: E.D.R., L.P.; methodology: E.D.R., L.P., G.F., M.R.; software: L.P.; validation: E.D.R., L.P., G.F., M.R.; formal analysis: E.D.R., L.P.; investigation: E.D.R., L.P.; resources: E.D.R., L.P.; data curation: E.D.R., L.P., G.F., M.R.; writing—original draft preparation: E.D.R., L.P.; writing—review and editing: E.D.R., L.P., G.F., M.R. visualization: E.D.R., L.P.; supervision: E.D.R.; project administration: E.D.R., L.P.; funding acquisition: E.D.R., G.F. All authors have read and agreed to the published version of the manuscript."

Funding: This research did not receive any specific grant from any funding agency in the public, commercial or not-profit sectors.

Conflicts of Interest: The authors have no conflict of interests.

References

1. Al Dawish, M.A.; Rober, A.A.; Thabet, M.A.; Braham, R. Thyroid nodule management: Thyroid-stimulating hormone, ultrasound and cytological classification system for predicting malignancy. *Cancer Inform.* **2018**, *17*, 1–9. [CrossRef]
2. Grani, G.; Sponziello, M.; Pecce, V.; Ramundo, V.; Durante, C. Contemporary thyroid evaluation and management. *J. Clin. Endocrinol. Metab.* **2020**, *105*, 2869–2883. [CrossRef]
3. Ardakani, A.A.; Mohammadzadeh, A.; Yaghoubi, N.; Ghaemmaghami, Z.; Reiazi, R.; Jafari, A.H.; Hekmat, S.; Shiran, M.B.; Bitarafa-Rajabi, A. Predictive quantitative sonographic features on classification of hot and cold thyroid nodules. *Eur. J. Radiol.* **2018**, *101*, 170–177. [CrossRef] [PubMed]
4. Tappouni, R.R.; Itri, J.N.; McQueen, T.S.; Lalwani, N.; Ou, J.J. ACR TI-RADS: Pitfalls, solutions and future directions. *Radiographics* **2019**, *39*, 2040–2052. [CrossRef] [PubMed]
5. Grant, E.G.; Tessler, F.N.; Hoang, J.K.; Langer, J.E.; Beland, M.D.; Berland, L.L.; Cronan, J.J.; Desser, T.S.; Frates, M.C.; Hamper, U.M.; et al. Thyroid ultrasound reporting lexicon: White paper of the ACR thyroid imaging reporting and data system (TIRADS) committee. *J. Am. Coll. Radiol.* **2015**, *12*, 1272–1279. [CrossRef] [PubMed]
6. Tessler, F.N.; Middleton, W.D.; Grant, E.G.; Hoang, J.K.; Berland, L.L.; Teefey, S.A.; Cronan, J.J.; Beland, M.D.; Desser, T.S.; Frates, M.C.; et al. ACR Thyroid Imaging, Reporting and Data System (TI-RADS): White Paper of the ACR TI-RADS Committee. *J. Am. Coll. Radiol.* **2019**, *14*, 587–595. [CrossRef] [PubMed]
7. Hauger, B.R.; Alexander, E.K.; Bible, K.C.; Doherty, G.M.; Mandel, S.J.; Nikiforov, Y.E.; Pacini, F.; Randolph, G.W.; Sawka, A.M.; Schlumberger, M.; et al. 2015 American thyroid association management guidelines for adult patients with thyroid nodules and differentiated thyroid cancer: The American thyroid association guidelines task force on thyroid nodules and differentiated thyroid cancer. *Thyroid* **2016**, *26*, 1–33.
8. Shin, J.H.; Back, J.H.; Chung, J.; Ha, E.J.; Kiim, J.H.; Lee, Y.H.; Lim, H.K.; Moon, W.J.; Na, D.G.; Park, J.S.; et al. Ultrasonography diagnosis and imaging-based management of thyroid nodules: Revised Korean society of thyroid radiology consensus statement and recommendations. *Korean J. Radiol.* **2016**, *17*, 370–395. [CrossRef]
9. Ali, S.; Cibas, E.S. *The Bethesda System for Reporting Thyroid Cytopathology*, 2nd ed.; Springer: Berlin, Germany, 2018.
10. Nardi, F.; Basolo, F.; Crescenzi, A.; Fadda, G.; Frasoldati, A.; Orlandi, F.; Palombini, L.; Papini, E.; Zini, M.; Pontecorvi, A.; et al. Italian consensus for the classification and reporting of thyroid cytology. *J. Endocrinol. Investig.* **2014**, *37*, 593–599. [CrossRef]
11. Fadda, G.; Basolo, F.; Bondi, A.; Bussolati, G.; Crescenzi, A.; Nappi, O.; Nardi, F.; Papotti, M.; Taddei, G.; Palombini, L.; et al. Cytological classification of thyroid nodules. Proposal of the SIAPEC-IAP italian consensus working group. *Pathologica* **2010**, *102*, 405–406.
12. Horvarth, E.; Majlis, S.; Rossi, R.; Franco, C.; Niedmann, J.P.; Castro, A.; Dominguez, M.S.L. An ultrasonogram reporting system for thyroid nodules stratifying cancer risk for clinical management. *J. Clin. Endocrinol. Metab.* **2009**, *94*, 1748–1751. [CrossRef]
13. Park, J.Y.; Lee, H.J.; Jang, H.W.; Kim, H.K.; Yi, J.H.; Lee, W.; Kim, S.H. A proposal for a thyroid imaging reporting and data system for ultrasound features of thyroid carcinoma. *Thyroid* **2009**, *19*, 1257–1264. [CrossRef] [PubMed]
14. Kwak, J.Y.; Han, K.H.; Yoon, J.H.; Moon, H.J.; Son, E.J.; Park, S.H.; Jung, H.K.; Choi, J.S.; Kim, B.M.; Kim, E.K. Thyroid imaging reporting and data system for US features of nodules: A step in establishing better stratification of cancer risk. *Radiology* **2011**, *260*, 892–899. [CrossRef]
15. Na, D.G.; Back, J.H.; Sung, J.Y.; Kim, J.H.; Kim, J.K.; Choi, Y.J.; Seo, H. Thyroid imaging reporting and data system risk stratification of thyroid noduels: Categorization based on solidity and echogenicity. *Thyroid* **2016**, *26*, 562–572. [CrossRef]
16. Russ, G.; Bonnema, S.J.; Erdogan, M.F.; Durant, C.; Ngu, R.; Leenhardt, L. European thyroid association guidelines for ultrasound malignancy risk stratification of thyroid nodules in adults: The EU-TIRADS. *Eur. Thyroid. J.* **2017**, *6*, 225–237. [CrossRef]
17. Frates, M.C.; Benson, C.B.; Charboneau, J.W.; Cibas, E.S.; Clark, O.H.; Coleman, B.G.; Cronan, J.J.; Doubilet, P.M.; Evans, D.B.; Goellner, J.R.; et al. Management of thyroid nodules detected at US: Society of radiologists in ultrasound consensus conference statement. *Radiology* **2005**, *237*, 794–800. [CrossRef]
18. Gharib, H.; Papini, E.; Garber, J.R.; Duick, D.S.; Harrell, R.M.; Hegedüs, L.; Paschke, R.; Valcavi, R.; Vitti, P. AACE/ACE/AME Task Force on Thyroid Nodules American association of clinical endocrinologist, american college of endocrinology, and associazione medici endocrinologi medical guidelines for clinical practice for the diagnosis and management of thyroid nodules: 2016 update. *Endocrin. Pract.* **2016**, *22*, 622–639.
19. National comprehensive Cancer Network. *NCCN Clinical Practice Guidelines in Oncology and (NCCN Guidelines) and Thyroid Carcinoma (Version 2.2014)*; National Comprehensive Cancer Network: Washington, DC, USA, 2014.
20. Atilla, F.D.; Saydam, B.O.; Erarslan, N.A.; Unlu, A.G.; Yasar, H.Y.; Ozer, M.; Akinci, B. Does the ACR TIRADS scoring allow us to safely avoid nnecessary thyroid biopsy? single center analysis in a large cohort. *Endocrine* **2018**, *61*, 398–402. [CrossRef]
21. Ha, E.J.; Na, D.G.; Back, J.H.; Sung, J.Y.; Kim, J.H.; Kang, S.Y. US fine needle aspiration biopsy for thyroid malignancy: Diagnostic performance of seven society guidelines applied to 2000thyroid nodules. *Radiology* **2018**, *287*, 893–900. [CrossRef]
22. Eze, O.P.; Cai, G.; Baloch, Z.W.; Khan, A.; Virk, R.; Hammers, L.W.; Udelsman, R.; Roman, S.A.; Sosa, J.A.; Carling, T.; et al. Vanishing thyroid tumors. A diagnostic dilemma after ultrasonography-guided fine needle aspiration. *Thyroid* **2013**, *23*, 194–200. [CrossRef] [PubMed]
23. Bhatia, P.; Deniwar, A.; Mohamed, H.E.; Sholl, A.; Murad, F.; Aslam, R.; Kandil, E.; Bhatia, P. Vanishing tumors of thyroid: Histological variations after fine needle aspiration. *Gland Surg.* **2016**, *5*, 270–277. [CrossRef] [PubMed]

24. Kholová, I. Vanishing thyroid gland tumors: Infarction as consequence of FNA? *Diagn. Cytopathol.* **2016**, *44*, 568–573. [CrossRef] [PubMed]
25. Shayganfar, A.; Hashemi, P.; Esfahani, M.M.; Ghanei, A.M.; Moghadam, N.A.; Ebrahimian, S. Prediction of thryoid nodule malignncy using thyroid imaging reporting and data system (TI-RADS) and nodule size. *Clin. Imag.* **2020**, *60*, 232–237. [CrossRef] [PubMed]
26. Barbosa, T.L.M.; Junior, C.O.M.; Graf, H.; Cavalvanti, T.; Trippia, M.A.; da Silveira Ugino, R.T.; de Oliveira, G.L.; Granella, V.H.; de Carvalho, G.A. ACR TI-RADS and ATA US scores are helful for the management of thyroid nodules with indeterminate cytology. *BMC Endocr. Disord.* **2019**, *19*, 112. [CrossRef] [PubMed]
27. Zhang, Y.; Zhou, P.; Tian, S.M. Usefulness of combined use of contrast-enhanced ultrasound and TI-RADS classification for the differentiation of benign from malignant lesions of thyroid nodules. *Eur. Radiol.* **2017**, *27*, 1527–1536. [CrossRef]
28. Maia, F.F.R.; Matos, P.S.; Pavin, E.J.; Vassallo, J.; Zantut-Wittmann, D.E. Thyroid imaging reporting and data system score combined with Bethesda system for malignncy risk stratification in thyroid nodules with indeterminate results on cytology. *Clin. Endocrinol.* **2015**, *82*, 439–444. [CrossRef] [PubMed]
29. Rocha, T.G.; Rosario, P.W.; Silva, A.L.; Nunes, M.B.; Calsolari, M.R. Ultrasonography classification of the american thyroid association for predicting malignancy in thyroid nodules >1cm with indterminate cytology: A proscpective study authors. *Horm. Metab. Res.* **2018**, *50*, 597–601.
30. Chaigeau, R.; Russ, G.; Royer, B.; Bigorgne, C.; Bienvenu-Perrard, M.; Rouxel, A.; Leenhardt, L.; Belin, L.; Buffet, C. TI-RADS score is of limited clinical value for risk stratification of indeterminate cytological reslults. *Eur. J. Endocrinol.* **2018**, *179*, 13–20. [CrossRef] [PubMed]
31. Valderrabano, P.; Mcgettigan, M.J.; Iam, C.A. Thyroid nodules with indeterminate cytology: Utility of the american thyroid association sonographic patterns for cancer risk. *Thyroid* **2018**, *28*, 1–29. [CrossRef]
32. Rahal, A.J.; Falsarella, P.M.; Rocha, R.D.; Lima, J.P.; Iani, M.J.; Vieira, F.A.; Queiroz, M.R.; Hidal, J.T.; Francisco Neto, M.J.; Garcia, R.G.; et al. Correlation of thyroid imaging reporting and data system (TI-RADS) and fine needle aspiration: Experience in 1000 nodules. *Einstein* **2016**, *14*, 119–123. [CrossRef] [PubMed]
33. Grani, G.; Lamartina, L.; Ascoli, V.; Bosco, D.; Biffoni, M.; Giacomelli, L.; Maranghi, M.; Falcone, R.; Ramundo, V.; Cantisani, V.; et al. Reducing the number of unnecessary thyroid biopsies while improving diagnostic accuracy: Toward the right TIRADS. *J. Clin. Endocrinol. Metab.* **2019**, *104*, 95–102. [CrossRef]
34. Friedrich-Rust, M.; Meyer, G.; Dauth, N.; Berner, C.; Bogdanou, D.; Herrmann, E.; Zeuzem, S.; Bojunga, J. Interobserver agreement of thyroid imaging reporting and data system (TI-RADS) and strain elastography for the assessment of thyroid nodules. *PLoS ONE* **2013**, *8*, e77927. [CrossRef]
35. Middleton, W.D.; Teefey, S.A.; Reading, C.C.; Langer, J.E.; Beland, M.D.; Szabunio, M.M.; Desser, T.S. Comparison of performance characteristics of American college of radiology TI-RADS, Korean society of thyroid radiology TIRADS, and American thyroid association guidelines. *Am. J. Roentgenol.* **2018**, *210*, 1148–1154. [CrossRef] [PubMed]
36. Lee, Y.H.; Kim, D.W.; In, H.S.; Park, J.S.; Kim, S.H.; Eom, J.W.; Kim, B.; Lee, E.J.; Rho, M.H. Differentation between benign and malignant solid thyroid nodules using an US classification system. *Korean J. Radiol.* **2011**, *12*, 559–567. [CrossRef] [PubMed]
37. Yang, G.C.H.; Fried, K.O.; Scognamiglio, T. Can cytology and the Thyroid Imaging, Reporting, and Data System (TI-RADS) identify noninvasive follicular thyroid neoplasm with papillary-like nuclear features (NIFTP) before surgery. *J. Am. Soc. Cytopathol.* **2020**, *9*, 159–165. [CrossRef] [PubMed]
38. Yang, G.C.; Fried, K.O.; Scognamiglio, T. Sonographic and cytologic differences of NIFTP from infiltrative or invasive encapsulated follicular variant of papillary thyroid carcinoma. A Review of 179 Cases. *Diagn. Cytopath.* **2017**, *45*, 533–541. [CrossRef] [PubMed]
39. Wu, M. A correlation study between thyroid imaging report and data systems and the Bethesda system for reporting thyroid cytology with surgical follow-up—An ultrasound-trained cytopathologist's experience. *Diagn. Cytopathol.* **2020**. [CrossRef]
40. Weller, A.; Sharif, B.; Qarib, M.H.; St Leger, D.; De Silva, H.S.; Lingam, R.K. British thyroid association 2014 classification ultrasound scoring of thyroid nodules in predicting malignncy: Diagnostic performance and inter-observer agreement. *Ultrasound* **2020**, *28*, 4–13. [CrossRef]
41. Cross, P.; Chandra, A.; Giles, T.; Johnson, S.; Kocjan, G.; Poller, D.; Stephenson, T. *Guidance on the Reporting of Thyroid Cytologyspecimens*; Royal College of Pathologists: London, UK, 2009. Available online: http://wwwrcpathorg/Resources/RCPath/ (accessed on 1 January 2016).
42. Brophy, C.; Mehanna, R.; McCarthy, J.; Tuthill, A.; Murphy, M.S.; Sheahan, P. Outcome of subclassification of indeterminate (Thy 3) thyroid cytology into Thy 3a and Thy 3f. *Eur. Thyroid. J.* **2015**, *4*, 246–251. [CrossRef]
43. Maia, F.F.; Matos, P.S.; Pavin, E.J.; Zantut-Wittmann, D.E. Thyroid imaging reporting and data system score combined with the new italian classification for thyroid cytology improves the clinical management of indeterminate nodules. *Int. J. Endocrinol.* **2017**. [CrossRef]
44. Chng, C.L.; Kurzawinski, T.R.; Beale, T. Value of sonographic features in predicting malignancy in thyroid nodules diagnosed as follicular neoplasm on cytology. *Clin. Endocrinol.* **2015**, *83*, 711–716. [CrossRef]
45. Moon, W.J.; Baek, J.H.; Jung, S.L.; Kim, D.W.; Kim, E.K.; Kim, J.Y.; Kwak, J.Y.; Lee, J.H.; Lee, J.H.; Lee, Y.H.; et al. Ultrasonography and the ultrasound-based management of thyroid nodules: Consensus statement and recommendations. *Korean J. Radiol.* **2011**, *12*, 1–14. [CrossRef] [PubMed]

46. Rosario, P.W.; da Silva, A.L.; Nunes, M.B.; Borges, M.A.R. Risk of Malignancy in Thyroid Nodules Using the American College of Radiology Thyroid Imaging Reporting and Data System in the NIFTP Era. *Horm. Metab. Res.* **2018**, *50*, 735–737. [CrossRef] [PubMed]
47. Singaporewalla, R.M.; Hwee, J.; Lang, T.U.; Desai, V. Clinico-pathological Correlation of Thyroid Nodule Ultrasound and Cytology Using the TIRADS and Bethesda Classifications. *World J. Surg.* **2017**, *41*, 1807–1811. [CrossRef] [PubMed]
48. Tan, H.; Li, Z.; Li, N.; Qian, J.; Fan, F.; Zhong, H.; Feng, J.; Xu, H.; Li, Z. Thyroid imaging reporting and data system combined with Bethesda classification in qualitative thyroid nodule diagnosis. *Medicine* **2019**, *98*, 50. [CrossRef] [PubMed]

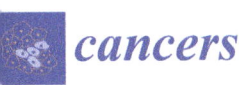

Systematic Review

Current Status and Challenges of US-Guided Radiofrequency Ablation of Thyroid Nodules in the Long Term: A Systematic Review

Stella Bernardi [1,2,*], Andrea Palermo [3], Rosario Francesco Grasso [4], Bruno Fabris [1,2], Fulvio Stacul [5] and Roberto Cesareo [6]

1. Department of Medical Sciences, University of Trieste, 34149 Trieste, Italy; b.fabris@fmc.units.it
2. U.C.O. Medicina Clinica, ASUGI (Azienda Sanitaria Universitaria Giuliano Isontina), Cattinara Hospital, 34149 Trieste, Italy
3. Unità di Endocrinologia e Diabete, Policlinico Universitario Campus Bio-Medico, 00128 Roma, Italy; a.palermo@unicampus.it
4. U.O.S. Radiologia Interventistica, Policlinico Universitario Campus Bio-Medico, 00128 Roma, Italy; r.grasso@unicampus.it
5. S.C. Radiologia, ASUGI (Azienda Sanitaria Universitaria Giuliano Isontina), Maggiore Hospital, 34125 Trieste, Italy; stacul.fulvio@gmail.com
6. U.O.S. Malattie Metaboliche, Ospedale Santa Maria Goretti, 04100 Latina, Italy; robertocesareo@libero.it
* Correspondence: stella.bernardi@asugi.sanita.fvg.it or shiningstella@gmail.com; Tel.: +39-04-0399-4318

Simple Summary: Ultrasound (US)-guided minimally-invasive techniques, such as radiofrequency ablation (RFA) have emerged as an alternative treatment to surgery for benign and malignant thyroid nodules. Based on a systematic literature search, here we report the long-term outcomes of thyroid RFA. Available data show that US-guided RFA significantly reduced benign thyroid nodules and destroyed most PTMC, and this was generally maintained for at least 5 years after the initial treatment. Further studies addressing the risk of regrowth in patients with benign thyroid nodules, as well as the risk of recurrence in patients with PTMC are needed.

Abstract: Background: US-guided minimally-invasive techniques, such as radiofrequency ablation (RFA) have emerged as an alternative treatment for benign and malignant thyroid nodules. This systematic review aims to provide an overview on the long-term outcomes of US-guided RFA in patients with benign and malignant thyroid nodules. Methods: We systematically searched PubMed/MEDLINE, EMBASE, and Scopus to identify articles reporting the outcomes of thyroid RFA after a follow-up of at least 3 years. Results: A total of 20 studies met the inclusion criteria and were included in the review. In patients with benign thyroid nodules, RFA significantly reduced nodule volume and this was generally maintained for the following 5 years. However, a small but not negligible proportion of nodules regrew and some of them required further treatments over time. In patients with malignant nodules, RFA has been used not only to treat differentiated thyroid cancer (DTC) neck recurrences, but also to treat papillary thyroid microcarcinoma (PTMC). In most patients with PTMC, RFA led to complete disappearance of the tumor. When it was compared to surgery, RFA was not inferior in terms of oncologic efficacy but it had a lower complication rate. However, RFA did not allow for final pathology, disease staging and accurate risk stratification. Conclusions: US-guided RFA significantly reduces benign thyroid nodules and destroys most PTMC, and this is generally maintained for at least 5 years after the initial treatment. Further studies addressing the risk of regrowths in patients with benign thyroid nodules, as well as the risk of recurrence in patients with PTMC are needed.

Keywords: US-guided minimally invasive techniques; radiofrequency ablation; RFA; benign thyroid nodules; thyroid cancer; DTC recurrences; PTMC; long term; follow-up; regrowth

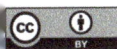

1. Introduction

Since the 80s, ultrasound (US) has played an increasingly important role in thyroid nodule assessment [1]. Beside thyroid nodule diagnosis, US has also been used for therapeutic purposes. In the last decade, US-guided minimally invasive techniques have been introduced into clinical practice as an alternative treatment for benign thyroid nodules as well as selected cases of differentiated thyroid cancer (DTC) [2–6]—such as neck recurrences or cases of low risk disease. These techniques go far beyond ethanol ablation, which has been the first technique to be introduced in the 90s [7], and they include laser, radiofrequency and microwave ablation, as well as HIFU [8]. A recent European survey on the use of US-guided minimally invasive techniques for thyroid nodules [9] showed that today RFA is the most frequently chosen, and so far it has been the most thoroughly assessed one.

US-guided RFA is an outpatient procedure, which is generally performed under local anesthesia [10,11]. It requires the US-guided insertion of a probe through the skin of the neck into the thyroid nodule. The probe tip generates heat which induces rapid heating and destruction of the target zone (i.e., one part of the nodule). Then, in order to treat an entire nodule, RFA is usually performed with the moving-shot technique, whereby the probe tip is sequentially moved from the medial to the lateral parts of the nodule, while it is slowly withdrawn towards the surface. Treatment is accompanied by the formation of coagulative necrosis, and over time, by fibrotic changes and progressive nodule shrinkage [5,11].

Several studies have demonstrated that this procedure is safe and effective, as it induces a significant reduction of benign thyroid nodule volume with improvement of local symptoms and cosmetic concerns [12,13], while in case of low-risk thyroid cancer, it is able to destroy the entire target zone [14–17]. In addition, in case of DTC neck recurrences or papillary thyroid microcarcinoma (PTMC), RFA has a similar efficacy and lower rate of complications than surgery [18–20]. Based on this background, accumulating evidence suggests that US-guided RFA could be used as a first line therapy not only for benign thyroid nodules but also for low-risk thyroid cancer.

Last year, one of the main focuses of the original articles that were published on thyroid RFA were its long-term outcomes [3,16,17,20–23], namely the volume reduction ratio and/or regrowths in patients with benign nodules and the recurrence rates in patients with malignant ones. Based on this, the aim of this systematic review was to provide an overview on these long-term outcomes of US-guided RFA in patients with either benign or malignant thyroid nodules, as well as to discuss its strengths and limitations.

2. Materials and Methods

The aim of this systematic review was to describe RFA long-term outcomes. Our primary outcome measure was volume reduction ratio. Our secondary outcome measures were regrowths in benign nodules and recurrence rates in malignant nodules. Based on the available literature on this topic, RFA long-term follow-up has been defined as a period of at least 3 years [24].

This systematic review was conducted following the PRISMA checklist. We conducted a systematic literature search on PubMed/Medline, EMBASE, Scopus to select all the studies reporting the follow-up of patients treated with RFA. The query included the terms "Radiofrequency", "RFA", "Thyroid" and "Follow-up". To expand our search, references of the retrieved articles were also screened for other data. Further literature search was done based on these result and from the PubMed option "Related Articles". The search was last updated on 28 February 2021.

Figure 1 shows the stepwise procedure for study selection. We retrieved a total of 421 results. Studies were examined and selected for inclusion independently by two investigators (S.B. and A.P.) and a third one (R.C.) was consulted in case of controversy. Investigators were not blinded to authors, institutions, journals, or interventions while selecting studies. Inclusion criteria were as follows: (i) original studies; (ii) thyroid RFA; (iii) follow-up of at least three years. Exclusion criteria of studies were as follows: (i) studies not written in English; (ii) wrong publication types (reviews, meta-analysis, study protocols, case reports, letters, errata, conference proceedings, book chapters); (iii) wrong population (i.e., RFA performed on other tissues and organs); (iv) wrong outcome (i.e., follow-up shorter than three years). Studies were also excluded if relevant information regarding the study design or outcomes was unclear or if there was any doubt regarding duplicate publications. At the end of our qualitative analysis, we identified 20 studies. The paper by Kim et al. was included in our analysis because initial follow-up after RFA was 37.7 ± 10.8 months [18].

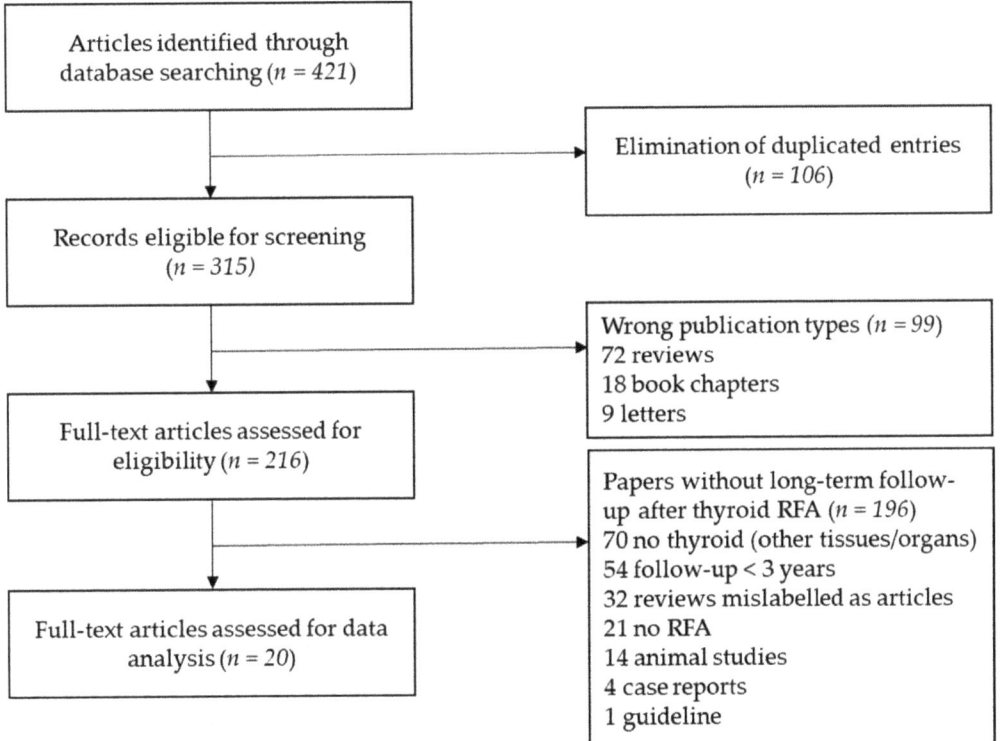

Figure 1. Stepwise procedure for study selection.

In order to assess the risk of bias of the included studies, we used the Cochrane Collaboration tool, namely the RoBANS [24]. Two authors (S.B. and B.F.) independently extracted data on study design, patient characteristics, RFA technique, volume reduction ratio, and follow-up and assessed risk of bias of included studies. Disagreements were resolved through discussion. The RoBANS assesses six domains of bias, specifically (D1) bias due to selection of participants, (D2) bias due to confounding variables, (D3) bias due to measurement of intervention, (D4) bias due to blinding of outcome assessment, (D5) incomplete outcome data follow-up, (D6) selective outcome reporting. In case of D1 we took into account if age, sex, nodule volume and cytology/pathology were specified. In case of D2 we took into account if RFA technique, number of RFA, and energy delivered were specified, in case of D3 we took into account if volume reduction ratio was specified, in case of D5 we took into account the number (proportion) of patient that were seen during follow-up. Traffic-light plots of risk of bias were designed using the robvis visualization tool [25].

3. Results

3.1. Long-Term Outcomes of RFA on Benign Thyroid Nodules

We identified a total of nine articles reporting the outcomes of RFA on benign thyroid nodules after a follow-up of at least three years (Tables 1 and 2). Eight studies were retrospective and one study was prospective. Overall, these studies showed that RFA-induced volume reduction ratio ranged between 66.9% and 97.9% after three years from the procedure. Regrowth was observed in 4.1–24.1% of nodules. Bias assessment is reported in Figure 2.

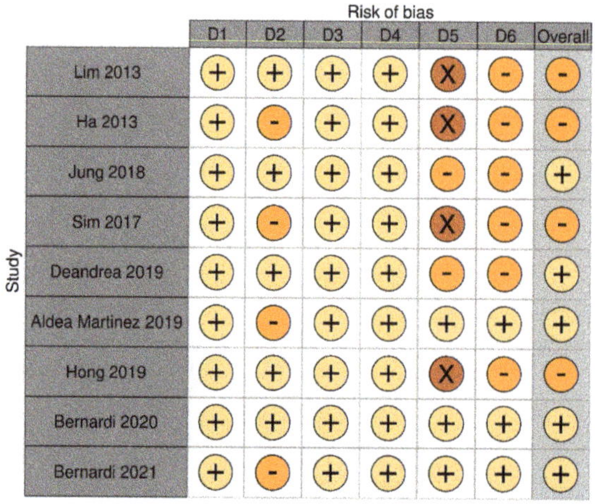

Figure 2. Bias assessment of studies on RFA long-term outcomes in patients with benign thyroid nodules. Risk of bias was classified as low (+) (pale yellow), unclear (-) (orange) or high (x) (brown). Risk of bias was based on the judgement of domains D1–D6. D1 is for selection of participants; D2 is for confounding variables; D3 is for measurement of intervention (VRR); D4 is for blinding of outcome assessment; D5 is for incomplete outcome data during follow-up; D6 is for selective outcome reporting. Risk of bias was judged unclear in D2 when number of RFA sessions or energy delivered were not specified. Risk of bias was judged high in D5 when the number of patients seen at specific follow-up time points was not specified. Risk of bias was judged unclear in D5 when the number of patients was lower than 80% of patients enrolled. Risk of bias in D6 was based on D5.

Table 1. Main findings of studies on RFA long-term outcomes in patients with benign thyroid nodules.

Study	Main Findings
Lim 2013 [26]	RFA was effective in reducing nodule volume and nodule-related problems such as symptoms and cosmetic concerns (mean VRR was 93.4% at last follow-up). Regrowth rate was 5.6%.
Ha 2013 [27]	RFA reduced nodule volume by 87.2% at last follow-up and it did not affect thyroid function in patients with previous lobectomy.
Jung 2018 [28]	Nodule volume was reduced by 80.3% after 1 year (n = 276) and by 95.3% after 5 years (n = 6). Solidity and applied energy predicted final volume reduction.
Sim 2017 [29]	RFA reduced nodule volume by 97.9% at last follow-up. Regrowth was observed in 24.1% of the nodules.
Deandrea 2019 [30]	The VRR that was found at 1 year (63% in 197/215 patients) was maintained at 5 years (67% in 71/215 patients). The best results were obtained in nodules with baseline volume < 10 mL. A total of 4.1% of nodules regrew.
Aldea Martinez 2019 [31]	RFA reduced nodule volume by 76.8% after 3 years (in 24/24 patients).
Hong 2019 [32]	RFA reduced nodule volume by 92.1% at last follow-up in children and adolescents with no complications.
Bernardi 2020 [21]	After propensity score matching, RFA was associated with greater 5-year VRR (75% vs. 56%) and technique efficacy (82% vs. 66%), as well as lower regrowth (17% vs. 34%) and retreatment rate (14% vs. 32%) as compared to LA. Young age, large volume, low 1-year VRR, and low energy delivered were associated with retreatments.
Bernardi 2021 [22]	RFA reduced nodule volume by 79% after 5 years (in 78/78 patients). IAR was significantly associated with technique efficacy, VRR, and the likelihood of retreatment but not with regrowth. IAR cut-off were >49% for technique efficacy and >73% for no retreatment.

IAR initial ablation ratio, LA is for laser ablation, RFA is for radiofrequency ablation, VRR is for volume reduction ratio.

Table 2. Main characteristics of studies on RFA long-term outcomes in patients with benign thyroid nodules.

Study	Design	Patients/Nodules *	Age (yrs)	Sex (F%)	Volume (mL)	Diameter (mm)	RFA (n)	Energy (J/mL)	VRR (%)	Follow-Up (Months)
Lim 2013 [26]	Retrospective	111/126	37.9 ± 10.6 (9–69)	91	9.8 ± 8.5 (2–43)	33 ± 10 (20–60)	1–6	2936 ± 1995 (271–9943)	93.5 ± 11.7 (17–100)	49.4 ± 13.6 (36–81)
Ha 2013 [27]	Retrospective	11/14	44.2 (30–64)	100	9.7 ± 36.3 (0.9–57.6)	29 ± 24 (15–60)	n.s	n.s.	87.2	43.7 ± 30.7 (7–92)
Jung 2018 [28]	Prospective	276/276	46.3 ± 12.8 (15–79)	88	14.2 ± 13.2 (1.1–80.8)	38 ± 11 (19–80)	1–2	4161 ± 2993 (656–22,031)	95.3 ± 4.3 (88.5–100)	60
Sim 2017 [29]	Retrospective	52/54	44.1 ± 13.2 (20–78)	91	14 ± 12.7 (3.1–56.6)	38 ± 11 (19–77)	1–?	n.s.	97.9	39.4 ± 21.7 (13–87)
Deandrea 2019 [30]	Retrospective	215/215	66# (60–88)	85	20.9# (15–33)	n.s.	1	2210# (1400–3080)	66.9#	60
Aldea Martinez 2019 [31]	Prospective	24/24	50.2 ± 13.6	83	36.3 ± 59.8 (0.7–231.6)	n.s.	1–?	1180 ± 716	76.8 ± 15.9	36
Hong 2019 [32]	Retrospective	15/15	15.7 ± 2.3 (12–19)	71	14.6 ± 13.3 (1.6–49.8)	37 ± 11 (20–56)	1–5	3153 ± 2065 (782–7504)	92.1 ± 11.4 (6–69)	36.9 ± 21.7
Bernardi 2020 [21]	Retrospective	216/216	57# (17–87)	75	17.2# (0.4–179)	n.s.	1	1398# (176–2410)	77.1# (−34.5–100)	60
Bernardi 2021 [33]	Retrospective	78/82	59.5# (18–86)	76	11.3# (0.4–54.6)	23.5# (17.3–30.1)	1	n.s.	79	60

Continuous variables are reported as mean ± SD [min—max] or median# [min—max]. "n" is for number, "n.s." is for not specified, VRR is for volume reduction ratio (at last follow-up). # Median values. * The number of patients/nodules refers to the groups treated with RFA (before matching).

The first retrospective study of this series was that of Lim et al. [26], who reported the outcomes of thyroid RFA on 111 patients (with 126 benign non-functioning nodules) after a follow-up duration of at least 3 years (mean follow-up length was 49.4 months, range 36–81 months). After a mean number of 2.2 ± 1.4 sessions, the Authors found that nodule volume was reduced by 70%, 90%, 90%, 90%, and 93.5% after 6 months, 1 year, 2 years, 3 years, and at last follow-up. This was associated with a significant amelioration of local symptoms and cosmetic concerns. Baseline nodule volume and solidity were independently associated with final volume reduction. Regrowth rate (i.e., an increase in nodule volume > 50% as compared with previous US examination) was 5.6%. Complication rate was 3.6% (4/111 patients), and they included voice change, brachial plexus injury, bruising and vomiting. The authors concluded that RFA is a safe and effective method and it can be used as a non-surgical treatment for patients with non-functioning benign thyroid nodules [26].

The subsequent studies confirmed most of these findings [26,28,30,31]. In particular, the efficacy and safety of RFA for the treatment of benign thyroid nodules have been confirmed by a prospective study [28] reporting RFA outcomes on 276 patients (with 276 nodules) treated on average with 1.3 sessions and followed for 46 months (range 15–79). In this study, nodule volume was reduced by 80%, 89%, 92%, and 95%, after 1, 2, 3, and 4 years from the procedure. Solidity and energy delivered were independent factors that predicted the final volume reduction. The overall complication rate was 5.1% (major complication rate was 1.1%), while side-effects occurred in 4.7% of the patients [28].

Contrary to the first studies evaluating the effects of multiple RFA sessions, Deandrea et al. reported the outcomes of one single session of RFA on 215 patients (with 215 nodules) followed for at least 3 years, showing that nodule volume was reduced by 67% at last follow-up. In this study, the nodules with a baseline volume < 10 mL showed the best response as their volume was reduced by 81% at last follow-up. This was associated with a significant amelioration of symptom and cosmetic scores. Regrowth, which was defined according to Lim et al. [26], occurred in 4.1% of nodules. There were no major complications, but only minor occurrences and side-effects, whose rates were 8.8% and 10%. Minor occurrences included hypotension, swelling, bruising, neck pain, fever and cough [30].

Other studies have extended these findings, showing that RFA does not modify thyroid function even in patients with previous lobectomy [34], such that the authors concluded that it can be considered as a first-line treatment for symptomatic benign thyroid nodules in order to preserve thyroid function. In addition, it has also been shown that RFA is effective and safe for non-functioning thyroid nodules in children and adolescents [32].

As opposed to the first long-term follow-up studies that focused primarily on the efficacy and safety of the technique, the most recent ones have brought up the issue of retreatment and regrowth [21,22,29], as defined by a recent proposal for standardization of terminology and reporting criteria [35]. Based on this proposal, nodule regrowth should be defined as a $\geq 50\%$ increase compared to the minimum recorded volume measured at a given follow-up time point [35]. In the work by Sim et al., 52 patients (54 nodules) were followed for 39 months (range 13–87 months) after thyroid RFA. Mean volume reduction ratio (VRR) after the first procedure was 77% and 97.9% at last follow-up. Complication rate was 3.6% and side effect rate was 3.6%. In this study, 24.1% of the nodules regrew after a mean time of approximately 40 months, as assessed by the new definition [35]. The authors suggested that it is the residual vital volume increase what may cause/precede regrowth [29].

Consistent with these findings, we have recently evaluated the 5-year outcomes of one RFA and compared it to laser ablation (LA) in a cohort of 406 patients, 216 of whom were treated with RFA and the remaining 190 with LA [21]. It has to be noted that in this study, all patients were followed for at least five years after the procedure. Overall, RFA significantly reduced nodule volume, which decreased by 72%, 75%, 76%, 76% and 77% after 1, 2, 3, 4, and 5 years after the ablation. Regrowth was observed in 20% of patients treated with RFA (43/216), however only 12% of the patients were retreated, due to the fact that regrowth is not always associated with symptom relapse. After propensity score matching analysis, RFA was associated with greater volume reduction ratio (75% vs. 56%), technique efficacy (82% vs. 66%), as well as lower regrowth (17% vs. 34%) and retreatment rate (14% vs. 32%) as compared to LA. On logistic regression model analyses, energy delivered was the only parameter that was associated with technique inefficacy (cut-off was 1360 J/mL) and with regrowth (but the low AUC did not allow to elaborate any cut-off). Younger age, larger baseline volume, lower amount of energy (cut-off 918 J/mL) were associated with likelihood of retreatment [21].

Given that in the aforementioned work, we could not identify predictors of regrowth, we evaluated if the initial ablation ratio (IAR), which is a semiquantitative index that measures the amount of the ablated area, could predict regrowth [22]. For this reason, we analysed RFA outcomes on 78 patients (82 nodules) that were followed for 5 years after the procedure. Technique efficacy (i.e., volume reduction > 50% after 1 year) was achieved in 92% of patients, 23% of nodules regrew and 12% of nodules were retreated. Median IAR was 83%. IAR was significantly associated with technique efficacy, VRR, and with the likelihood of retreatment, but not with nodule regrowth [22]. In particular, an IAR > 49% was a good predictor of technique efficacy and an IAR > 73% was a good predictor of no retreatment in the five years following the procedure [22].

3.2. Long-Term Outcomes of RFA on Malignant Thyroid Nodules

We identified a total of 11 articles reporting the outcomes of RFA on malignant thyroid nodules after a follow-up of at least 3 years (Tables 3–5). All these studies were retrospective. Five studies evaluated RFA outcomes on differentiated thyroid cancer (DTC) neck recurrences, while the remaining six studies evaluated it on papillary thyroid microcarcinomas (PTMC), low risk papillary carcinoma, and small follicular neoplasms. Overall, these studies showed that RFA-induced volume reduction ratio ranged between 81.2% and 99.5% in DTC neck recurrences, between 98.5% and 100% in PTMC, and that it was 99.5% in follicular neoplasms. With respect to local recurrences, they ranged between 6.25% and 27% in DTC neck recurrences, and 0% and 4% in PTMC. Bias assessment is reported in Figure 3.

Table 3. Main findings of studies on RFA long-term outcomes in patients with malignant thyroid nodules.

Study	Main Findings
	DTC Neck Tecurrences
Monchik 2006 [36]	No recurrent disease was detected at the treatment site in 14/16 patients.
Kim 2015 [18]	After IPTW adjustement, the 3-year recurrence-free survival rate after RFA was comparable to surgery (92.6% vs. 92.2%).
Choi 2019 [19]	After PSM, the recurrence-free survival rate after RFA was comparable to surgery (98% vs. 95%).
Chung 2019 [37]	RFA reduced DTC recurrences by 99.5% at 5 years and 91.3% of them disappeared. Local recurrences were seen in 27% of patients.
Chung 2021 [38]	RFA reduced nodule volume by 81.2% and made disappear 124/172 recurrences (72.1%) after 48 months.
	Small Follicular Neoplasm
Ha 2017 [34]	RFA reduced the volume of follicular neoplasms by 99.5% after 5 years. 8 out of 10 lesions (80%) disappeared.
	Low-Risk Papillary Carcinomas/PTMC
Kim 2017 [14]	RFA reduced the volume of papillary carcinoma by 98.5%. 4 out of 6 lesions (66.7%) disappeared. There were no recurrences.
Lim 2019 [15]	RFA led to complete disappearance of 91.4% of PTMC, and the remaining PTMC did not regrow. There were no recurrences.
Zhang 2020 [20]	RFA was not inferior to surgery in terms of recurrences (1.1% vs. 1.3%). The surgery group had a higher complication rate and a lower quality of life than the RFA group.
Cho 2020 [17]	RFA resulted in complete disappearance of all ablated tumors, with no local tumor progression, no lymph-node or distant metastases. 3 patients developed 4 new cancers (4%).
Yan 2021 [16]	VRR was 98%. A total of 88.4% of tumors disappeared. Local tumor progression rate was 3.62%. Recurrence rate was 3.4%.

DTC is for differentiated thyroid cancer, IPTW is for inverse probability of treatment weights, PSM is for propensity score matching, PTMC is for papillary thyroid microcarcinoma, RFA is for radiofrequency ablation, VRR is for volume reduction ratio.

Table 4. Studies on RFA long-term outcomes in patients with DTC neck recurrences.

Study	Design	Patients/Nodules *	Age (yrs)	Sex (F%)	Volume (mL)	Diameter (mm)	RFA (n)	E (J/mL)	VRR (%)	Recur-Rence	Follow-Up (Months)
					DTC Neck Recurrences						
Monchik 2006 [36]	Retrospective	16/16	53 (28–84)	75	n.s.	17 (8–40)	1–6	n.s.	n.s.	1/16 (6.25%)	40.7 (10–68)
Kim 2015 [18]	Retrospective (vs. surgery)	27/36	42.4 ± 10.3	74	n.s.	21.1 ± 1.01	1–2	n.s.	98.4 ± 6.2 (77–100)	3/26 (11.5%)	37.7 ± 10.2
Choi 2019 [19]	Retrospective (vs. surgery)	96/115	47.4 ± 14.1	72	n.s	10 ± 8	1–3	n.s.	n.s.	12/96 (12.5%)	76.9 ± 23
Chung 2019 [37]	Retrospective	29/46	51.8 ± 15 (21–84)	59	0.25 ± 0.4 (0.001–2.3)	8.4 ± 4.7 (3.1–21)	1–3	n.s.	99.5 ± 2.9 (81–100)	8/29 (27%)	80 ± 17.3 (60–114)
Chung 2021 [38]	Retrospective	119/172	50.7 ± 16 (14–83)	72	0.4 ± 1.4 (0.001–12.6)	9 ± 6 (3–41)	1–5	n.s.	81.2 ± 55.7	n.s.	47.9 ± 35.4 (6–128)

Continuous variables are reported as mean ± SD [min-max]. DTC is for differentiated thyroid cancer, "n" is for number, "n.s." is for not specified, RFA is for radiofrequency ablation, VRR is for volume reduction ratio (at last follow-up). * The number of patients/nodules refers to the groups treated with RFA (before matching).

Table 5. Studies on RFA long-term outcomes in patients with low-risk thyroid cancers.

Study	Design	Patients/Nodules *	Age (yrs)	Sex (F%)	Volume (mL)	Diameter (mm)	RFA (n)	E (J/mL)	VRR (%)	Recur-rence	Follow-Up (Months)
					Small Follicular Neoplasm						
Ha 2017 [34]	Retrospective	10/10	45 ± 10.5 (27–74)	100	0.6 ± 0.4 (0.2–1.6)	14 ± 3 (10–19)	1–2	9245 ± 5409 (3976–19,332)	99.5 ± 1 (97–100)	0/10 (0%)	66.4 ± 5.1 (60–76)
					Low-Risk Papillary Carcinomas/PTMC						
Kim 2017 [14]	Retrospective	6/6	72 (64–79)	66	0.3 ± 0.2 (0.05–0.4)	9.2 (6–13)	1–2	n.s.	98.5 ± 3.3 (92–100)	0/6 (0%)	48.5 ± 12.3 (36–65)
Lim 2019 [15]	Retrospective	133/152	46 ± 12 (19–79)	85.7	0.03 ± 0.04 (0.001–0.3)	4.3 ± 1.4 (3–10)	1–2	3169 ± 1423 (600–11,550)	100	0/133 (0%)	39 ± 25 (6–104)
Zhang 2020 [20]	Retrospective (vs surgery)	94/94	45 ± 10.8	74.5	0.17 ± 0.23	6.14 ± 2.54	1	n.s.	n.s.	1/94 (1.1%)	64.2 ± 2.8
Cho 2020 [17]	Retrospective	74/84	46 ± 12	89	0.02 (0.001–0.23)	4 (3–9.9)	1–2	185,237 (13,088–4,716,379)	100	3/74 (4%)	72 ± 18 (60–124)
Yan 2021 [16]	Retrospective	414/414	43.6 ± 9.8 (18–73)	78	0.09 ± 0.08 (0.001–0.5)	5.22 ± 1.59 (2–10)	1–?	n.s.	98.8 ± 6.4 (50–100)	15/414 (3.62%)	42.1 ± 11.9 (24–69)

Continuous variables are reported as mean ± SD [min-max]. "n" is for number, "n.s." is for not specified, PTMC is for papillary thyroid microcarcinoma, RFA is for radiofrequency ablation, VRR is for volume reduction ratio (at last follow-up). * The number of patients/nodules refers to the groups treated with RFA (before matching).

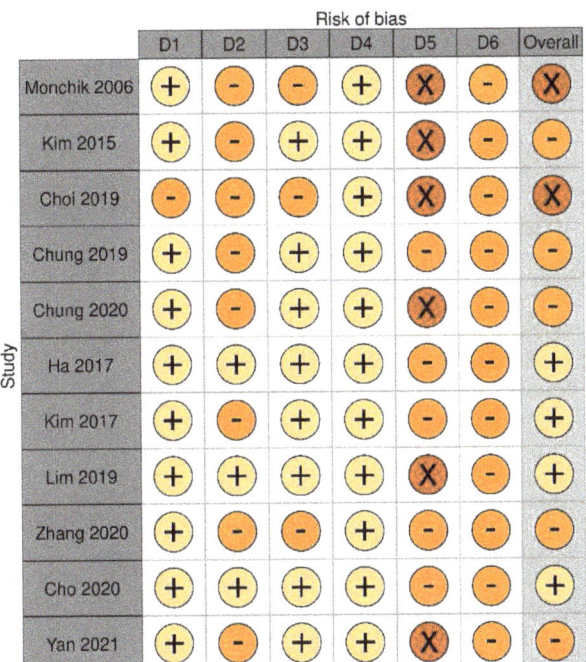

Figure 3. Bias assessment of studies on RFA long-term outcomes in patients with malignant thyroid nodule. Risk of bias was classified as low (+) (pale yellow), unclear (-) (orange) or high (x) (brown). Risk of bias was based on the judgement of domains D1-D6. D1 is for selection of participants; D2 is for confounding variables; D3 is for measurement of intervention (VRR); D4 is for blinding of outcome assessment; D5 is for incomplete outcome data during follow-up; D6 is for selective outcome reporting. Risk of bias was judged unclear in D1 when histology was not specified. Risk of bias was judged unclear in D2 when energy delivered was not specified. Risk of bias was judged unclear in D3 when VRR was not specified. Risk of bias was judged high in D5 when the number of patients seen at specific follow-up time points was not specified, but it was judged unclear if shorter follow-up time was >3 years. Risk of bias in D6 was based on D5.

The use of RFA for the treatment of DTC neck recurrences dates back to the early 2000s [39], and it remains the only indication for thyroid RFA by some authoritative guidelines [40]. In 2006, Monchik et al. reported the outcomes of one or more RFA sessions on DTC neck recurrences in 16 patients that were followed for 41 months (range 10–68 months), showing that only one patient presented with a new recurrence in the neck. RFA caused laryngeal nerve injury in one patient and a 5-mm skin burn in another, as well as neck swelling and regional discomfort [36]. The authors concluded that RFA was a promising alternative to surgical treatment of DTC recurrence in patients with difficult reoperations [36]. Almost a decade after, Chung et al. confirmed that RFA is an effective and safe method for local control of DTC recurrences, as they reported that RFA reduced tumor volume by 99.5% and it induced its disappearance in 91.3% of patients after a mean follow-up of 80 months (range 60–114 months), with no delayed complications [37]. Local recurrences were seen in 27% of patients (8/29) and distant metastases in 6.9% of patients (2/29). Recently, the same authors have demonstrated that in DTC recurrences invading the airways [38], RFA reduced tumor volume by 81.2%, leading to its complete disappearance in 72% of the cases with an overall complication rate of 21.4%. The rate of volume reduction, tumor disappearance and complications were different as those reported previously, due to the inclusion of patients who were treated for curative and palliative purposes for recurrent tumors which were more likely to adhere or invade critical adjacent structures, increasing the complications rate during RFA [38].

A few papers have compared the efficacy and safety of RFA to surgery in the treatment of DTC neck recurrences. In particular, in the first study evaluating recurrences smaller than 2 cm, a total of 27 patients were treated with RFA, which induced a 98.4% volume reduction ratio and made 86% of lesions disappear. Overall, 12.5% of patients had a recurrence after 38 months. Recurrence free-survival rate was 93% and 88% at 1 and 3-year follow-up. After IPTW adjustement, 24 patients treated with RFA were compared to 40 patients treated with surgery and in the end the overall survival rate, as well as the 1- and 3-year recurrence-free survival rates, did not differ between groups, after a follow-up of almost 3 years (32 months) [18]. More recently, 96 patients with DTC neck recurrences were followed for 77 months after being treated with RFA. A total of 11.2% of them had a recurrence. The 3-year and 6-year recurrence-free survival rate was 91% and 89%. A subgroup of 70 patients was compared to 70 patients surgically treated. In this study, the recurrence-free survival rates were comparable between these groups, but the surgery group had a significantly higher rate of hypocalcemia [19].

Only very recently has RFA been used to treat low-risk PTMC. In the first study reporting RFA outcomes on low-risk small papillary thyroid carcinomas after a long-term follow-up, 66.7% lesions (4 out of 6) completely disappeared, while the remaining ones exhibited only small calcified residues [14]. No recurrences were reported after a mean follow-up of 4 years. More recently, in a cohort of 139 patients with 152 PTMC, RFA completely destroyed as many as 91.4% of ablated PTMC, while the remaining ones did not display any sign of regrowth after a mean follow-up duration of 39 months (6–104 months) [15]. When looking at the patients of this cohort with follow-up data of more than 5 years, 74 patients with 84 PTMC were selected for a subsequent study [17]. In these patients, RFA led to complete disappearance of all PTMC. There was no local tumor progression and no lymphnode or distant metastasis. There were four new PTMC in three patients in the remaining thyroid gland, which were ablated by RFA. The rate of minor complications was 4.1% (two hematomas and one first-degree skin burn) and that of major complications was 1.4% (one case of voice change) [17]. Likewise, in a cohort of 414 patients with unifocal PTMC, Yan et al. have recently demonstrated that RFA effectively reduced the target lesion by 98.8% and destroyed it in 88.4% of cases with no significant complications after a follow-up of 42 ± 12 months. In this study, the overall rate of local tumor progression was 3.62% (one persistent PTMC, four lymph node metastasis and 10 cases of new PTMC) [16]. It has to be noted that in a study retrospectively comparing RFA to surgery in case of unifocal PTMC, the Authors did not found any difference in terms of oncologic outcomes after 5 years of follow-up, but surgery took longer, had a longer hospitalization time, and was costlier than RFA [20].

4. Discussion

4.1. The Use of RFA to Treat Benign Thyroid Nodules

The advent of thyroid thermal ablations is likely to significantly change our conventional approach to thyroid nodules. In case of a benign thyroid nodule, patients are generally referred to surgery when they complain of symptoms or cosmetic concerns, while they are followed by US in case they do not. Thyroid thermal ablations, and RFA, represent a new therapeutic alternative in this conventional dichotomous scenario [3]. Randomized clinical trials have shown that RFA significantly reduces thyroid nodule volume and relieves from nodule-related clinical problems, such as local symptoms and cosmetic concerns [12,13]. The procedure does not affect thyroid function in euthyroid patients, and it is safe and extremely well tolerated. Our systematic review shows that RFA induces a volume reduction ratio ranging between 66.9% and 97.9% after 3 years from the procedure. Altogether, these data support the use of RFA to treat benign thyroid nodules, particularly when the target is a single, cold, benign, and symptomatic nodule [5,6,41]. Today, several scientific societies have included the use of minimally invasive techniques among the therapeutic options for symptomatic benign thyroid nodules [4,6,42]. In this new scenario, where observation, surgery and RFA are all viable options, we believe that RFA and surgery are not overlapping techniques, but they should be used to treat different types of nodules as well as different patients. Surgery for example is more effective than one RFA session for treating autonomously functioning nodules or very large nodules [10] (i.e., nodules with volumes > 20 mL). On the other hand, surgery may be unnecessary for treating small but symptomatic benign thyroid nodules that can be effectively managed with an outpatient procedure. This distinction applies also to the other minimally invasive technique, namely laser and microwave ablation or high-intensity focused ultrasound, whose choice depends also on local availability and physician expertise.

In case of benign thyroid nodules, one of the main differences between surgery and RFA is that surgery removes the entire nodule, while RFA reduces it (whereby it reduces patient symptoms). The follow-up studies that have been summarized in this review demonstrate that nodule volume reduction induced by RFA is generally maintained for (at least) 5 years. However, patients should be informed that in the vast majority of the cases a relatively small nodule persists. Some of the studies reviewed have tried to identify predictors of initial volume reduction and retreatment after RFA. These studies have demonstrated that baseline nodule volume, solidity, and applied energy predicted final volume reduction (and the likelihood of any retreatment). Deandrea et al. observed that the best response occurred in nodules with a volume < 10 mL, which were reduced by 82% and remained stable over time. By contrast, nodules with a volume between 10 and 20 mL and with a volume >20 mL were reduced by 75% and 65% respectively [30]. This is consistent with the study by Lim et al., where patients with nodules < 10 mL were treated with 1.7 RFA sessions, while patients with nodules between 10 and 20 mL were treated with 2.8 RFA sessions and patients with nodules > 20 mL were treated with 3.8 RFA sessions [26]. In our multicenter retrospective study, where RFA reduced nodule volume by 72% and 77% after 1 and 5 years from the procedure, and 12% of patients were retreated [21], large baseline volume was significantly associated with the likelihood of being retreated [21]. Of note, in this work, the baseline volume cut-off that predicted retreatment after RFA was 22.1 mL but it had an area under the curve indicating poor accuracy. By contrast, we found that a 1-year volume reduction <66% was a better predictor of nodule retreatment over time [21].

Energy delivered is another parameter that correlates with the volume reduction of benign thyroid nodules (as well as retreatments) [28,43–45]. In our multicenter study, an amount of energy delivered of 1360 J/mL was a moderately accurate predictor of technique efficacy (i.e., volume reduction > 50% after 1 year) and an amount of energy < 918 J/mL was a good predictor of retreatment in the five years following the procedure [21]. Our data are consistent with the recent observation that delivering 756 J/mL, 1311 J/mL, 2109 J/mL was associated with a 50%, 75%, and 95% likelihood of technique efficacy [45].

Recent studies have shown that also the initial ablation ratio (IAR) [46] or the residual vital ratio (RVR) [47] might help predict volume reduction and/or retreatment after RFA [22,33,46,47]. The IAR is a semiquantitative index that measures the amount of ablation after 1–3 months from RFA and it is calculated as follows: IAR = (ablated volume/total volume) × 100 [46]. It has been shown that an IAR > 49% is a good predictor of technique efficacy and an IAR > 73% is a good predictor of no retreatment in the five years that follow the first procedure [22]. On the other hand, the RVR is a similar index that takes into account the viable volume instead of the ablated volume and it is calculated as follows: RVR = (viable volume/total volume) × 100 [33]. As opposed to the IAR, the greater the RVR the lower the likelihood of technique efficacy and the higher the likelihood of being retreated. We have recently found that a RVR > 73% was a moderately accurate predictor of technique inefficacy (i.e., volume reduction < 50% after 1 year) and a RVR > 60% was a good predictor of being retreated in the five years that follow the first procedure [33].

In contrast, the issue that remains to be fully understood is nodule regrowth [48,49]. There are several reasons that might explain such difficulty. First of all, nodule regrowth has been defined in different ways, which makes the existing follow-up studies difficult to compare. In addition, the majority of these studies have incomplete follow-ups, leading to an under or overestimate of regrowth. According to Mauri et al., regrowth is a $\geq 50\%$ nodule volume increase compared to the minimum recorded volume measured at a given follow-up time point [35]. Taking into account this definition, regrowth seems to occur in 20% of patients treated with RFA after 5 years from initial treatment [21,29]. However, we do not know yet if this definition is too broad and might include regrowths that will never become clinically relevant problems. Second, most of the parameters related to volume reduction and retreatment (i.e., baseline volume, energy, IAR) have failed to predict nodule regrowth, apart from the RVR [47].

These data suggest that regrowth may be a distinct process from nodule shrinkage, and there might be other factors accounting for it, such as additional patient characteristics (ethnicity and iodine status for instance), as well as the nodule behaviour and/or technical issues. These technical issues include the operator experience, the lack of treatment of the nodule's margins [29,48] or the lack of treatment of the feeding artery [50] and the draining vein, the latter of which is usually located at the nodule margins. Also the size and the position of the nodule influence the quality of an RFA treatment, given that the moving-shot technique (i.e., the probe repositioning) is tailored to the patient nodule and in large nodules or nodules whose location is close to critical structures it is difficult to treat the entire nodule [47]. In these cases, contrast-enhanced rather than non-enhanced ultrasound might provide useful information on the treatment outcome [51,52]. Additional classifiers based not only on clinical and US features, but also on molecular markers [53] and artificial intelligence might help predict treatment response as well as nodule behaviour over time [54].

4.2. The Use of RFA to Treat Differentiated Thyroid Cancer

The use of RFA is recommended by current guidelines in patients with suspected structural DTC neck recurrences [4,40]. In this circumstance, the use of RFA has been associated with volume reductions ranging from 55% to 95% and complete disappearance of metastatic foci in 40–90% of cases [36,55]. The few long-term follow-up studies that are available demonstrate that RFA is a promising alternative to surgical treatment in this setting, and this is confirmed by the fact that RFA and surgery have shown comparable recurrence-free survival rates [19].

By contrast, the use of RFA to treat PTMC or low-risk thyroid carcinoma has only recently been explored. The possibility to treat with RFA patients with PTMC or low-risk thyroid carcinoma unable or unwilling to undergo surgery has been introduced for the first time by the 2017 Korean Society of Thyroid Radiology guidelines [4]. Available studies show that when RFA is used to treat PTMC, it can effectively destroy the entire nodule, such that after 5 years from the procedure the ablation site reliably and consistently demonstrates no evidence of viable tumor [17]. In addition, Zhang et al. have recently shown that recurrence rates did not differ between RFA and surgery and that RFA had a lower complication rate and a higher quality of life than surgery [20]. Based on this ground, RFA could become a third therapeutic option in a scenario where the choices are either active surveillance or surgery.

The basic goals of initial therapy for patients with differentiated thyroid cancer are not only to improve overall and disease-specific survival and reduce the risk of persistent/recurrent disease, but also to permit accurate disease staging and risk stratification [40]. Surgery is the only approach that can remove the primary tumor and permit accurate staging and risk stratification of the disease [40].

Nevertheless, the ATA guidelines have recently introduced the possibility of chosing an active surveillance approach in case of patients with very low risk tumors, such as PTMC without clinically evident metastases or local invasion and no cytologic/genetic evidence of aggressive disease [40]. This is based on the observation that loco-regional recurrence rates, distant recurrence rates, and mortality rates do not differ between patients with PTMC who underwent surgery and those who were only followed up [40]. Ito et al. followed 1235 patients with PTMC for an average 5–6 years (up to 15 years), and 1.5% of them showed lymph node metastases, 3.5% showed progression to clinical disease, 4.6% showed tumor size enlargement [56], indicating that PTMC have an indolent nature.

Having said that, if RFA became a third option for PTMC, it would have some limitations/drawbacks. As compared to surgery, for example, RFA does not allow for identification of additional foci of PTMC as well as micrometastases in the central neck compartment [3]. As compared to active surveillance, on the other hand, if patients with PTMC were treated with RFA, it is not entirely clear how to monitor them, given that during active surveillance, the primary biomarker to signal that surgical intervention is warranted is the change in size of the primary tumor [23]. On this ground, we believe that studies on larger cohorts of patients followed for a longer period of time are needed to understand if the risk of disease recurrence and metastatic spread after RFA will not differ from surgery or the active surveillance approach [23].

4.3. What Do the Guidelines State about the Use of RFA

Based on some of these and other pioneering studies, several authoritative international societies have included RFA among the treatment modalities for thyroid nodule management and/or have established specific recommendations for the use of RFA.

In 2016, the American Association of Clinical Endocrinologists (AACE) introduced the possibility to use laser or radiofrequency ablation for the treatment of solid or complex thyroid nodules that progressively enlarge or are symptomatic or cause cosmetic concerns, after repeating fine-needle aspiration for cytology confirmation [42]. On the other hand, in the same years, the American Thyroid Associations (ATA) suggested the use of RFA only in case of structural neck recurrences of DTC (particularly in case of lesions measuring > 10 mm), in high-risk surgical patients or patients refusing additional surgery [40]. Here RFA was also taken into account in case of liver, lung, and bone metastases in patients iodine-refractory metastatic DTC [40].

A few scientific societies and national working groups have developed also specific practice guidelines on the use of thermal ablations for the treatment of thyroid nodules. The principal and most recent statements have been issued by the following groups: the Korean Society of Thyroid Radiology (KSThR) [4], the Italian working group on minimally invasive treatments of the thyroid (MITT) [5], interdisciplinary working groups of German and Austrian professional associations [57,58], and the European Thyroid Association (ETA) [6,59]. The principal indication is the treatment of non-functioning benign nodules that are symptomatic, although the use of RFA can be taken into account in case of autonomously functioning thyroid nodules when radioiodine or surgery are contraindicated or unwanted. The Korean and Austrian statements include also the treatment of local recurrences of iodine-refractory thyroid carcinoma, while the use of RFA in "low-risk" papillary PTMC is taken into account by the KSThR as well as by the ETA [59], while it remains an area "under discussion" [58] for the Austrian working group.

As far as benign thyroid nodules are concerned, this systematic review shows that the best RFA results have been generally obtained in nodules with baseline volume < 10–20 mL [21,26,30]. Therefore, we believe that RFA should be used to treat preferentially symptomatic benign lesions if their volume does not exceed 20–30 mL (unless they are cystic or predominantly cystic). Our results highlight also that the best RFA results have been generally obtained when energy delivered was >1300 J/mL. Therefore, guidelines should emphasize the importance of energy delivered as a key to successful treatment.

As far as malignant thyroid nodules are concerned, our systematic review show that recurrence-free survival rates do not differ between RFA and surgery in patients with DTC recurrences, which is in line with the concept that RFA can be used to treat DTC recurrences in patients in high-risk surgical patients or patients refusing additional surgery. On the other hand, we believe that further (and longer) studies are needed before extending RFA to "low-risk" papillary microcarcinomas. In particular, the lack of definite histopathological information in the absence of diagnostic surgery will represent a significant impediment to its use in this setting.

4.4. Strenghts and Limitations

This systematic review addresses what is currently seen as an open question [58], namely the regrowth/recurrence rates in the long-term follow-up after RFA. The limitations include the fact that regrowth has been defined in many ways, studies are heterogeneous in terms of number of treatments and energy delivered, and -most importantly- the majority of them has incomplete follow-ups and in many cases the number of patients seen over time is not specified.

5. Conclusions

Current scientific literature indicates that RFA is an effective treatment of benign thyroid nodules. The ideal target appears to be a single, cold, benign, and symptomatic thyroid nodule, with a baseline volume below 20 mL. In this nodule, RFA should deliver more than 1300 J/mL, in order to achieve a satisfactory volume reduction and avoid retreatments in the following 5 years. Nodule regrowth remains poorly understood, and patients should be followed after initial procedure. RFA represents a therapeutic option in patients with DTC neck recurrences that have a high surgical risk, or refuse additional surgery. On the other hand, it might become a treatment for PTMC in the future, particularly once the issue of accurate staging and risk stratification of the disease as well as removal of micrometastases have been resolved.

Author Contributions: Conceptualization S.B., A.P. and R.C.; systematic literature search S.B., A.P. and R.C.; writing—original draft preparation, S.B. and B.F.; writing—review and editing, A.P., R.F.G., F.S. and R.C.; supervision R.C. All authors have read and agreed to the published version of the manuscript.

Funding: This research received no external funding.

Conflicts of Interest: F.S. is a consultant for HS AMICA (LT, Italy). All the other authors declare no conflict of interest. The funders had no role in the design of the study; in the collection, analyses, or interpretation of data; in the writing of the manuscript, or in the decision to publish the results.

References

1. Trimboli, P. Ultrasound: The Extension of Our Hands to Improve the Management of Thyroid Patients. *Cancers* **2021**, *13*, 567. [CrossRef] [PubMed]
2. Mauri, G.; Sconfienza, L.M. Image-guided thermal ablation might be a way to compensate for image deriving cancer overdiagnosis. *Int. J. Hyperth.* **2017**, *33*, 489–490. [CrossRef]
3. Rangel, L.; Volpi, L.M.; Stabenow, E.; Steck, J.H.; Volpi, E.; Russell, J.O.; Tufano, R.P. Radiofrequency for benign and malign thyroid lesions. *World J. Otorhinolaryngol. Head Neck Surg.* **2020**, *6*, 188–193. [CrossRef] [PubMed]
4. Kim, J.H.; Baek, J.H.; Lim, H.K.; Ahn, H.S.; Baek, S.M.; Choi, Y.J.; Choi, Y.J.; Chung, S.R.; Ha, E.J.; Hahn, S.Y.; et al. 2017 Thyroid Radiofrequency Ablation Guideline: Korean Society of Thyroid Radiology. *Korean J. Radiol.* **2018**, *19*, 632–655. [CrossRef]
5. Papini, E.; Pacella, C.M.; Solbiati, L.A.; Achille, G.; Barbaro, D.; Bernardi, S.; Cantisani, V.; Cesareo, R.; Chiti, A.; Cozzaglio, L.; et al. Minimally-invasive treatments for benign thyroid nodules: A Delphi-based consensus statement from the Italian minimally-invasive treatments of the thyroid (MITT) group. *Int. J. Hyperth.* **2019**, *36*, 376–382. [CrossRef]
6. Papini, E.; Monpeyssen, H.; Frasoldati, A.; Hegedus, L. 2020 European Thyroid Association Clinical Practice Guideline for the Use of Image-Guided Ablation in Benign Thyroid Nodules. *Eur. Thyr. J.* **2020**, *9*, 172–185. [CrossRef] [PubMed]
7. Monzani, F.; Caraccio, N.; Basolo, F.; Iacconi, P.; LiVolsi, V.; Miccoli, P. Surgical and pathological changes after percutaneous ethanol injection therapy of thyroid nodules. *Thyroid* **2000**, *10*, 1087–1092. [CrossRef] [PubMed]
8. Dietrich, C.F.; Muller, T.; Bojunga, J.; Dong, Y.; Mauri, G.; Radzina, M.; Dighe, M.; Cui, X.W.; Grunwald, F.; Schuler, A.; et al. Statement and Recommendations on Interventional Ultrasound as a Thyroid Diagnostic and Treatment Procedure. *Ultrasound Med. Biol.* **2018**, *44*, 14–36. [CrossRef]
9. Hegedus, L.; Frasoldati, A.; Negro, R.; Papini, E. European Thyroid Association Survey on Use of Minimally Invasive Techniques for Thyroid Nodules. *Eur. Thyr. J.* **2020**, *9*, 194–204. [CrossRef]
10. Bernardi, S.; Dobrinja, C.; Fabris, B.; Bazzocchi, G.; Sabato, N.; Ulcigrai, V.; Giacca, M.; Barro, E.; De Manzini, N.; Stacul, F. Radiofrequency ablation compared to surgery for the treatment of benign thyroid nodules. *Int. J. Endocrinol.* **2014**, *2014*, 934595. [CrossRef]

1. Bernardi, S.; Stacul, F.; Zecchin, M.; Dobrinja, C.; Zanconati, F.; Fabris, B. Radiofrequency ablation for benign thyroid nodules. *J. Endocrinol. Investig.* **2016**, *39*, 1003–1013. [CrossRef] [PubMed]
2. Cesareo, R.; Pasqualini, V.; Simeoni, C.; Sacchi, M.; Saralli, E.; Campagna, G.; Cianni, R. Prospective study of effectiveness of ultrasound-guided radiofrequency ablation versus control group in patients affected by benign thyroid nodules. *J. Clin. Endocrinol. Metab.* **2015**, *100*, 460–466. [CrossRef]
3. Deandrea, M.; Sung, J.Y.; Limone, P.; Mormile, A.; Garino, F.; Ragazzoni, F.; Kim, K.S.; Lee, D.; Baek, J.H. Efficacy and Safety of Radiofrequency Ablation Versus Observation for Nonfunctioning Benign Thyroid Nodules: A Randomized Controlled International Collaborative Trial. *Thyroid* **2015**, *25*, 890–896. [CrossRef] [PubMed]
4. Kim, J.H.; Baek, J.H.; Sung, J.Y.; Min, H.S.; Kim, K.W.; Hah, J.H.; Park, D.J.; Kim, K.H.; Cho, B.Y.; Na, D.G. Radiofrequency ablation of low-risk small papillary thyroidcarcinoma: Preliminary results for patients ineligible for surgery. *Int. J. Hyperth.* **2017**, *33*, 212–219. [CrossRef] [PubMed]
5. Lim, H.K.; Cho, S.J.; Baek, J.H.; Lee, K.D.; Son, C.W.; Son, J.M.; Baek, S.M. US-Guided Radiofrequency Ablation for Low-Risk Papillary Thyroid Microcarcinoma: Efficacy and Safety in a Large Population. *Korean J. Radiol.* **2019**, *20*, 1653–1661. [CrossRef]
6. Yan, L.; Lan, Y.; Xiao, J.; Lin, L.; Jiang, B.; Luo, Y. Long-term outcomes of radiofrequency ablation for unifocal low-risk papillary thyroid microcarcinoma: A large cohort study of 414 patients. *Eur. Radiol.* **2021**, *31*, 685–694. [CrossRef] [PubMed]
7. Cho, S.J.; Baek, S.M.; Lim, H.K.; Lee, K.D.; Son, J.M.; Baek, J.H. Long-Term Follow-Up Results of Ultrasound-Guided Radiofrequency Ablation for Low-Risk Papillary Thyroid Microcarcinoma: More than 5-Year Follow-Up for 84 Tumors. *Thyroid* **2020**, *30*, 1745–1751. [CrossRef] [PubMed]
8. Kim, J.H.; Yoo, W.S.; Park, Y.J.; Park, D.J.; Yun, T.J.; Choi, S.H.; Sohn, C.H.; Lee, K.E.; Sung, M.W.; Youn, Y.K.; et al. Efficacy and Safety of Radiofrequency Ablation for Treatment of Locally Recurrent Thyroid Cancers Smaller than 2 cm. *Radiology* **2015**, *276*, 909–918. [CrossRef] [PubMed]
9. Choi, Y.; Jung, S.L.; Bae, J.S.; Lee, S.H.; Jung, C.K.; Jang, J.; Shin, N.Y.; Choi, H.S.; Ahn, K.J.; Kim, B.S. Comparison of efficacy and complications between radiofrequency ablation and repeat surgery in the treatment of locally recurrent thyroid cancers: A single-center propensity score matching study. *Int. J. Hyperth.* **2019**, *36*, 359–367. [CrossRef] [PubMed]
10. Zhang, M.; Tufano, R.P.; Russell, J.O.; Zhang, Y.; Zhang, Y.; Qiao, Z.; Luo, Y. Ultrasound-Guided Radiofrequency Ablation Versus Surgery for Low-Risk Papillary Thyroid Microcarcinoma: Results of over 5 Years' Follow-Up. *Thyroid* **2020**, *30*, 408–417. [CrossRef]
11. Bernardi, S.; Giudici, F.; Cesareo, R.; Antonelli, G.; Cavallaro, M.; Deandrea, M.; Giusti, M.; Mormile, A.; Negro, R.; Palermo, A.; et al. Five-Year Results of Radiofrequency and Laser Ablation of Benign Thyroid Nodules: A Multicenter Study from the Italian Minimally Invasive Treatments of the Thyroid Group. *Thyroid* **2020**, *30*, 1759–1770. [CrossRef] [PubMed]
12. Bernardi, S.; Cavallaro, M.; Colombin, G.; Giudici, F.; Zuolo, G.; Zdjelar, A.; Dobrinja, C.; De Manzini, N.; Zanconati, F.; Cova, M.A.; et al. Initial Ablation Ratio Predicts Volume Reduction and Retreatment after 5 Years from Radiofrequency Ablation of Benign Thyroid Nodules. *Front. Endocrinol.* **2020**, *11*, 582550. [CrossRef]
13. Hegedus, L.; Miyauchi, A.; Tuttle, R.M. Nonsurgical Thermal Ablation of Thyroid Nodules: Not if, but Why, When, and How? *Thyroid* **2020**, *30*, 1691–1694. [CrossRef]
14. Cho, S.J.; Baek, J.H.; Chung, S.R.; Choi, Y.J.; Lee, J.H. Long-Term Results of Thermal Ablation of Benign Thyroid Nodules: A Systematic Review and Meta-Analysis. *Endocrinol. Metab.* **2020**, *35*, 339–350. [CrossRef]
15. Bernardi, S.; Giudici, F.; Barbato, V.; Zanatta, L.; Grillo, A.; Fabris, B. Meta-analysis on the Effect of Mild Primary Hyperparathyroidism and Parathyroidectomy upon Arterial Stiffness. *J. Clin. Endocrinol. Metab.* **2021**, *106*, 1832–1843. [CrossRef]
16. Lim, H.K.; Lee, J.H.; Ha, E.J.; Sung, J.Y.; Kim, J.K.; Baek, J.H. Radiofrequency ablation of benign non-functioning thyroid nodules: 4-year follow-up results for 111 patients. *Eur. Radiol.* **2013**, *23*, 1044–1049. [CrossRef] [PubMed]
17. Ha, E.J.; Baek, J.H.; Lee, J.H.; Sung, J.Y.; Lee, D.; Kim, J.K.; Shong, Y.K. Radiofrequency ablation of benign thyroid nodules does not affect thyroid function in patients with previous lobectomy. *Thyroid* **2013**, *23*, 289–293. [CrossRef]
18. Jung, S.L.; Baek, J.H.; Lee, J.H.; Shong, Y.K.; Sung, J.Y.; Kim, K.S.; Lee, D.; Kim, J.H.; Baek, S.M.; Sim, J.S.; et al. Efficacy and Safety of Radiofrequency Ablation for Benign Thyroid Nodules: A Prospective Multicenter Study. *Korean J. Radiol.* **2018**, *19*, 167–174. [CrossRef] [PubMed]
19. Sim, J.S.; Baek, J.H.; Lee, J.; Cho, W.; Jung, S.I. Radiofrequency ablation of benign thyroid nodules: Depicting early sign of regrowth by calculating vital volume. *Int. J. Hyperth.* **2017**, *33*, 905–910. [CrossRef]
20. Deandrea, M.; Trimboli, P.; Garino, F.; Mormile, A.; Magliona, G.; Ramunni, M.J.; Giovanella, L.; Limone, P.P. Long-Term Efficacy of a Single Session of RFA for Benign Thyroid Nodules: A Longitudinal 5-Year Observational Study. *J. Clin. Endocrinol. Metab.* **2019**, *104*, 3751–3756. [CrossRef]
21. Aldea Martinez, J.; Aldea Viana, L.; Lopez Martinez, J.L.; Ruiz Perez, E. Radiofrequency Ablation of Thyroid Nodules: A Long-Term Prospective Study of 24 Patients. *J. Vasc. Interv. Radiol.* **2019**, *30*, 1567–1573. [CrossRef] [PubMed]
22. Hong, M.J.; Sung, J.Y.; Baek, J.H.; Je, M.S.; Choi, D.W.; Yoo, H.; Yang, S.J.; Nam, S.Y.; Yoo, E.Y. Safety and Efficacy of Radiofrequency Ablation for Nonfunctioning Benign Thyroid Nodules in Children and Adolescents in 14 Patients over a 10-Year Period. *J. Vasc. Interv. Radiol.* **2019**, *30*, 900–906. [CrossRef] [PubMed]
23. Bernardi, S.; Giudici, F.; Colombin, G.; Cavallaro, M.; Stacul, F.; Fabris, B. Residual vital ratio predicts 5-year volume reduction and retreatment after radiofrequency ablation of benign thyroid nodules but not regrowth. *Int. J. Hyperth.* **2021**, *38*, 111–113. [CrossRef] [PubMed]

34. Ha, S.M.; Sung, J.Y.; Baek, J.H.; Na, D.G.; Kim, J.H.; Yoo, H.; Lee, D.; Whan Choi, D. Radiofrequency ablation of small follicular neoplasms: Initial clinical outcomes. *Int. J. Hyperth.* **2017**, *33*, 931–937. [CrossRef]
35. Mauri, G.; Pacella, C.M.; Papini, E.; Solbiati, L.; Goldberg, S.N.; Ahmed, M.; Sconfienza, L.M. Image-Guided Thyroid Ablation: Proposal for Standardization of Terminology and Reporting Criteria. *Thyroid* **2019**, *29*, 611–618. [CrossRef]
36. Monchik, J.M.; Donatini, G.; Iannuccilli, J.; Dupuy, D.E. Radiofrequency ablation and percutaneous ethanol injection treatment for recurrent local and distant well-differentiated thyroid carcinoma. *Ann. Surg.* **2006**, *244*, 296–304. [CrossRef]
37. Chung, S.R.; Baek, J.H.; Choi, Y.J.; Lee, J.H. Longer-term outcomes of radiofrequency ablation for locally recurrent papillary thyroid cancer. *Eur. Radiol.* **2019**, *29*, 4897–4903. [CrossRef]
38. Chung, S.R.; Baek, J.H.; Choi, Y.J.; Sung, T.Y.; Song, D.E.; Kim, T.Y.; Lee, J.H. Efficacy of radiofrequency ablation for recurrent thyroid cancer invading the airways. *Eur. Radiol.* **2021**, *31*, 2153–2160. [CrossRef]
39. Dupuy, D.E.; Monchik, J.M.; Decrea, C.; Pisharodi, L. Radiofrequency ablation of regional recurrence from well-differentiated thyroid malignancy. *Surgery* **2001**, *130*, 971–977. [CrossRef]
40. Haugen, B.R.; Alexander, E.K.; Bible, K.C.; Doherty, G.M.; Mandel, S.J.; Nikiforov, Y.E.; Pacini, F.; Randolph, G.W.; Sawka, A.M.; Schlumberger, M.; et al. 2015 American Thyroid Association Management Guidelines for Adult Patients with Thyroid Nodules and Differentiated Thyroid Cancer: The American Thyroid Association Guidelines Task Force on Thyroid Nodules and Differentiated Thyroid Cancer. *Thyroid* **2016**, *26*, 1–133. [CrossRef]
41. Lupo, M.A. Radiofrequency Ablation for Benign Thyroid Nodules–a Look Towards the Future of Interventional Thyroidology. *Endocr. Pract.* **2015**, *21*, 972–974. [CrossRef]
42. Gharib, H.; Papini, E.; Garber, J.R.; Duick, D.S.; Harrell, R.M.; Hegedus, L.; Paschke, R.; Valcavi, R.; Vitti, P.; Nodules, A.A.A.T.F.o.T. American Association of Clinical Endocrinologists, American College of Endocrinology, and Associazione Medici Endocrinologi Medical Guidelines for Clinical Practice for the Diagnosis and Management of Thyroid Nodules—2016 Update. *Endocr. Pract.* **2016**, *22*, 622–639. [CrossRef] [PubMed]
43. Trimboli, P.; Deandrea, M. Treating thyroid nodules by radiofrequency: Is the delivered energy correlated with the volume reduction rate? A pilot study. *Endocrine* **2020**, *69*, 682–687. [CrossRef] [PubMed]
44. Cesareo, R.; Pacella, C.M.; Pasqualini, V.; Campagna, G.; Iozzino, M.; Gallo, A.; Lauria Pantano, A.; Cianni, R.; Pedone, C.; Pozzilli, P.; et al. Laser Ablation Versus Radiofrequency Ablation for Benign Non-Functioning Thyroid Nodules: Six-Month Results of a Randomized, Parallel, Open-Label, Trial (LARA Trial). *Thyroid* **2020**, *30*, 847–856. [CrossRef] [PubMed]
45. Deandrea, M.; Trimboli, P.; Mormile, A.; Cont, A.T.; Milan, L.; Buffet, C.; Giovanella, L.; Limone, P.P.; Poiree, S.; Leenhardt, L.; et al. Determining an energy threshold for optimal volume reduction of benign thyroid nodules treated by radiofrequency ablation. *Eur. Radiol.* **2021**. [CrossRef]
46. Sim, J.S.; Baek, J.H.; Cho, W. Initial Ablation Ratio: Quantitative Value Predicting the Therapeutic Success of Thyroid Radiofrequency Ablation. *Thyroid* **2018**, *28*, 1443–1449. [CrossRef]
47. Yan, L.; Luo, Y.; Xie, F.; Zhang, M.; Xiao, J. Residual vital ratio: Predicting regrowth after radiofrequency ablation for benign thyroid nodules. *Int. J. Hyperth.* **2020**, *37*, 1139–1148. [CrossRef] [PubMed]
48. Sim, J.S.; Baek, J.H. Long-Term Outcomes Following Thermal Ablation of Benign Thyroid Nodules as an Alternative to Surgery: The Importance of Controlling Regrowth. *Endocrinol. Metab.* **2019**, *34*, 117–123. [CrossRef]
49. Negro, R.; Trimboli, P. Thermal ablation for benign, non-functioning thyroid nodules: A clinical review focused on outcomes, technical remarks, and comparisons with surgery. *Electromagn. Biol. Med.* **2020**, *39*, 347–355. [CrossRef]
50. Offi, C.; Garberoglio, S.; Antonelli, G.; Esposito, M.G.; Brancaccio, U.; Misso, C.; D'Ambrosio, E.; Pace, D.; Spiezia, S. The Ablation of Thyroid Nodule's Afferent Arteries Before Radiofrequency Ablation: Preliminary Data. *Front. Endocrinol.* **2020**, *11*, 565000. [CrossRef]
51. Yan, L.; Luo, Y.; Xiao, J.; Lin, L. Non-enhanced ultrasound is not a satisfactory modality for measuring necrotic ablated volume after radiofrequency ablation of benign thyroid nodules: A comparison with contrast-enhanced ultrasound. *Eur. Radio.* **2020**. [CrossRef]
52. Schiaffino, S.; Serpi, F.; Rossi, D.; Ferrara, V.; Buonomenna, C.; Alì, M.; Monfardini, L.; Sconfienza, L.M.; Mauri, G. Reproducibility of Ablated Volume Measurement Is Higher with Contrast-Enhanced Ultrasound than with B-Mode Ultrasound after Benign Thyroid Nodule Radiofrequency Ablation—A Preliminary Study. *J. Clin. Med.* **2020**, *9*, 1504. [CrossRef]
53. Colombo, C.; Muzza, M.; Pogliaghi, G.; Palazzo, S.; Vannucchi, G.; Vicentini, L.; Persani, L.; Gazzano, G.; Fugazzola, L. The thyroid risk score (TRS) for nodules with indeterminate cytology. *Endocr. Relat. Cancer* **2021**, *28*, 225–235. [CrossRef] [PubMed]
54. Negro, R.; Trimboli, P. Placing Thermal Ablation for Benign Thyroid Nodules into Context. *Eur. Thyr. J.* **2020**, *9*, 169–171. [CrossRef] [PubMed]
55. Park, K.W.; Shin, J.H.; Han, B.K.; Ko, E.Y.; Chung, J.H. Inoperable symptomatic recurrent thyroid cancers: Preliminary result of radiofrequency ablation. *Ann. Surg. Oncol.* **2011**, *18*, 2564–2568. [CrossRef] [PubMed]
56. Ito, Y.; Miyauchi, A.; Inoue, H.; Fukushima, M.; Kihara, M.; Higashiyama, T.; Tomoda, C.; Takamura, Y.; Kobayashi, K.; Miya, A. An observational trial for papillary thyroid microcarcinoma in Japanese patients. *World J. Surg.* **2010**, *34*, 28–35. [CrossRef]
57. Feldkamp, J.; Grunwald, F.; Luster, M.; Lorenz, K.; Vorlander, C.; Fuhrer, D. Non-Surgical and Non-Radioiodine Techniques for Ablation of Benign Thyroid Nodules: Consensus Statement and Recommendation. *Exp. Clin. Endocrinol. Diabetes* **2020**, *128*, 687–692. [CrossRef] [PubMed]

68. Dobnig, H.; Zechmann, W.; Hermann, M.; Lehner, M.; Heute, D.; Mirzaei, S.; Gessl, A.; Stepan, V.; Hofle, G.; Riss, P.; et al. Radiofrequency ablation of thyroid nodules: "Good Clinical Practice Recommendations" for Austria: An interdisciplinary statement from the following professional associations: Austrian Thyroid Association (OSDG), Austrian Society for Nuclear Medicine and Molecular Imaging (OGNMB), Austrian Society for Endocrinology and Metabolism (OGES), Surgical Endocrinology Working Group (ACE) of the Austrian Surgical Society (OEGCH). *Wien Med. Wochenschr.* **2020**, *170*, 6–14. [CrossRef]

69. Mauri, G.; Hegedüs, L.; Bandula, S.; Cazzato, R.L.; Czarniecka, A.; Dudeck, O.; Fugazzola, L.; Netea-Maier, R.; Russ, G.; Wallin, G.; et al. European Thyroid Association and Cardiovascular and Interventional Radiological Society of Europe 2021 Clinical Practice Guideline for the Use of Minimally Invasive Treatments in Malignant Thyroid Lesions. *Eur. Thyr. J.* **2021**. [CrossRef]

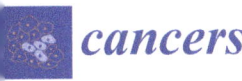

Article

Diagnostic Algorithm for Metastatic Lymph Nodes of Differentiated Thyroid Carcinoma

Sae Rom Chung [1], Jung Hwan Baek [1,*], Young Jun Choi [1], Tae-Yon Sung [2], Dong Eun Song [3], Tae Yong Kim [4] and Jeong Hyun Lee [1]

1. Department of Radiology and Research Institute of Radiology, University of Ulsan College of Medicine, Asan Medical Center, Seoul 05505, Korea; jserom@naver.com (S.R.C.); jehee23@gmail.com (Y.J.C.); jeonghlee@amc.seoul.kr (J.H.L.)
2. Department of Surgery, University of Ulsan College of Medicine, Asan Medical Center, Seoul 05505, Korea; tysung@amc.seoul.kr
3. Department of Pathology, University of Ulsan College of Medicine, Asan Medical Center, Seoul 05505, Korea; hipuha@hanmail.net
4. Department of Endocrinology and Metabolism, University of Ulsan College of Medicine, Asan Medical Center, Seoul 05505, Korea; tykim@amc.seoul.kr
* Correspondence: radbaek@naver.com; Tel.: +82-2-3010-4348; Fax: +82-2-476-0090

Citation: Chung, S.R.; Baek, J.H.; Choi, Y.J.; Sung, T.-Y.; Song, D.E.; Kim, T.Y.; Lee, J.H. Diagnostic Algorithm for Metastatic Lymph Nodes of Differentiated Thyroid Carcinoma. *Cancers* **2021**, *13*, 1338. https://doi.org/10.3390/cancers13061338

Academic Editor: Riccardo Vigneri

Received: 19 February 2021
Accepted: 11 March 2021
Published: 16 March 2021

Publisher's Note: MDPI stays neutral with regard to jurisdictional claims in published maps and institutional affiliations.

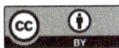

Copyright: © 2021 by the authors. Licensee MDPI, Basel, Switzerland. This article is an open access article distributed under the terms and conditions of the Creative Commons Attribution (CC BY) license (https://creativecommons.org/licenses/by/4.0/).

Simple Summary: Fine-needle aspiration cytology (FNAC) with measurement of thyroglobulin concentrations obtained through aspiration (FNA-Tg) is routinely used for the diagnosis of metastatic lymph nodes (LNs) from differentiated thyroid carcinomas. However, some areas of uncertainty remain, including the optimal FNA-Tg cutoff and its interpretation based on ultrasound (US) features. In this study, we evaluated the appropriate strategies for interpreting FNAC and FNA-Tg results based on the sonographic features of LNs. We confirmed that the malignancy rate of LNs found to be malignant by FNAC or elevated FNA-Tg was sufficiently high to be diagnosed as metastasis, regardless of the sonographic features. The malignancy rate of LNs with indeterminate or benign FNAC findings and low FNA-Tg were stratified according to their sonographic features. We propose a diagnostic algorithm, based on combined FNAC, FNA-Tg, and US features of LNs, for diagnosing metastatic LNs of differentiated thyroid carcinomas.

Abstract: We aimed to evaluate appropriate strategies for interpreting fine-needle aspiration cytology (FNAC) and thyroglobulin concentrations obtained through aspiration (FNA-Tg) results based on the sonographic features of lymph nodes (LNs). Consecutive patients who underwent ultrasound-guided FNAC and FNA-Tg for metastatic LNs from differentiated thyroid carcinomas (DTCs) from January 2014 to December 2018 were reviewed retrospectively. LNs were categorized sonographically as suspicious, indeterminate, or benign. The optimal FNA-Tg cutoff for metastatic LNs was evaluated preoperatively, after lobectomy, and after total thyroidectomy. The diagnostic performances of FNA-Tg, FNAC, and their combination were analyzed based on the sonographic features of LNs. The malignancy rates of LNs were analyzed based on the sonographic features, FNAC, and FNA-Tg results. Of the 1543 LNs analyzed, 528 were benign, whereas 1015 were malignant. FNA-Tg increased the sensitivity and accuracy of FNAC for LNs. The malignancy rate of LNs found to be malignant by FNAC or elevated FNA-Tg ranged from 82% to 100%, regardless of the sonographic features. The malignancy rate of LNs with indeterminate or benign FNAC findings and low FNA-Tg were stratified according to their sonographic features. We propose a diagnostic algorithm, based on combined FNAC, FNA-Tg, and ultrasound features of LNs, for diagnosing metastatic LNs of DTCs.

Keywords: papillary thyroid carcinoma; neoplasm metastasis; ultrasonography; biopsy; fine-needle; thyroglobulin

1. Introduction

Patients with differentiated thyroid carcinoma (DTC) have an excellent prognosis. However, despite their relatively indolent clinical and biological behaviors, DTCs are frequently associated with cervical lymph node (LN) metastases at the time of diagnosis or during the postoperative follow-up period [1]. Accurate diagnosis of LN metastasis is important for patients with DTCs, with likely LN involvement taken into consideration when deciding whether to perform neck dissection or not and when predicting the patient prognosis. Particularly, lateral LN metastasis increases the risk of locoregional recurrence and decreases the rate of tumor-free survival among patients with PTC [2]. Thus, detection of lateral LN metastases during the initial operation is important for reducing reoperation rates and complications of reoperation [3].

Ultrasound (US)-guided fine aspiration cytology (FNAC) is the most useful technique for diagnosing nodal metastases, although inadequate cellularity or nonrepresentative sampling precludes diagnosis in up to 20% of specimens, including small metastatic lesions or those with partial involvement or cystic changes [4–6]. The diagnostic yield of FNA could improve by directly measuring the thyroglobulin (Tg) concentration in the washout fluid of the fine-needle aspirate (FNA-Tg) [7]. Current guidelines recommend that patients with DTC undergo biopsy of sonographically suspicious LNs to obtain cytology results and determine the FNA-Tg concentration [8–10].

Although FNA-Tg is important in assessing lesions suspected of being recurrent or metastatic, some areas of uncertainty remain, including the optimal FNA-Tg cutoff and its interpretation based on US features. Therefore, the aim of the present study was to determine the optimal FNA-Tg cutoff detecting malignant LNs based on the patient's surgical status, compare the diagnostic performance of this cutoff with that of FNAC based on the US features of LNs, and propose a diagnostic algorithm to detect metastatic LNs of DTCs using combined FNAC, FNA-Tg, and US features of LNs.

2. Results

2.1. Study Population

A total of 1543 LNs in 1173 patients were included in our study. Of these 1543 LNs, 528 (34.2%) were benign and 1015 (65.8%) were metastatic, including 997 from classic-type papillary thyroid carcinoma, 15 from follicular variant papillary thyroid carcinoma, and 3 from follicular carcinoma. Of the 1543 LNs, 865 (56.0%) were obtained preoperatively, 63 (4.1%) were obtained after hemithyroidectomy, and 615 (39.9%) were obtained after total thyroidectomy. LN characteristics according to the final diagnosis are shown in Table 1. The mean FNA-Tg level was $45{,}266.8 \pm 191{,}378.6$ ng/mL for metastatic LNs and 21.3 ± 465.7 ng/mL for benign LNs. The mean serum Tg concentration was also significantly higher in patients with metastatic LNs than in those with benign LNs.

2.2. Optimal FNA-Tg Cutoff Values

Boxplots showing the distribution of FNA-Tg levels in the benign and metastatic LNs obtained preoperatively, after lobectomy, and after total thyroidectomy are shown in Figure 1. The median FNA-Tg levels for metastatic and benign LNs were 3005 and 0.16 ng/mL, 1760 and 0.08 ng/mL, and 890 and 0.08 ng/mL in patients preoperatively, after lobectomy, and after total thyroidectomy, respectively.

The optimal FNA-Tg cutoff for detecting metastatic LNs were determined using the receiver operating characteristic (ROC) analysis. The optimal cutoff for LNs obtained preoperatively, after lobectomy, and after total thyroidectomy FNA-Tg were 8.3, 0.97, and 1.1 ng/mL, respectively, with area under the curve of 0.962, 0.958, and 0.974, respectively (Figure 2).

Table 1. Demographic and clinical characteristics of patients and lymph nodes.

Characteristic	Benign	Metastatic	p-Value
No. of patients	418	755	
Age (years)	50.8 ± 13.2	49.4 ± 14.7	0.003
Sex Male Female	 107 (25.6%) 311 (74.4%)	 266 (35.2%) 489 (64.8%)	0.0004
No. of nodules	528	1015	
Preoperative evaluation Lobectomy Total thyroidectomy	261 (49.4%) 18 (3.4%) 249 (47.2%)	604 (59.5%) 45 (4.4%) 366 (36.1%)	0.0001
Sonographic diagnosis Benign Indeterminate Suspicious	 78 (14.8%) 371 (70.2%) 79 (15.0%)	 2 (0.2%) 143 (14.1%) 870 (85.7%)	<0.0001
Size Short axis diameter Longest diameter	 0.5 ± 0.2 1.1 ± 0.5	 0.6 ± 0.5 1.1 ± 0.7	 <0.0001 0.242
FNA cytology Benign Malignant Indeterminate	 472 (89.4%) 1 (0.2%) 55 (10.4%)	 92 (9.1%) 804 (79.2%) 119 (11.7%)	<0.0001
FNA-Tg, ng/mL	21.3 ± 465.7	45,266.8 ± 191,378.6	<0.0001
Serum Tg, ng/mL	9.2 ± 34.8	37.9 ± 201.0	0.001

FNA, fine-needle aspiration; Tg, thyroglobulin.

2.3. Comparison of the Diagnostic Performance of FNAC, FNA-Tg, and Combined FNAC and FNA-Tg

Table 2 compares the diagnostic performances of FNAC and combined FNAC and FNA-Tg according to the sonographic features of LNs. Only 2 of the 80 sonographically benign LNs were diagnosed as metastatic.

The positive predictive values of FNAC and FNA-Tg were 99.8–100% and 97.5–100%, respectively. Combined FNA-Tg to FNAC increases sensitivity of FNAC in the diagnosis of metastatic LNs, regardless of US features of LNs ($p \leq 0.004$). Their specificities did not differ significantly ($p \geq 0.059$). The negative predictive value of FNAC for LNs with cystic change, suspicious LNs without cystic change, and indeterminate LNs were 1.5%, 47.2%, and 86.7%, respectively. The combination of FNA-Tg and FNAC improved these values to 50%, 74.0%, and 95.6%, respectively.

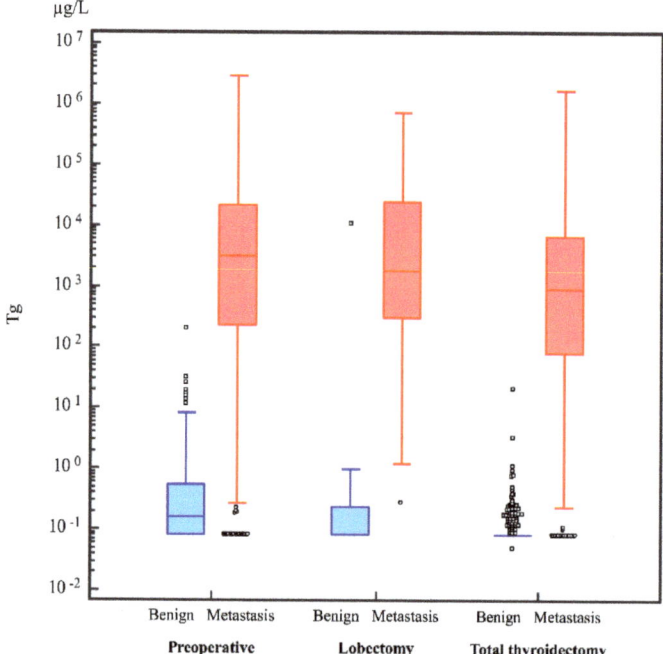

Figure 1. The distribution of FNA-Tg in benign and metastatic LNs obtained preoperatively, after lobectomy, and after total thyroidectomy. Boxplots represent median (line within box), 25th percentile (lower hinge) and its lower adjacent value (lower adjacent line), 75th percentile (upper hinge) and its upper adjacent value (upper adjacent line), and outside values (dots). FNA, fine-needle aspiration; LN, lymph node; Tg, thyroglobulin.

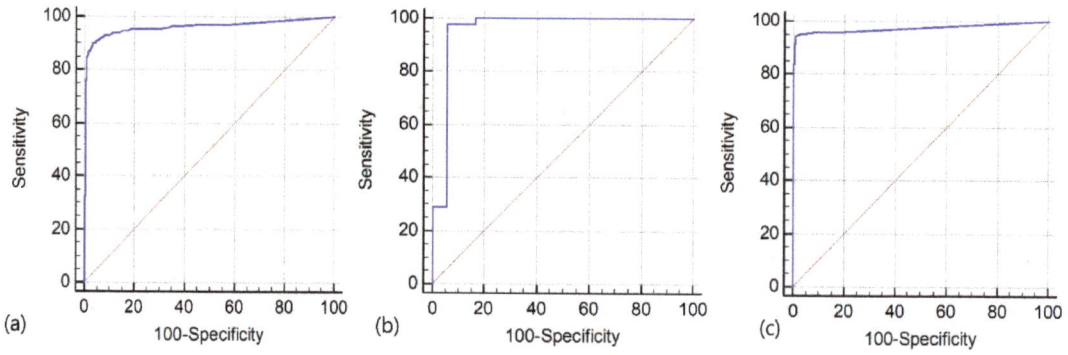

Figure 2. Receiver operating characteristic curves for FNA-Tg measurements in patients assessed preoperatively (**a**), after lobectomy (**b**), and after total thyroidectomy (**c**). The areas under the curves were 0.962, 0.958, and 0.974, respectively and $p < 0.001$; FNA, fine-needle aspiration; Tg, thyroglobulin.

Only one lesion was a false-positive on FNAC, with surgery confirming that this lesion was a suture granuloma with a foreign body reaction. There are nine LNs with false-positive results on FNA-Tg. Eight of nine LNs were obtained at the preoperative evaluation, and the false-positive result of FNA-Tg may be associated with elevated serum Tg levels in some preoperative patients with thyroid cancer.

Table 2. Diagnostic performances of fine-needle aspiration and thyroglobulin measurements for the diagnosis of lymph node metastases according to sonographic features.

Variables	Suspicious LN with Cystic Changes			Suspicious LN without Cystic Changes			Indeterminate Lymph Nodes		
	FNAC	FNA-Tg	Combined	FNAC	FNA-Tg	Combined	FNAC	FNA-Tg	Combined
Sensitivity	70.9 (161/227) [64.6–76.7]	99.6 * (226/227) [97.6–9.99]	99.6 † (226/227) [97.6–9.99]	86.6 (557/643) [83.8–89.2]	91.0 * (585/643) [88.5–93.1]	96.1 † (618/643) [94.3–97.5]	60.1 (86/143) [51.6–68.2]	81.8 * (117/143) [74.5–87.8]	88.1 † (126/143) [81.7–92.9]
Specificity	100 (1/1) [2.5–100]	100 (1/1) [2.5–100]	100 (1/1) [2.5–100]	98.7 (77/78) [93.1–100]	92.3 (72/78) [84.0–97.1]	91.0 (71/78) [82.4–96.3]	100 (371/371) [99.0–100]	99.2 (368/371) [97.7–99.8]	99.1 (368/371) [97.7–99.8]
PPV	100 (161/161) [100–100]	100 (226/226) [100–100]	100 (226/226) [100–100]	99.8 (557/558) [98.8–100]	99.0 (585/591) [97.8–99.5]	98.9 (618/625) [97.8–99.4]	100 (86/86) [100–100]	97.5 (117/120) [92.7–99.2]	97.7 (126/129) [93.1–99.2]
NPV	1.5 (1/67) [1.2–1.8]	50 (1/67) [12.4–87.6]	50 (1/2) [12.4–87.6]	47.2 (77/163) [42.3–52.2]	55.4 (72/130) [49.1–61.5]	74.0 (71/96) [65.8–80.8]	86.7 (371/428) [84.2–88.8]	93.4 (368/394) [90.9–95.3]	95.6 (368/385) [93.3–97.1]
Diagnostic accuracy	71.1 (162/228) [64.7–96.9]	99.6 * (227/228) [97.6–100]	99.6 † (227/228) [97.6–100]	87.9 (634/721) [85.3–90.2]	91.1 (657/721) [88.8–93.1]	95.6 † (689/721) [93.8–96.9]	88.9 (457/514) [85.9–91.5]	94.4 * (485/514) [92.0–96.2]	96.1 † (494/514) [94.1–97.6]
False-positive	0 (0/161)	0 (0/226)	0 (0/226)	0.2% (1/558)	1% (6/591)	1.1% (7/625)	0 (0/86)	2.5% (3/120)	2.3% (3/129)
False-negative	1.5% (1/67)	50% (1/2)	50% (1/2)	52.8% (86/163)	44.6% (58/130)	26% (25/96)	13.3% (57/428)	6.6% (26/394)	4.4% (17/385)

Data are percentage with proportion in parentheses and 95% confidence index in brackets unless otherwise indicated. Cutoff for Tg-FNA were 8.3 μg/L preoperatively, 0.97 μg/L following lobectomy, and 1.1 μg/L following total thyroidectomy. * $p < 0.025$ for comparisons of FNAC and FNA-Tg. † $p < 0.025$ for comparisons of FNAC and combined FNAC and FNA-Tg. LN, lymph node; FNA, fine-needle aspiration; Tg, thyroglobulin; PPV, positive predictive value; NPV, negative predictive value.

There was only a single false-negative case on FNAC and FNA-Tg for LNs with cystic change, which was likely caused by mistargeting of the LN during FNA. For suspicious LNs without cystic change and indeterminate LNs, FNAC showed false-negative results of 52.8% and 13.3%, respectively. Combination of FNA-Tg and FNAC reduced these false-negative rates to 26% and 4.44%, respectively.

2.4. Malignancy Rates of LNs Based on Sonographic Features, FNAC, and FNA-Tg

Table 3 shows the malignancy rate of FNAC according to sonographic features, as well as the FNA-Tg results of the LNs. Of the 805 LNs diagnosed as malignant by FNAC, 804 (99.9%) were metastatic LNs with the malignancy rate ranging from 97.1% to 100%. The malignancy rates of LNs with elevated FNA-Tg were higher than 87.0%, regardless of FNAC or sonographic feature of LNs. The malignancy rate of LNs with cytologically indeterminate results and low FNA-Tg was 8.9–46.7%. The malignancy rates of LNs with cytologically benign results and low FNA-Tg with sonographically suspicious and indeterminate were 22.9% and 3.8%, respectively.

Table 3. Malignancy rate of lymph nodes (LNs) according to the sonographic feature, fine-needle aspiration cytology results, and washout thyroglobulin levels.

FNA Result	Sonographic Feature of LN	Malignancy Rate		
		Total	FNA-Tg > Cutoff	FNA-Tg < Cutoff
Malignant	Suspicious	99.9% (718/719)	100% (685/685)	97.1% (33/34)
	Indeterminate	100% (86/86)	100% (77/77)	100% (9/9)
Benign	Suspicious	45.7% (59/129)	87.0% (40/46)	22.9% (19/83)
	Indeterminate	9.1% (33/363)	87.0% (20/23)	3.8% (13/340)
Indeterminate	Suspicious	92.1% (93/101)	100% (86/86)	46.7% (7/15)
	Indeterminate	36.9% (24/65)	100% (20/20)	8.9% (4/45)

Cutoff values for Tg-FNA were 8.3 µg/L preoperatively, 0.97 µg/L after lobectomy, and 1.1 µg/L after total thyroidectomy. FNA, fine-needle aspiration; LN, lymph node; Tg, thyroglobulin.

3. Discussion

This study showed that the optimal cutoffs for LNs obtained preoperatively, after lobectomy, and after total thyroidectomy FNA-Tg were 8.3, 0.97, and 1.1 µg/L. Adding FNA-Tg to FNAC improved the sensitivity and accuracy for the diagnosis of LNs that were sonographically indeterminate and suspicious. The analysis of malignancy rates of LNs based on their sonographic features, FNAC results, and FNA-Tg cutoff resulted in stratification of the risk of malignancy. Based on these results, we propose an algorithm, based on a combination of FNAC, FNA-Tg, and US features of LNs, for the diagnosis of metastatic LNs of DTCs.

Tg is a glycoprotein produced specifically by the follicular cells of the thyroid, regardless of whether the cells are benign or malignant [11]. This association of Tg concentration with thyroid follicular cells allows for the postoperative monitoring and diagnosis of metastatic LNs in patients with DTCs. Although FNA-Tg has been found to improve the evaluation of suspicious LNs in DTC patients, the cutoff for FNA-Tg varies among studies [7,12–21]. Serum Tg is a potential source of bias because Tg in the peripheral blood can contaminate aspirated fluid during FNA [12,22]. Because serum Tg is associated with the presence of follicular cells and tumor burden, even when not indicative of pathological status [23,24], FNA-Tg cutoff should reflect the surgical status of patients and the presence of residual thyroid tissue. Although the FNA-Tg cutoffs have been determined for detecting metastatic LNs, previous studies have been limited by small numbers of included participants [12,17,18,22,25] or because they did not consider the patients' surgical status [13,19]. Thus, the present study determined separate FNA-Tg cutoff preoperatively, after lobectomy, and after total thyroidectomy in a large study population. The optimal FNA-Tg cutoff was higher for patients evaluated preoperatively (8.3 µg/L) than after surgery, which was consistent with previous studies [16,21,22,25], but was similar after lobectomy (0.97 µg/L) and after total thyroidectomy (1.1 µg/L).

The cystic appearance of LNs is a characteristic finding of metastatic DTC. Cystic metastatic LNs have shown high false-negative rates on FNAC, which can be reduced by the addition of FNA-Tg measurements [13,14,26]. However, the ability of FNA-Tg for the diagnosis of sonographically suspicious LNs without cystic changes or indeterminate LNs has not been investigated. Metastatic LNs with suspicious features on US are distinguished by gross tumor cell implantation, whereas metastatic LNs with indeterminate sonographic features are likely to contain micrometastases that are not large enough to produce any characteristic changes on US [8]. Consequently, the diagnostic performances of FNAC and FNA-Tg may differ according to the sonographic appearance of LNs. In our study, we found that adding FNA-Tg increased the sensitivity and accuracy of FNAC in the diagnosis of sonographically suspicious and indeterminate LNs. These results are consistent with findings showing that FNA-Tg increased the accuracy of the diagnosis of LNs without suspicious features [14]. By contrast, another study reported that FNA-Tg did not enhance the ability of diagnosing LNs without suspicious features, suggesting that FNA-Tg is not useful for diagnosing LNs without suspicious features [13]. This discrepancy may be a result of the application of the same cutoff for pre- and postoperative patients in that study.

The malignancy rates of LNs were analyzed based on the sonographic features, FNAC results, and FNA-Tg cutoff, resulting in the development of the diagnostic algorithm shown in Figure 3. First, because sonographically benign LNs have a very low malignancy rate (2.5%), FNA is not recommended. This is consistent with several current guidelines [8–10]. Sonographically suspicious and indeterminate LNs with cytologically malignant or with elevated FNA-Tg can be diagnosed as metastatic LNs. The malignancy rates of LNs with cytologically indeterminate or benign results and low FNA-Tg were further stratified according to the sonographic features of LNs. Re-aspiration is recommended for LNs with cytologically indeterminate results and low FNA-Tg, because the malignancy rate ranges from 8.9% to 46.7%. LNs with cytologically benign results, low FNA-Tg, and sonographically indeterminate characteristics should undergo observation because of their low malignancy rates of 3.8%. However, if these LNs have suspicious sonographic findings, re-aspiration is recommended because their malignancy rate is 22.9%.

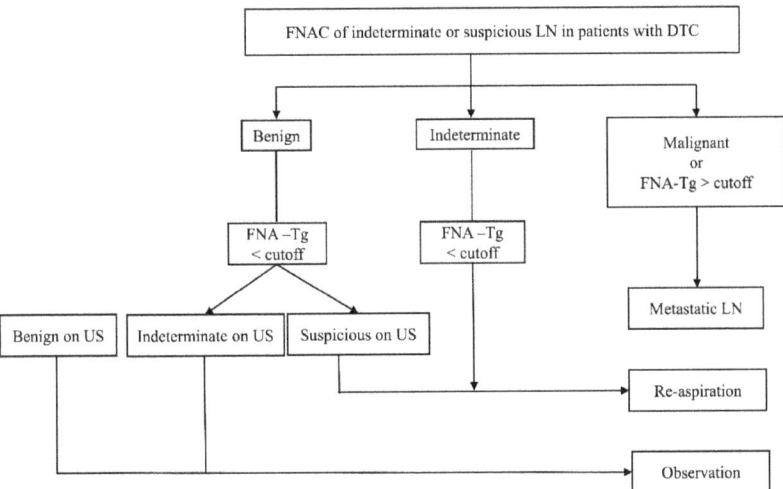

Figure 3. Diagram showing the algorithm for the diagnosis and management of metastatic LNs from DTC. DTC, differentiated thyroid carcinoma; FNA, fine-needle aspiration; LN, lymph node; Tg, thyroglobulin; US, ultrasound.

One of the limitations of the present study was its retrospective design. In addition, although our study included large numbers of patients and LNs, all patients were recruited at a single tertiary referral center. This could result in selection bias among the study population. It should also be noted that different devices for measuring FNA-Tg among institutions and tissue samples obtained by FNA can contain variable cell content and that diluting volumes of saline may not always precisely correspond to 1 mL. Therefore, our cutoff may not be applicable to patients from other institutions, and it may be difficult to compare results from different studies. Finally, there may have been interobserver variability in categorizing LNs as benign, indeterminate, and suspicious based on US. Prospective, multicenter studies would help to validate the generalizability of our findings.

4. Materials and Methods

4.1. Patient Selection

This retrospective study was approved by the Institutional Review Board of our institution approval (No. 2020-1508, 24 February 2020), and patient consent was waived due to retrospective study. Consecutive patients who had undergone US-guided FNA of LNs with measurement of FNA-Tg at our institution from January 2014 to December 2018 were included. Patients were included if they (i) were diagnosed with DTC and (ii) had metastatic LNs at final diagnosis. Patients were excluded if (i) they were not diagnosed with DTC, (ii) LNs were diagnosed as metastatic from other malignancies, (iii) evaluated lesions were not LNs, or (iv) they did not undergo subsequent surgical resection or follow-up imaging for at least 1 year. Finally, 1543 LNs from 1174 patients were included in the study population (Figure 4).

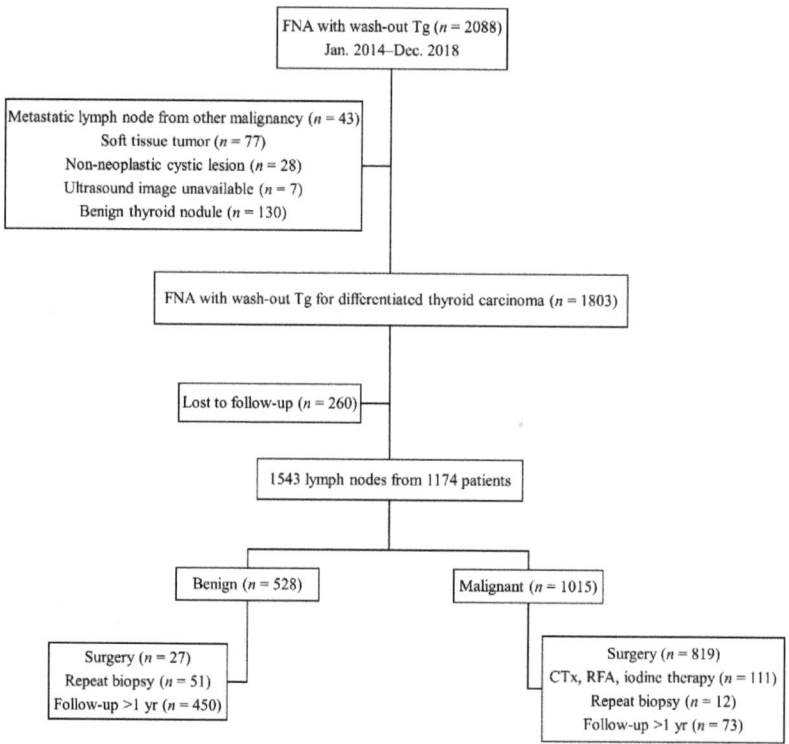

Figure 4. Flowchart showing the study population.

4.2. US and US-FNA

All patients underwent US examination of the neck using the HDI 5000 or IU22 scanner (Philips Medical Systems, Bothell, WA, USA) with a 12.5-MHz linear phased-array transducer. US-guided FNA of suspicious or indeterminate LNs, regardless of their size, was performed by radiologists. Sonographically benign LNs were defined by the presence of echogenic hilum or hilar vascularity in the absence of suspicious findings. Sonographically suspicious LNs were diagnosed if any of the following features was present: calcification, cystic change, hyperechogenicity, or peripheral or diffuse increased vascularity on color Doppler imaging. Sonographically indeterminate LNs did not have benign or suspicious LN imaging features (neither echogenic hilum nor hilar vascularity in the absence of suspicious findings), according to the Korean Society of Thyroid Radiology guidelines. Sonographically benign LNs were examined at the clinician's request, mainly because of their enlarged size.

FNA was performed under US guidance with the free hand technique using a 23-gauge needle connected to a 10-mL syringe. FNA specimens were prepared from direct smears or liquid-based cytology. The specimen was smeared onto a slide and immediately fixed in 95% ethanol using the direct smear method. With the liquid-based cytology method, specimens were prepared using the ThinPrep 2000 Processor (Hologic Co., Marlborough, MA, USA). The same needle and syringe were rinsed with 1 mL normal saline, and Tg was measured in the washout fluid (FNA-Tg). If aspirates were serous fluid, Tg was measured in this fluid without adding saline [18,27]. Cytology findings were interpreted by cytopathologists specialized in thyroid cytology. The cytology results were grouped into three categories: malignant, benign, and indeterminate [15].

4.3. Measurement of Tg

Serum Tg and FNA-Tg were measured using the immunoradiometric method (Tg-PluS RIA kit; BRAHMS AG, Henningsdorf, Germany) with a functional sensitivity (coefficient of variation of 20%) of 0.2 µg/L and an analytical sensitivity of 0.08 µg/L.

4.4. Reference Standard

LNs were finally diagnosed as metastatic if they showed malignant FNA cytology satisfying at least one of the following criteria: (i) confirmation based on the surgical specimen, (ii) subsequent repeat FNA or core-needle biopsy, or (iii) follow-up with imaging after more than 1 year. LNs with benign or indeterminate FNA cytology and deemed free of metastatic disease by the same criteria were finally diagnosed as benign.

4.5. Statistical Analysis

Continuous variables were compared by Student's *t*-tests, and categorical variables by the chi-square or Fisher's exact test. Optimal FNA-Tg cutoff concentrations determining malignant LNs were evaluated preoperatively, after lobectomy, and after total thyroidectomy by ROC curve analysis and maximization of the Youden index (sensitivity + specificity $-$ 1).

The diagnostic performances of FNAC, FNA-Tg, and their combination, including their sensitivity, specificity, and diagnostic accuracy, according to the sonographic characteristic of LNs, were compared by McNemar's test. Associations were considered statistically significant at an α level of 0.025 (0.05/2); i.e., using a Bonferroni correction due to multiple comparisons issue. The malignancy rates of LNs were analyzed based on their sonographic features, FNAC results, and FNA-Tg cutoff.

All statistical analyses were performed using SAS, version 9.4 (SAS Institute, Cary, NC, USA) and MedCalc version 19.1 (MedCalc Software, Mariakerke, Belgium).

5. Conclusions

In conclusion, measuring FNA-Tg is useful for improving the detection of metastatic LNs from DTCs, regardless of their sonographic features. The evaluation of these metastatic

LNs based on FNA-guided biopsy should include needle-wash Tg measurements. We propose a diagnostic algorithm for the diagnosis of metastatic LNs from DTCs. This algorithm, which includes FNAC, FNA-Tg, and US features of LNs, is applicable to most patients with this disease.

Author Contributions: Conceptualization, S.R.C. and J.H.B.; data curation, S.R.C., Y.J.C., T.-Y.S., D.E.S., T.Y.K., and J.H.L.; formal analysis, S.R.C.; investigation, S.R.C., J.H.B., Y.J.C., T.-Y.S., D.E.S., T.Y.K., and J.H.L.; methodology, S.R.C. and J.H.B.; writing—original draft preparation, S.R.C. and J.H.B.; writing—review and editing, S.R.C., J.H.B., Y.J.C., T.-Y.S., D.E.S., T.Y.K., and J.H.L. All authors have read and agreed to the published version of the manuscript.

Funding: This research received no external funding.

Institutional Review Board Statement: This retrospective study was approved by the Institutional Review Board of Asan Medical Center (No. 2020-1508, 24 February 2020).

Informed Consent Statement: Patient consent was waived due to retrospective study.

Data Availability Statement: Data sharing not applicable.

Conflicts of Interest: No conflicting relationship exists for any of the authors.

References

1. Grani, G.; Fumarola, A. Thyroglobulin in lymph node fine-needle aspiration washout: A systematic review and meta-analysis of diagnostic accuracy. *J. Clin. Endocrinol. Metab.* **2014**, *99*, 1970–1982. [CrossRef] [PubMed]
2. Liu, Z.; Lei, J.; Liu, Y.; Fan, Y.; Wang, X.; Lu, X. Preoperative predictors of lateral neck lymph node metastasis in papillary thyroid microcarcinoma. *Medicine* **2017**, *96*, e6240. [CrossRef] [PubMed]
3. Watkinson, J.C.; Franklyn, J.A.; Olliff, J.F. Detection and surgical treatment of cervical lymph nodes in differentiated thyroid cancer. *Thyroid* **2006**, *16*, 187–194. [CrossRef]
4. Orija, I.B.; Hamrahian, A.H.; Reddy, S.S. Management of nondiagnostic thyroid fine-needle aspiration biopsy: Survey of endocrinologists. *Endocr. Pract.* **2004**, *10*, 317–323. [CrossRef]
5. Florentine, B.D.; Staymates, B.; Rabadi, M.; Barstis, J.; Black, A. The reliability of fine-needle aspiration biopsy as the initial diagnostic procedure for palpable masses: A 4-year experience of 730 patients from a community hospital-based outpatient aspiration biopsy clinic. *Cancer* **2006**, *107*, 406–416. [CrossRef] [PubMed]
6. Hall, T.L.; Layfield, L.J.; Philippe, A.; Rosenthal, D.L. Sources of diagnostic error in fine needle aspiration of the thyroid. *Cancer* **1989**, *63*, 718–725. [CrossRef]
7. Pacini, F.; Fugazzola, L.; Lippi, F.; Ceccarelli, C.; Centoni, R.; Miccoli, P.; Elisei, R.; Pinchera, A. Detection of thyroglobulin in fine needle aspirates of nonthyroidal neck masses: A clue to the diagnosis of metastatic differentiated thyroid cancer. *J. Clin. Endocrinol. Metab.* **1992**, *74*, 1401–1404.
8. Shin, J.H.; Baek, H.J.; Chung, J.; Ha, J.E.; Kim, H.J.; Lee, H.Y.; LIm, H.K.; Moon, W.-J.; Na, D.G.; Park, J.S.; et al. Ultrasonography Diagnosis and Imaging-Based Management of Thyroid Nodules: Revised Korean Society of Thyroid Radiology Consensus Statement and Recommendations. *Korean J. Radiol.* **2016**, *17*, 370–395. [CrossRef] [PubMed]
9. Haugen, B.R.; Alexander, E.K.; Bible, K.C.; Doherty, G.M.; Mandel, S.J.; Nikiforov, Y.E.; Pacini, F.; Randolph, G.W.; Sawka, A.M.; Schlumberger, M.; et al. 2015 American Thyroid Association Management Guidelines for Adult Patients with Thyroid Nodules and Differentiated Thyroid Cancer: The American Thyroid Association Guidelines Task Force on Thyroid Nodules and Differentiated Thyroid Cancer. *Thyroid. Off. J. Am. Thyroid. Assoc.* **2016**, *26*, 1–133. [CrossRef] [PubMed]
10. Russ, G.; Bonnema, S.J.; Erdogan, M.F.; Durante, C.; Ngu, R.; Leenhardt, L. European Thyroid Association Guidelines for Ultrasound Malignancy Risk Stratification of Thyroid Nodules in Adults: The EU-TIRADS. *Eur. Thyroid. J.* **2017**, *6*, 225–237. [CrossRef]
11. Whitley, R.J.; Ain, K.B. Thyroglobulin: A specific serum marker for the management of thyroid carcinoma. *Clin. Lab Med.* **2004**, *24*, 29–47. [CrossRef] [PubMed]
12. Moon, J.H.; Kim, Y.I.; Lim, J.A.; Choi, H.S.; Cho, S.W.; Kim, K.W.; Park, H.J.; Paeng, J.C.; Park, Y.J.; Yi, K.H.; et al. Thyroglobulin in washout fluid from lymph node fine-needle aspiration biopsy in papillary thyroid cancer: Large-scale validation of the cutoff value to determine malignancy and evaluation of discrepant results. *J. Clin. Endocrinol. Metab.* **2013**, *98*, 1061–1068. [CrossRef]
13. Jung, J.Y.; Shin, J.H.; Han, B.K.; Ko, E.Y. Optimized cutoff value and indication for washout thyroglobulin level according to ultrasound findings in patients with well-differentiated thyroid cancer. *AJNR Am. J. Neuroradiol.* **2013**, *34*, 2349–2353. [CrossRef] [PubMed]
14. Chung, J.; Kim, E.K.; Lim, H.; Son, E.J.; Yoon, J.H.; Youk, J.H.; Kim, J.-A.; Moon, H.J.; Kwak, J.Y. Optimal indication of thyroglobulin measurement in fine-needle aspiration for detecting lateral metastatic lymph nodes in patients with papillary thyroid carcinoma. *Head Neck* **2014**, *36*, 795–801. [CrossRef]

15. Giovanella, L.; Bongiovanni, M.; Trimboli, P. Diagnostic value of thyroglobulin assay in cervical lymph node fine-needle aspirations for metastatic differentiated thyroid cancer. *Curr. Opin. Oncol.* **2013**, *25*, 6–13. [CrossRef] [PubMed]
16. Pak, K.; Suh, S.; Hong, H.; Cheon, G.J.; Hahn, S.K.; Kang, K.W.; Kim, E.E.; Lee, D.S.; Chung, J.-K. Diagnostic values of thyroglobulin measurement in fine-needle aspiration of lymph nodes in patients with thyroid cancer. *Endocrine* **2015**, *49*, 70–77. [CrossRef]
17. Kim, D.W.; Jeon, S.J.; Kim, C.G. Usefulness of thyroglobulin measurement in needle washouts of fine-needle aspiration biopsy for the diagnosis of cervical lymph node metastases from papillary thyroid cancer before thyroidectomy. *Endocrine* **2012**, *42*, 399–403. [CrossRef]
18. Kim, M.J.; Kim, E.K.; Kim, B.M.; Kwak, J.Y.; Lee, E.J.; Park, C.S.; Cheong, W.Y.; Nam, K.H. Thyroglobulin measurement in fine-needle aspirate washouts: The criteria for neck node dissection for patients with thyroid cancer. *Clin. Endocrinol. Oxf.* **2009**, *70*, 145–151. [CrossRef] [PubMed]
19. Cunha, N.; Rodrigues, F.; Curado, F.; Ilhéu, O.; Cruz, C.; Naidenov, P.; Rascão, M.J.; Ganho, J.; Gomes, I.; Pereira, H.; et al. Thyroglobulin detection in fine-needle aspirates of cervical lymph nodes: A technique for the diagnosis of metastatic differentiated thyroid cancer. *Eur. J. Endocrinol.* **2007**, *157*, 101–107. [CrossRef] [PubMed]
20. Snozek, C.L.; Chambers, E.P.; Reading, C.C.; Sebo, T.J.; Sistrunk, J.W.; Singh, R.J.; Grebe, S.K. Serum thyroglobulin, high-resolution ultrasound, and lymph node thyroglobulin in diagnosis of differentiated thyroid carcinoma nodal metastases. *J. Clin. Endocrinol. Metab.* **2007**, *92*, 4278–4281. [CrossRef]
21. Zhao, H.; Wang, Y.; Wang, M.-J.; Zhang, Z.-H.; Wang, H.-R.; Zhang, B.; Guo, H.-Q. Influence of presence/absence of thyroid gland on the cutoff value for thyroglobulin in lymph-node aspiration to detect metastatic papillary thyroid carcinoma. *BMC Cancer* **2017**, *17*, 296. [CrossRef] [PubMed]
22. Boi, F.; Baghino, G.; Atzeni, F.; Lai, M.L.; Faa, G.; Mariotti, S. The diagnostic value for differentiated thyroid carcinoma metastases of thyroglobulin (Tg) measurement in washout fluid from fine-needle aspiration biopsy of neck lymph nodes is maintained in the presence of circulating anti-Tg antibodies. *J. Clin. Endocrinol. Metab.* **2006**, *91*, 1364–1369. [CrossRef]
23. Kim, H.; Kim, Y.N.; Kim, H.I.; Park, S.Y.; Choe, J.H.; Kim, J.H.; Kim, J.S.; Chung, J.H.; Kim, T.H.; Kim, S.W. Preoperative serum thyroglobulin predicts initial distant metastasis in patients with differentiated thyroid cancer. *Sci. Rep.* **2017**, *7*, 16955. [CrossRef] [PubMed]
24. Bachelot, A.; Cailleux, A.F.; Klain, M.; Baudin, E.; Ricard, M.; Bellon, N.; Caillou, B.; Travagli, J.P.; Schlumberger, M. Relationship between tumor burden and serum thyroglobulin level in patients with papillary and follicular thyroid carcinoma. *Thyroid* **2002**, *12*, 707–711. [CrossRef]
25. Frasoldati, A.; Toschi, E.; Zini, M.; Flora, M.; Caroggio, A.; Dotti, C.; Valcavi, R. Role of thyroglobulin measurement in fine-needle aspiration biopsies of cervical lymph nodes in patients with differentiated thyroid cancer. *Thyroid* **1999**, *9*, 105–111. [CrossRef] [PubMed]
26. Cignarelli, M.; Ambrosi, A.; Marino, A.; Lamacchia, O.; Campo, M.; Picca, G.; Giorgino, F. Diagnostic Utility of Thyroglobulin Detection in Fine-Needle Aspiration of Cervical Cystic Metastatic Lymph Nodes from Papillary Thyroid Cancer with Negative Cytology. *Thyroid* **2003**, *13*, 1163–1167. [CrossRef]
27. Suh, Y.J.; Son, E.J.; Moon, H.J.; Kim, E.K.; Han, K.H.; Kwak, J.Y. Utility of thyroglobulin measurements in fine-needle aspirates of space occupying lesions in the thyroid bed after thyroid cancer operations. *Thyroid* **2013**, *23*, 280–288. [CrossRef] [PubMed]

Article

Sonographic Features Differentiating Follicular Thyroid Cancer from Follicular Adenoma–A Meta-Analysis

Martyna Borowczyk [1,*,†], Kosma Woliński [1,†], Barbara Więckowska [2], Elżbieta Jodłowska-Siewert [1], Ewelina Szczepanek-Parulska [1], Frederik A. Verburg [3] and Marek Ruchała [1]

1 Department of Endocrinology, Metabolism and Internal Medicine, Poznan University of Medical Sciences, 61-701 Poznan, Poland; kosma@ump.edu.pl (K.W.); jodlela@wp.pl (E.J.-S.); ewelina@ump.edu.pl (E.S.-P.); mruchala@ump.edu.pl (M.R.)
2 Department of Computer Science and Statistics, Poznan University of Medical Sciences, 61-701 Poznan, Poland; barbara.wieckowska@ump.edu.pl
3 Department of Radiology and Nuclear Medicine, Erasmus MC, 3015 Rotterdam, The Netherlands; f.verburg@erasmusmc.nl
* Correspondence: martyna.borowczyk@ump.edu.pl; Tel.: +48-512131285
† Martyna Borowczyk and Kosma Woliński equally contributed to this work.

Simple Summary: The risk of thyroid malignancy assessment may include certain ultrasound features. The analysis is lacking for the differentiation of follicular thyroid adenomas and cancers (FTAs and FTCs). Our meta-analysis aimed to identify sonographic features suggesting malignancy in the case of follicular lesions, potentially differentiating FTA and FTC. Based on twenty studies describing sonographic features of 10,215 nodules, we found that the most crucial feature associated with an increased risk of FTC were tumor protrusion (odds ratios—OR = 10.19), microcalcifications or mixed type of calcifications: 6.09, irregular margins: 5.11, marked hypoechogenicity: 4.59, and irregular shape: 3.6.

Abstract: Certain ultrasound features are associated with an increased risk of thyroid malignancy. However, they were studied mainly in papillary thyroid cancers (PTCs); these results cannot be simply extrapolated for the differentiation of follicular thyroid adenomas and cancers (FTAs and FTCs). The aim of our study was to perform a meta-analysis to identify sonographic features suggesting malignancy in the case of follicular lesions, potentially differentiating FTA and FTC. We searched thirteen databases from January 2006 to December 2020 to find all relevant, full-text journal articles written in English. Analyses assessed the accuracy of malignancy detection in case of follicular lesions, potentially differentiating FTA and FTC included the odds ratio (OR), sensitivity, specificity, positive and negative predictive values. A random-effects model was used to summarize collected data. Twenty studies describing sonographic features of 10,215 nodules met the inclusion criteria. The highest overall ORs to increase the risk of malignancy were calculated for tumor protrusion (OR = 10.19; 95% confidence interval: 2.62–39.71), microcalcifications or mixed type of calcifications (coexisting micro and macrocalcifications): 6.09 (3.22–11.50), irregular margins: 5.11 (2.90–8.99), marked hypoechogenicity: 4.59 (3.23–6.54), and irregular shape: 3.6 (1.19–10.92). The most crucial feature associated with an increased risk of FTC is capsule protrusion, followed by the presence of calcifications, irrespectively of their type.

Keywords: thyroid; ultrasonography; follicular neoplasm; follicular lesion of unknown significance; follicular thyroid cancer

1. Introduction

Ultrasound-guided fine-needle aspiration biopsy (FNAB) is a widely used procedure and a gold standard for the evaluation of thyroid nodules [1]. However, despite its utility, it has certain limitations, particularly when it comes to follicular lesions [2]. Then the cytological diagnosis is often consistent with "atypia of undetermined significance" (AUS) or "follicular lesion of undetermined significance" (FLUS), the III diagnostic category of the Bethesda System for Reporting Thyroid Cytopathology, or IV diagnostic category being follicular neoplasm or suspicion of follicular neoplasm [3]. The malignancy risk for the III category is estimated at 10–30%, while it is slightly higher in the IV category, being equal to 25–40% [3]. However, the risk may differ according to the population studied, i.e., in previously iodine-deficient countries, the estimated malignancy risk for these categories may be 2.4–5.2% and 8.2–19%, respectively [4]. Therefore, it is of considerable significance to find accessible tools or criteria that would allow distinguishing between benign and malignant lesions in case of inconclusive biopsy results. The estimation of the malignancy risk preoperatively is of enormous importance as it allows doctors to decide on surgical treatment or follow-up.

Despite increasing accessibility of novel imaging methods, e.g., positron emission tomography with computed tomography, they were not demonstrated to result in a dramatic reduction of unnecessary thyroidectomies performed among patients with FNAB Bethesda IV category. Another option is the identification of particular genetic markers obtained from cytological material [2]. However, results of genetic studies so far have not yielded satisfactory sensitivity and specificity while still being an invasive procedure, considerably expensive, and not widely available [5]. Unlike them, thyroid ultrasound is nowadays a routine examination, which is quick, non-invasive, cheap, and reproducible [6]. Ultrasound features could potentially be used to stratify the risk of malignancy in Bethesda III and IV categories. According to the results of several research and meta-analyses, there are certain ultrasound features associated with increased risk of malignancy [7,8]. Among them, the most useful were "taller than wide shape", decreased elasticity, irregular margins, microcalcifications, lack of halo, and hypoechogenicity [7,9,10]. However, these concern mainly the most common type of thyroid neoplasm-papillary thyroid cancer (PTC), i.e., two large meta-analyses by Brito et al. and Wolinski et al. took into account all types of thyroid cancer, but with definite predominance (84% and 89%, respectively) of PTC [7,9]. Still, little is known about the features of other thyroid cancer types, i.e., follicular (FTC) or medullary thyroid cancer (MTC). We hypothesize that conclusions drawn from meta-analyses taking into account in majority PTCs cannot be extrapolated and used for the estimation of malignancy risk of FTCs or MTCs. There was one meta-analysis published to date, aiming to summarize the characteristics of the ultrasound picture of MTCs [11]. However, to the best of the authors' knowledge, there has been no meta-analysis concerning ultrasound features indicating FTC. It has already been observed that PTCs and FTCs differ in terms of size, contour" and echogenicity of the lesion evaluated preoperatively by conventional ultrasonography [12]. There were only a few studies devoted to sonographic characteristics of FTC [13–15]. Other studies report the sonographic features of thyroid lesions according to the exact histopathological diagnosis, instead of only distinguishing between benign and malignant lesions, and include, among other FTCs and follicular thyroid adenomas (FTAs). However, they represent a limited number of follicular lesions; indicated sonographic features vary greatly and may not be useful in the differentiation of follicular lesions [16–19]. Another promising method potentially differentiating FTA and FTC are elastography and tridimensional Doppler [20,21]. Our study aimed to perform a meta-analysis of so far conducted studies and identify sonographic features suggesting malignancy in the case of follicular lesions, potentially differentiating FTA and FTC.

2. Results

After a complete systematic review was performed, 20 studies met the inclusion criteria. They covered analyses of 10,215 nodules. The search results and steps of selection are shown in the flowchart (Figure 1 and Table 1). The overall odds ratios for particular features giving a risk of FTC varied from 1.44 to 10.19 (Table 2 and Figure 2).

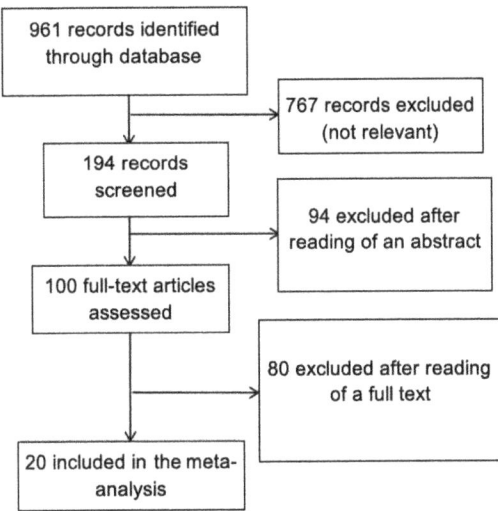

Figure 1. Methodological flow diagram of the meta-analysis for sonographic features differentiating follicular thyroid cancer from follicular adenoma utility.

Table 1. The list of included studies.

Author	Year	Number of Nodules (FTC/FTA); Malignancy Rate (%)	1	2	3	4	5	6	7	8	9	10	11	12	13	14
Seo HS et al. [15]	2009	126 (66/60) 52.4														
Sillery JC et al. [13]	2010	102 (50/52); 49.0														
Lee EK et al. [22]	2012	110 (33/77); 30.0														
Lai X et al. [23]	2013	111 (37/74); 33.3														
Lee KH et al. [24]	2013	75 (11/64); 14.7														
Lee SH et al. [25]	2013	66 (16/50); 24.2														
Pompili G et al. [26]	2013	102 (14/88); 13.7														
Kamran SC et al. [27]	2013	7348 (927/6421); 12.6														
Tutuncu J et al. [28]	2014	88 (6/82); 6.8														
Cordes M et al. [12]	2014	57 (24/33); 42.1														
Yoon JH et al. [29]	2014	177 (25/152); 14.1														
Zhang JZ et al. [14]	2014	88 (36/52); 40.9														
Cordes M et al. [30]	2016	200 (100/100); 50														
Jeong SH et al. [31]	2016	178 (22/156); 12.4														
Kobayashi K et al. [32]	2016	531 (184/347); 34.7														
Yang GCH et al. [33]	2016	279 (6/273); 2.2														
Kuru B. et al. [34]	2018	139 (51/88). 36.7														
Kim M et al. [35]	2018	160 (50/110); 31.3														
Kuo TC et al. [36]	2020	188 (49/139); 26.1														
Liu BJ et al. [37]	2020	90 (28/62); 31.1														

1-Tumor protrusion; 2-Microcalcifications or mixed type (coexisting micro- and macrocalcifications); 3-Irregular margins; 4-Hypoechogenicity or marked hypoechogenicity; 5-Irregular shape; 6-Lack of halo or presence of thick halo; 7-Macrocalcifications, eggshell or rim calcifications; 8-All types of calcifications; 9-Solitary nodule; 10-Taller than wide; 11-Solid or mainly solid structure; 12-Size over 4 cm; 13-Heterogenous echostructure; 14-Doppler pattern three or more. FTC: follicular thyroid cancer; FTA: follicular thyroid adenoma.

Table 2. Overall specificity, sensitivity, negative prognostic value (NPV), and positive predictive value (PPV) for sonographic features differentiating follicular thyroid cancer from follicular adenoma utility and their overall odds ratios (OR) with their 95% confidence intervals (95% CI).

Sonographic Feature	OR (95% CI)	Sensitivity (95% CI)	Specificity (95% CI)	PPV (95% CI)	NPV (95% CI)
Tumor protrusion Table S1	10.19 (2.62–39.71)	0.06 (0.03–0.09)	1.00 (0.99–1.00)	0.96 (0.7–1.00)	0.64 (0.61–0.68)
Microcalcifications or mixed type (coexisting micro- and macrocalcifications) Table S2	6.09 (3.22–11.5)	0.10 (0.03–0.19)	0.97 (0.95–0.99)	0.53 (0.19–0.86)	0.78 (0.69–0.85)
Irregular margins Table S3	5.11 (2.9–8.99)	0.24 (0.13–0.37)	0.94 (0.90–0.96)	0.53 (0.34–0.71)	0.80 (0.74–0.86)
Hypoechogenicity or marked hypoechogenicity Table S4	4.59 (3.23–6.54)	0.74 (0.6–0.86)	0.63 (0.53–0.73)	0.44 (0.35–0.53)	0.87 (0.81–0.92)
Irregular shape Table S5	3.6 (1.19–10.92)	0.13 (0.04–0.26)	0.97 (0.92–0.99)	0.60 (0.38–0.8)	0.75 (0.63–0.86)
Lack of halo or presence of thick halo Table S6	3.34 (1.95–5.73)	0.70 (0.64–0.76)	0.63 (0.43–0.82)	0.46 (0.29–0.63)	0.83 (0.75–0.90)
Macrocalcifications, eggshell or rim calcifications Table S7	3.28 (1.69–6.35)	0.21 (0.14–0.29)	0.92 (0.89–0.95)	0.44 (0.22–0.67)	0.79 (0.68–0.88)
All types of calcifications Table S8	3.26 (2.20–4.83)	0.35 (0.27–0.43)	0.88 (0.82–0.92)	0.54 (0.39–0.69)	0.76 (0.69–0.83)
Solitary nodule Table S9	2.72 (1.26–5.86)	0.74 (0.27–1.00)	0.48 (0.17–0.80)	0.38 (0.20–0.58)	0.83 (0.51–1.00)
Taller than wide Table S10	2.52 (1.02–6.19)	0.03 (0.00–0.10)	0.98 (0.97–1.00)	0.41 (0.14–0.70)	0.72 (0.58–0.84)
Solid or mainly solid structure Table S11	2.3 (1.27–4.17)	0.93 (0.87–0.97)	0.18 (0.08–0.31)	0.28 (0.20–0.37)	0.9 (0.81–0.96)
Size over 4 cm Table S12	1.73 (0.99–3.00)	0.19 (0.11–0.30)	0.89 (0.83–0.94)	0.47 (0.17–0.77)	0.69 (0.51–0.84)
Heterogenous echostructure Table S13	1.53 (1.02–2.30)	0.69 (0.33–0.96)	0.53 (0.41–0.65)	0.4 (0.16–0.67)	0.82 (0.63–0.96)
Doppler pattern 3 or more Table S14	1.44 (0.76–2.74)	0.60 (0.29–0.88)	0.48 (0.23–0.74)	0.28 (0.10–0.51)	0.80 (0.61–0.94)

Specificity to predict FTC for individual features varied from 18% to 100%, and the sensitivity ranged from 3% to 93%. Negative predictive value (NPV) was 64% to 90%, and positive predictive value (PPV) was 28% to 96% (Table 2 and Figure 2). All tables in the Supplementary files present the pooled estimates of sensitivity, specificity, PPV, NPV, and odds ratios obtained from the bivariate model.

The highest overall odds ratio in increasing the risk of malignancy was calculated for tumor protrusion odds ratio (OR) (95% confidence interval (CI)) = 10.19 (2.62–39.71), microcalcifications or mix type of calcifications (micro and macrocalcifications): 6.09 (3.22–11.50), irregular margins: 5.11 (2.90–8.99), marked hypoechogenicity: 4.59 (3.23–6.54), and irregular shape: 3.60 (1.19–10.92). The lowest OR was characteristic for a Doppler pattern of three or more: 1.44 (0.76–2.74).

The highest overall sensitivity with its 95% CI was 93% (87–97%) for solid or mainly solid structure, and the lowest was for taller than wide size: 3% (0–10%). The highest specificity was 100% (99–100%) for tumor protrusion, and the lowest was for solid or mainly solid structure: 18% (6–31%). Accordingly, the highest PPV was 96% (70–100%) for tumor protrusion; the lowest was for solid or mainly solid structure 28% (20–37%) and for a Doppler pattern of three or more 28% (10–51%). Furthermore, the highest NPV was 90% (81–96%) for solid or mainly solid structure, and the lowest was for tumor protrusion: 64% (61–68%). Table 2 and all Tables in the Supplementary files show detailed calculations of OR, sensitivity, specificity, PPV, and NPV for all analyzed features with their overall summaries, tests of heterogeneity, and Egger's asymmetry tests.

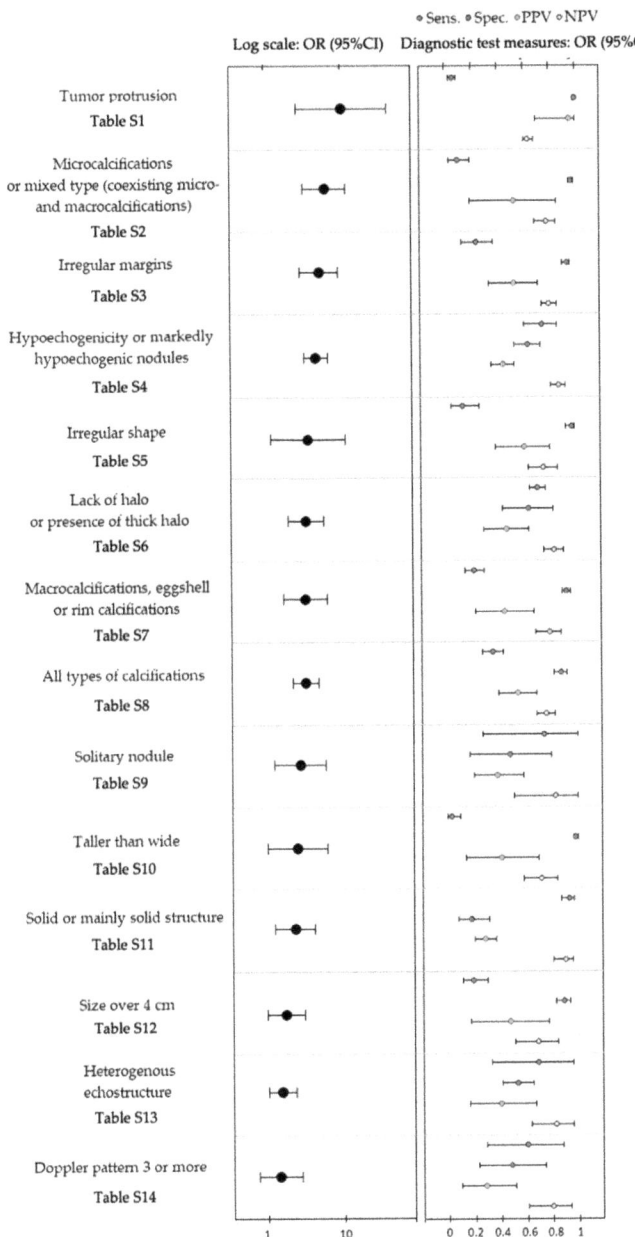

Figure 2. The graphic presentation of overall specificity, sensitivity, negative prognostic value (NPV), and positive predictive value (PPV) for sonographic features differentiating follicular thyroid cancer from follicular adenoma utility and their overall odds ratios (OR) with their 95% confidence intervals (95% CI).

Patients finally diagnosed with FTC were more than 10 times more likely to have a tumor protrusion (Figure 3)—OR (95% CI): 10.19 (2.62–39.71) (Tables S2 and S13a,b). The analysis included 633 patients and the group proved to be homogenous (test for heterogeneity: $I^2 = 0.0\%$, $p = 0.4350$. The specificity (95% CI) of this feature reached 1.00 (0.99–1.00) with low sensitivity (95% CI) of 0.06 (0.03–0.09).

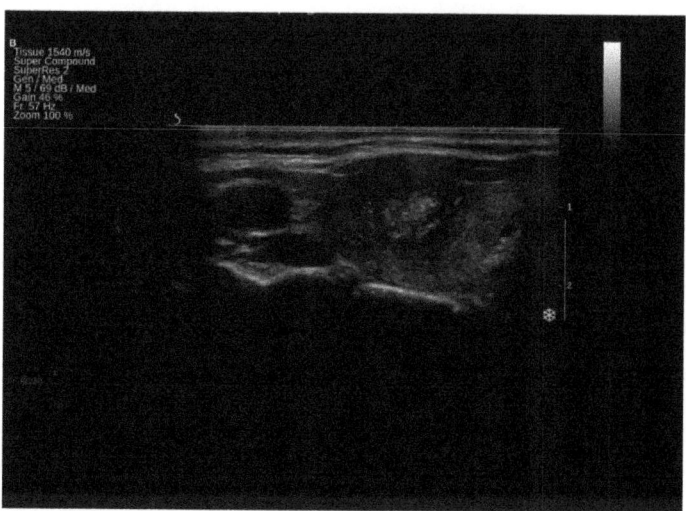

Figure 3. The result of ultrasound examination demonstrating thyroid lesion, which turned out to be follicular cancer on histopathological examination. The lesion presents tumor protrusion, irregular margins, microcalcifications, and heterogeneous echostructure.

The analysis of microcalcifications or mixed type (coexisting micro and macrocalcifications) was based on nine publications covering 1199 patients (Tables S1a,b and S2). No recent studies were located, and the group proved to be homogeneous (test for heterogeneity: $I^2 = 0\%$, p-value = 0.5494) and publication bias was not reported (Egger's p-value = 0.0800). Summary OR, presented as an overall OR (95% CI) = 6.09 (3.22–11.50), meaning that cancer patients are more than six times more likely to have a positive microcalcifications or mixed type (coexisting micro and macrocalcifications) than those with adenoma. There was relatively low overall sensitivity (95% CI) = 0.10 (0.03–0.19) and overall PPV (95% CI) = 0.53 (0.19–0.86) but quite high overall specificity (95% CI) = 0.97 (0.95–0.99) and overall NPV (95% CI) = 0.78 (0.69–0.88). Overall sensitivity and specificity determined jointly in the hierarchical summary receiver operating characteristic (HSROC) model was similar and amounted to overall sensitivity (95% CI) = 0.1 (0.04–0.21), overall specificity (95% CI) = 0.98 (0.95–0.99).

For irregular margins, initially, the analysis covered 14 papers and a total of 1721 patients (Tables S2 and S8a,b). Studies were distributed symmetrically (Egger's p-value = 0.0980). Strong study heterogeneity was detected ($I^2 = 75.3\%$, $p < 0.0001$) which resolved after excluding four outlier studies. As a result, outliers were identified based on sensitivity analysis and funnel plot inspection. After removal of the outlier, the group was more homogeneous ($I^2 = 36.59\%$, $p = 0.1156$) and based on 1227 patients. Originally overall OR (95% CI) was 3.49 (1.66–7.35) and after exclusion of the indicated study, the summary OR increased to the value of overall OR (95% CI) = 5.11 (2.90–8.99). Overall sensitivity (95% CI) was quite low = 0.24 (0.13–0.37) and overall NPV (95% CI) = 0.80 (0.74–0.86) and overall specificity (95% CI) was high = 0.94 (0.90–0.96) and overall PPV (95% CI) was = 0.53 (0.34–0.71). High specificity and quite low sensitivity were also confirmed by the HSROC curve analysis: overall specificity (95% CI) = 0.94 (0.89–0.96), HSROC overall sensitivity (95% CI) = 0.24 (0.15–0.37).

For hypo- and markedly hypoechogenic structure, initially, the analysis covered 16 papers and a total of 1864 patients (Tables S2 and S4a,b). Studies were distributed symmetrically (Egger's p-value = 0.2811). Strong study heterogeneity was detected (I^2 = 68.1%, $p < 0.0001$) which resolved after excluding two outlier studies. As a result, outliers were identified based on sensitivity analysis and funnel plot inspection. After removal of the outlier, the group was more homogeneous (I^2 = 34.96%, $p = 0.0955$) and based on 1610 patients. Originally overall OR (95% CI) was 3.69 (2.30–5.92) and after exclusion of the indicated study, the summary OR increased slightly to the value of overall OR (95% CI) = 4.59 (3.23–6.54). High overall sensitivity (95% CI) = 0.74 (0.60–0.86) and overall NPV (95% CI) = 0.87 (0.81–0.92) and quite high overall specificity (95% CI) = 0.63 (0.53–0.73) and overall PPV (95% CI) = 0.44 (0.35–0.53). High sensitivity and specificity values were also confirmed by the HSROC curve analysis: overall sensitivity (95% CI) = 0.74 (0.62–0.84), HSROC overall specificity (95% CI) = 0.63 (0.53–0.73).

3. Discussion

The incidence of differentiated thyroid cancer (DTC) has risen considerably over the past few decades. It is attributed mostly to the increasing rate of PTC, which constitutes the primary histological type of thyroid cancer [4]. The exact data on the changing rate of FTC is unavailable. However, American studies demonstrated an increase of 30% in the follow-up period from 1980 to 2009 [38]. On the other hand, the incidence of FTC was found to be reduced with the introduction of the iodination program in the previously iodine-deficient areas [39]. However, it may still account for up to 20% of differentiated thyroid cancers in the regions previously affected by iodine deficiency, constituting an important clinical problem.

The issue of sonographic features of malignancy has been covered in a few large meta-analyses. Brito et al., in their meta-analysis covering 31 studies including 18,288 focal lesions, indicated that the best predictor of malignancy was the shape of the lesion; "taller than wide" lesions were 11 times more likely to be diagnosed with thyroid cancer than those oval or round. The second important ultrasound feature that was most strongly associated with malignancy risk was the presence of microcalcifications (OR = 6.8) [9]. The size of the lesion did not correlate importantly with malignancy risk. On the other hand, the authors indicated that spongiform appearance and the presence of a cystic component were significantly associated with the benignity of a lesion. In another meta-analysis by Campanella et al., again, the shape of the lesion was found to correlate with malignancy risk (OR = 10.2). Other but less suspected features were lack of halo, presence of microcalcifications, and irregular borders [10]. According to recent European Thyroid Association guidelines, lesions presenting at least one of the following features: shape different than oval, irregular borders, microcalcifications, and deep hypoechogenicity, were at the highest malignancy risk, equal to 26–87%. The more malignancy features are present in the lesion, the highest malignancy risk is. This approach allows for the identification of thyroid cancer with high specificity at the level of 83–84% and moderate sensitivity equal to 26–59% [40]. Moreover, incomplete calcified capsule, thick halo, dominant central vascularization, and decreased elasticity of the lesion, increase the risk of moderately suspected lesions. On the other hand, thin halo, cystic component, comet-tail artifacts, peripheral vascularization, and high elasticity of the lesion were found to decrease malignancy risk. The results of a meta-analysis, including only prospective studies with histopathological verification previously performed by our team, were consistent with the findings as the most critical ultrasound feature associated with the highest malignancy risk (OR = 13.7) was the lesion shape [7]. Further essential features most strongly suggesting malignant character were decreased elasticity, irregular margins, and presence of microcalcifications. However, one must remember that in all of the mentioned meta-analyses, the predominant type of malignant lesions were PTCs. Moreover, many studies do not provide information on the histopathological type of thyroid cancer. In the studies in which the final histopathology is given, 89% of cancers were PTCs [7]. Thus, it is not clear whether the conclusions from these studies can be extrapolated on other types of thyroid cancers, i.e., follicular of medullary type. To the best of our knowledge, our research constitutes the first meta-analysis aiming to compare sonographic features differentiating FTC from follicular thyroid adenoma.

Our meta-analysis demonstrated that the sonographic feature the most strongly increasing the risk of FTC, but not underlined in the previous studies, was capsule protrusion. Although only two studies took into account this feature, it turned out to be the substantial differentiating factor between FTA and FTC, with an OR at the level of 10.19 [13,32]. Capsule protrusion towards the surrounding structures with or without visible capsule disruption can be considered as a risk factor for the extrathyroidal extension, which is equal to 61% in these subjects, while 31% for macroscopic invasion [40].

Many studies have identified the presence of calcifications as malignancy predictors. While microcalcifications are one of the features significantly associated with the diagnosis of PTC, our results demonstrated that malignancy of follicular lesion might be suggested by the presence of not only microcalcifications but also mixed calcifications of a different type. In our meta-analysis, the presence of entirely macrocalcifications (>1 mm) was associated with a moderate risk of FTC with ORs between 2–3. Quite similar results were obtained by Kunt et al., where authors aimed to identify the risk factors of malignancy in a group of nodules preoperatively diagnosed as suspicion of FTC, and intranodular calcifications increased by about three times the relative risk of malignancy when present [41]. The diagnostic utility of calcifications in the case of FTC is limited by its low sensitivity. In the study by Sillery et al. comparing the distribution of particular sonographic variables in 52 FTAs vs. 50 FTCs, the feature occurred only in 14% of FTCs [13]. However, the absence of calcifications may have a negative predictive value. In the study by Zhang et al., over 90% of FTAs did not present calcifications, while the diagnosis of FTC was more frequently associated with the presence of calcifications (not only microcalcifications but also macrocalcifications and peripheral type). Still, this was not a sensitive feature, as in 55.5% of FTCs, calcifications were absent [14]. In a Chinese group, punctuate calcifications were more prevalent in FTCs (40.5%) compared to 13.5% of FTAs [23]. In the study by Kuo et al., either type of calcification was present in about one-third of FTCs, compared to only 3.6% of FTAs [36], while Liu et al. noted that macrocalcifications were the type of calcifications most importantly differentiating FTCs from FTAs, with specificity equal to 90.3% [37].

Another essential feature confirmed to be associated with FTC risk was a solid character of a lesion as well as heterogeneous and hypoechogenic echostructure. Hypoechogenicity was the most frequent ultrasound feature, occurring in 82% of FTCs reported by Sillery et al. [13]. In another study, by Chng et al., evaluating lesions diagnosed as follicular neoplasm on cytology, hypoechogenicity was present in 74.3% of FTCs vs. 51.4% of FTAs [42], and 64.9% vs. 39.2%, respectively in a group by Lai et al. [23]. The latter group also reported that the absence of cystic component was more frequently associated with FTC than FTA (78.4% vs. 54.1%) [23]. Predominant (>50%) cystic component was a predictor of benignity and presence of FTA in the group by Sillery et al. [13]. Authors explain that hypoechogenicity and lack of cystic degeneration might be a consequence of the rapidity of growth of the tumor cells, resulting in a disturbed formation of follicles, more typical for malignant lesions [13]. In another study by Zhang et al., a previous observation was confirmed that cystic component was significantly more frequent prevalent in FTAs, while in all of the studied 36 FTCs, a cystic component comprised less than 25% of the nodule volume [14]. Another FTC feature confirmed in this study was hypoechogenicity, while other echogenicity shades were more typical of FTAs. Most FTCs (83.3%) presented with heterogeneous echogenicity, while 80.8% of FTAs characterized by homogeneous echotexture. Authors demonstrated that a predominantly solid pattern, a heterogeneous echogenicity, and presence of calcifications were factors independently associated with the risk of FTC. The observations were consistent with the results obtained by Seo et al. [15]. Their logistic regression analysis demonstrated that predominantly solid character, mixed echotexture, and presence of microcalcifications or rim calcifications significantly increased the relative risk for FTC. However, neither Kuo et al. nor Liu et al. found significant difference in terms of nodule composition between FTAs and FTCs [36,37]. In addition, Liu et al. demonstrated that FTCs are more often hypoechogenic, while FTAs isoechogenic or presenting mixed echogenicity [37].

Irregular (microlobulated or spiculated) margins [40] increased the malignancy rate by 2.92, according to our results. The study by Maia et al. aiming to evaluate the value of ultrasound retrospectively to predict malignancy in indeterminate thyroid nodules by cytology confirmed this observation. Multivariate analysis revealed that borders irregularity on sonographic examination predicted malignancy risk in indeterminate thyroid nodules with 76.9% accuracy [43]. In another study by Chng et al., evaluating lesions diagnosed as follicular neoplasm on cytology, irregular margins were found to be present in 20% of FTCs but no FTA [42]. The irregular margin was also one of the features more prevalent in FTCs (21.6%) vs. 1.4% FTAs in a group by Lai et al. [23]. Both Liu et al. and Kuo et al. found that spiculated, lobulated, or irregular margins were significantly more prevalent in FTCs, while FTAs presented with a rather smooth contour [36,37].

The characteristic "taller than wide" shape of a lesion, so strongly associated with malignancy rate if PTCs are concerned, does not seem to play an important role in the case of FTCs. Our results demonstrated that OR for this feature was equal to 2.81. In another study by Chng et al., evaluating lesions diagnosed as follicular neoplasm on cytology and taller than wide morphology was not very frequent in FTCs (17.1%) but occurred rarer in FTAs (0.9%) [42]. In the studies by Liu et al. and Kuo et al., the taller than wide shape was not a very important feature useful in differentiation between FTAs and FTCs [36,37].

An OR between 2–3 was yielded for lack of halo or presence of thick halo and solitary lesions. Our conclusions about the halo sign are consistent with the risk factors for thyroid malignancy in general. Recent European Thyroid Association Guidelines indicate that a thin halo decreases the malignancy risk by about three-times (OR = 0.3), while thick or lack of halo increase the malignancy risk, with ORs equal to 3.4 and 7.1, respectively [10,40,44]. Halo was not present in 64% of FTCs in a group reported by Sillery et al. [13], being the second (after hypoechogenicity) most common feature associated with the malignant follicular lesion. The presence of halo sign may be attributed to the preserved capsule of FTA, which continuity is a feature allowing pathologists to differentiate between FTA and FTC. The presence of a thin halo was almost three times more frequently observed in FTAs in comparison to FTCs in a study by Zhang et al., while incomplete or unevenly thick halo was a feature significantly more frequently occurring in FTCs [14]. In the Chinese study, the authors also noticed the almost twice more common absence of halo in FTC patients (67.6%) vs. the FTA group (36.5%) [23].

Less important feature suggesting the malignant character of follicular lesions in our meta-analysis was size > 4 cm. The median volume of FTC (11.75 mL) was larger than FTA (5.95 mL) in the study by Sillery et al. [13]. Previous studies comparing ultrasound features of lesions eventually diagnosed as PTC or FTC demonstrated that FTCs were significantly greater than PTCs [12,45]. This may be explained by the hypothesis also supported by some genetic studies [46], that FTC may result from the transformation from FTA and by the difficulties in cytological detection of malignant features in small FTC tumors [12]. Other studies did not report a significant difference in terms of size between FTAs and FTCs [36,37].

One of the less useful features of FTCs in our meta-analysis was the presence of central vascularization. The vascularization pattern on the Color Doppler examination was not a helpful feature in the differentiation of FTC and FTA by Sillery et al. [13]. In another study comparing ultrasound features of 37 FTCs with 74 FTAs, the incidence of intranodular vascularization did not differ significantly between the two groups [23]. This feature was also of limited value in the prediction of malignancy in the case of PTCs [7]. However, the reported results are not entirely consistent, as Kunt et al. indicated that intranodular vascularization (Doppler pattern three for a peripheral ring of flow and a small-to-moderate amount of internal flow, and four for extensive internal flow with or without a peripheral ring) [47], as the most useful predictor of malignancy with an OR at the level of 14.7, which is in contrast to our and previous observations [41].

Once sonoelastography was introduced to thyroid diagnostics, it raised hopes that it would be of value in presurgical and non-invasive differentiation of follicular lesions. Fukunari et al. analyzed 56 follicular lesions. Out of 51 FTAs, 48 (94.1%) presented with normal elasticity, while all FTCs demonstrated a characteristic pattern of elasticity, corresponding with an elastic central part and a stiff peripheral region. The authors concluded that sonoelastography might reflect the differences in the histopathological structure of follicular lesions and might be helpful in differentiation between benign and malignant follicular lesions. Another communication from this research group resulted in the conclusion that over 70% of FTCs present with such a sonoelastographic pattern [48]. Another paper by Rago et al. also postulated the potential usefulness of sonoelastography in the presurgical prediction of the character of thyroid lesions, in which cytological examination yielded inconclusive results [49]. However, future studies did not confirm the previous findings and usefulness of sonoelastography of differentiation of follicular lesions. As there was only one full-text paper encompassing the sonoelastographic picture of follicular lesions, we were not able to include this feature in our meta-analysis. In the study by Liu et al., the speed of shear waves propagation on sonoelastographic examination was greater for FTCs if compared to FTAs [37].

The most crucial feature associated with an increased risk of FTC is capsule protrusion, followed by the presence of calcifications, irrespectively of their type. The most important ultrasound malignancy risk factors for PTC were rather taller than wide (ORs = 13.7, 11.4, and 10.15), which was only the tenth feature in our analysis for FTC with an OR = 2.52. However, microcalcifications and irregular margins seem to be common malignancy ultrasound features both for FTC and PTC [7,9,50].

Currently, due to the inconsistency of ultrasound terminology and to enable easier risk of malignancy determination for thyroid nodules ultrasound assessment, there are many risk stratification models comprising conventional ultrasound and elastography characteristics. They enable a better combined evaluation of thyroid nodules and are considered an important step in endocrinology [40,51–55]. Although helpful in the assessment of cytologically equivocal thyroid nodules, according to some studies [56], they may have limited clinical values for risk stratification of intermediate cytological results according to the others [57]. Therefore, there is still a need for research in this field.

4. Materials and Methods

4.1. Search Strategy

We carried out the meta-analysis following the guidelines formulated in the Cochrane Handbook for Systematic Reviews of Interventions and the Preferred Reporting Items for Systematic Reviews and Meta-Analyses (PRISMA) guidelines [58]. We searched PubMed, MEDLINE, Academic Search Complete, CINAHL Complete, CINAHL, Scopus, Cochrane, Health Source: Nursing/Academic Edition, Web of Knowledge, MasterFILE Premier, Health Source-Consumer Edition, Agricola, Dentistry and Oral Science Source databases from January 2006 up to December 2020 to find all relevant, full-text journal articles written in English.

We included studies, regardless of their sample size, with the investigation of the association between one or more ultrasound feature and the risk of follicular thyroid malignancy, which did not have any restriction criteria for the inclusion of detected nodules in the study, such as nodule size or thyroid-stimulating hormone (TSH) levels [10]. We considered histopathological diagnosis after surgery to be the gold standard reference test and included only studies considering the histopathological result of FTA and FTC as the exclusive diagnoses, as well as within an analysis of different thyroid histopathological diagnoses. Studies were excluded if focusing only on particular subgroups of patients such as pediatric patients only, with a prior history of thyroid cancer or were clearly exposed to known risk factors for thyroid cancer, e.g., Chernobyl survivors or particular types of nodules (e.g., palpable, less than 1 cm, pure cystic or solid, etc.) [7,9,50].

The search strategy included Medical Subject Headings terms and keywords: "thyroid and ("follicular cancer" or "follicular carcinoma" or "follicular neoplasm" or "follicular adenoma" or "follicular nodule") and (ultrasound or ultrasonography or elastography or "color doppler" or "power doppler")". Reference lists of all the selected articles, previous meta-analyses, and reviews were hand-searched for any additional articles.

4.2. Data Extraction

Two authors (M.B. and E.J.S.) independently selected papers, which fulfilled the inclusion criteria and extracted data for the outcomes using a standardized data extraction form. Relevant data included articles assessing echogenicity, calcifications, presence of a "halo", size, shape, protrusion, margins, Doppler pattern, solitarity, and structure of nodules. Another author (E.S.P.) rechecked the extracted data.

4.3. Assessment of Methodological Quality

The risk of bias in the included studies was independently assessed by two authors (MB and ESP by the Cochrane risk of bias tool [20]. As recommended for diagnostic accuracy-test studies, the revised Quality Assessment of Diagnostic Accuracy Studies-2 (QUADAS-2) tool was also used. All included studies were assessed using the Newcastle-Ottawa Scale [59]. Studies with a result of seven stars or more were included.

4.4. Statistical Analysis

Analyses assessing the accuracy of malignancy detection in case of follicular lesions, potentially differentiating FTA and FTC included the odds ratio (OR), sensitivity, specificity, positive predictive values (PPV), and negative predictive values (NPV). A random-effects model described by DerSimonian and Laird was used to summarize collected data.

In the first stage, we calculated ORs and assessed studies' heterogeneity and publication bias. Statistical heterogeneity between the studies was examined using Cochrane's Q statistics and I^2 statistics. The publication bias was explored by visual inspection of funnel plots, and asymmetry was tested formally with Egger's regression test [60,61]. Furthermore, a sensitivity analysis was performed for parameters showing significant heterogeneity. In the case of high heterogeneity (i.e., $I^2 > 50\%$ and $p < 0.05$), outlying studies were identified. The meta-analysis was repeated to confirm the obtained results, excluding outliers and the overall OR, and the heterogeneity test results were given again. In the event of a zero outcome, continuity correction was performed by adding a correction factor of 0.5.

In the second stage, after outliers exclusion, based on the number of true positive (TP), true negative (TN), false positive (FP), and false negative (FN) results univariates of sensitivity, specificity, Negative Predictive Value (NPV), and Positive Predictive Value (PPV) with 95% confidence intervals were estimated using the exact binomial Clopper-Pearson method. In the meta-analysis, the pooled estimation was calculated after Freeman-Tukey Double Arcsine Transformation to stabilize the variances [62]. Additionally, for the analysis of traits that were based on more research and met the assumptions of the HSROC model (currently recommended by the Cochrane Collaboration), bivariate meta-analyses were performed to jointly models both sensitivity and specificity.

The significance level $p = 0.05$ was assumed in all analyzes. The analysis of the odds ratio was carried out in the PQStat v1.6.6 program, while the results regarding sensitivity, specificity, PPV, and NPV were obtained in the Stata v14 package, using the metaprop and metandi functions.

5. Conclusions

In conclusion, sonographic features associated with the malignancy of follicular lesions are distinct from those widely reported for all thyroid cancers, of which the predominant histological type is PTC. The most crucial feature associated with an increased risk of FTC is capsule protrusion, followed by the presence of calcifications, irrespective of their type. Less specific but more frequent are the irregular shape of the lesion, solid character of the lesion, and hypoechogenicity. On the other hand, a high probability of a diagnosis of FTA is suggested by an oval or round shape of the lesion and the presence of a cystic component. Less specific features suggesting benign lesions are a lack of calcifications and a visible halo.

Supplementary Materials: The following are available online at https://www.mdpi.com/2072-6694/13/5/938/s1, Table S1a: The results of odds rations (OR) of each study in increasing the risk of nodule malignancy for tumor protrusion with 95% confidence intervals and forest plots, Table S1b: The number of patients with true positive (TP), false negative (FN), false positive (FP), and true negative (TN) results presenting the estimates of sensitivity, specificity, positive predictive value (PPV), and negative predictive value (NPV with 95% confidence intervals of each study for tumor protrusion, Table S2a: The results of odds rations (OR) of each study in increasing the risk of nodule malignancy when microcalcifications or mixed type (coexisting micro- and macrocalcifications) are present in the ultrasound with 95% confidence intervals and forest plots, Table S2b: The number of patients with true positive (TP), false negative (FN), false positive (FP), and true negative (TN) results presenting the estimates of sensitivity, specificity, positive predictive value (PPV), and negative predictive value (NPV with 95% confidence intervals of each study for microcalcifications or mixed type (coexisting micro- and macrocalcifications) in the ultrasound, Table S3a: The results of odds rations (OR) of each study in increasing the risk of nodule malignancy for irregular margins with 95% confidence intervals and forest plots, Table S3b: The number of patients with true positive (TP), false negative (FN), false positive (FP), and true negative (TN) results presenting the estimates of sensitivity, specificity, positive predictive value (PPV), and negative predictive value (NPV with 95% confidence intervals of each study for irregular margins, Table S4a: The results of odds rations (OR) of each study in increasing the risk of nodule malignancy for hypoechogenicity markedly hypoechogenic nodules with 95% confidence intervals and forest plots, Table S4b: The number of patients with true positive (TP), false negative (FN), false positive (FP), and true negative (TN) results presenting the estimates of sensitivity, specificity, positive predictive value (PPV), and negative predictive value (NPV with 95% confidence intervals of each study for hypoechogenicity or markedly hypoechogenic nodules, Table S5a: The results of odds rations (OR) of each study in increasing the risk of nodule malignancy for irregular shape with 95% confidence intervals and forest plots, Table S5b: The number of patients with true positive (TP), false negative (FN), false positive (FP), and true negative (TN) results presenting the estimates of sensitivity, specificity, positive predictive value (PPV), and negative predictive value (NPV with 95% confidence intervals of each study for irregular shape, Table S6a: The results of odds rations (OR) of each study in increasing the risk of nodule malignancy for lack of halo or presence of thick halo with 95% confidence intervals and forest plots, Table S6b: The number of patients with true positive (TP), false negative (FN), false positive (FP), and true negative (TN) results presenting the estimates of sensitivity, specificity, positive predictive value (PPV), and negative predictive value (NPV with 95% confidence intervals of each study for lack of halo or presence of thick halo, Table S7a: The results of odds rations (OR) of each study in increasing the risk of nodule malignancy when macrocalcifications, eggshell or rim calcifications are present in the ultrasound with 95% confidence intervals and forest plots, Table S7b: The number of patients with true positive (TP), false negative (FN), false positive (FP), and true negative (TN) results presenting the estimates of sensitivity, specificity, positive predictive value (PPV), and negative predictive value (NPV with 95% confidence intervals of each study for macrocalcifications, eggshell or rim calcifications in the ultrasound, Table S8a: The results of odds rations (OR) of each study in increasing the risk of nodule malignancy when any type of calcifications is present in the ultrasound with 95% confidence intervals and forest plots, Table S8b: The number of patients with true positive (TP), false negative (FN), false positive (FP), and true negative (TN) results presenting the estimates of sensitivity, specificity, positive predictive value (PPV), and negative predictive value (NPV with 95% confidence intervals of each study for all types of calcifications in the ultrasound, Table S9a: The results of odds rations (OR) of each study in increasing the risk of nodule malignancy for solitary nodule with 95% confidence intervals and forest plots, Table S9b: The number of patients with true positive (TP), false negative (FN), false positive (FP), and true negative (TN) results presenting the estimates of sensitivity, specificity, positive predictive value (PPV), and negative predictive value (NPV with 95% confidence intervals of each study for solitary nodule, Table S10a: The results of odds rations (OR) of each study in increasing the risk of nodule malignancy for taller than wide feature in the ultrasound with 95% confidence intervals and forest plots, Table S10b: The number of patients with true positive (TP), false negative (FN), false positive (FP), and true negative (TN) results presenting the estimates of sensitivity, specificity, positive predictive value (PPV), and negative predictive value (NPV with 95% confidence intervals of each study for taller than wide feature in the ultrasound, Table S11a: The results of odds rations (OR) of each study in increasing the risk of nodule malignancy for solid or mainly solid structure with 95% confidence intervals and forest plots, Table S11b: The number of patients with true positive (TP), false negative (FN), false positive (FP), and true negative (TN) results presenting the estimates of sensitivity, specificity, positive predictive value (PPV), and negative predictive value (NPV with 95% confidence intervals of each study for solid or mainly solid structure, Table S12a: The results of odds rations (OR) of each study in increasing the risk of nodule malignancy for size over 4 cm with 95% confidence intervals and forest plots, Table S12b: The number of patients with true positive (TP), false negative (FN), false positive (FP), and true negative (TN) results presenting the estimates of sensitivity, specificity, positive predictive value (PPV), and negative predictive value (NPV with 95% confidence intervals of each study for size over 4 cm, Table S13a: The results of odds rations (OR) of each study in increasing the risk of nodule malignancy for heterogeoenous echostructure in the ultrasound with 95% confidence intervals and forest plots, Table S13b: The number of patients with true positive (TP), false negative (FN), false positive (FP), and true negative (TN) results presenting the estimates of sensitivity, specificity, positive predictive value (PPV), and negative predictive value (NPV with 95% confidence intervals of each study for heterogeoenous echostructure.

Author Contributions: Conceptualization, M.B., K.W. and E.S.-P.; methodology, M.B., K.W., B.W., E.J.-S. and E.S.-P.; formal analysis, K.W., E.S.-P., F.A.V. and M.R.; investigation, M.B., K.W., B.W., E.J.-S. and E.S.-P.; resources, M.B., B.W.; data curation, M.B., K.W., B.W., E.J.-S. and E.S.-P.; writing—original draft preparation, M.B., B.W., E.J.-S. and E.S.-P.; writing—review and editing, K.W., E.S.-P., F.A.V. and M.R.; visualization: M.B., B.W.; supervision, E.S.-P., F.A.V. and M.R.; project administration, M.B.; funding acquisition, M.B. All authors have read and agreed to the published version of the manuscript.

Funding: This study was supported by a PRELUDIUM Grant of the Polish National Center for Science, No. 2015/19/N/NZ5/02257, awarded to M.B.

Institutional Review Board Statement: Not applicable.

Informed Consent Statement: Not applicable.

Data Availability Statement: The data presented in this study are available in this article (and Supplementary Material).

Conflicts of Interest: The authors declare no conflict of interest.

References

1. Burman, K.D.; Wartofsky, L. CLINICAL PRACTICE. Thyroid Nodules. *N. Engl. J. Med.* **2015**, *373*, 2347–2356. [CrossRef]
2. Borowczyk, M.; Szczepanek-Parulska, E.; Olejarz, M.; Wieckowska, B.; Verburg, F.A.; Debicki, S.; Budny, B.; Janicka-Jedynska, M.; Ziemnicka, K.; Ruchala, M. Evaluation of 167 Gene Expression Classifier (GEC) and ThyroSeq v2 Diagnostic Accuracy in the Preoperative Assessment of Indeterminate Thyroid Nodules: Bivariate/HROC Meta-analysis. *Endocr. Pathol.* **2019**, *30*, 8–15. [CrossRef]
3. Cibas, E.S.; Ali, S.Z. The 2017 Bethesda System for Reporting Thyroid Cytopathology. *Thyroid* **2017**, *27*, 1341–1346. [CrossRef] [PubMed]
4. Jarzab, B.; Dedecjus, M.; Slowinska-Klencka, D.; Lewinski, A.; Adamczewski, Z.; Anielski, R.; Baglaj, M.; Baldys-Waligorska, A.; Barczynski, M.; Bednarczuk, T.; et al. Guidelines of Polish National Societies Diagnostics and Treatment of Thyroid Carcinoma. 2018 Update. *Endokrynol. Pol.* **2018**, *69*, 34–74. [CrossRef] [PubMed]

5. Munoz Perez, N.; Villar del Moral, J.M.; Muros Fuentes, M.A.; Lopez de la Torre, M.; Arcelus Martinez, J.I.; Becerra Massare, P.; Esteva Martinez, D.; Canadas Garre, M.; Coll Del Rey, E.; Bueno Larano, P.; et al. Could 18F-FDG-PET/CT avoid unnecessary thyroidectomies in patients with cytological diagnosis of follicular neoplasm? *Langenbecks Arch. Surg* **2013**, *398*, 709–716. [CrossRef]
6. Ruchala, M.; Szczepanek, E. Thyroid ultrasound—A piece of cake? *Endokrynol. Pol.* **2010**, *61*, 330–344. [PubMed]
7. Wolinski, K.; Szkudlarek, M.; Szczepanek-Parulska, E.; Ruchala, M. Usefulness of different ultrasound features of malignancy in predicting the type of thyroid lesions: A meta-analysis of prospective studies. *Pol. Arch. Med. Wewn* **2014**, *124*, 97–104. [CrossRef] [PubMed]
8. Szczepanek-Parulska, E.; Wolinski, K.; Stangierski, A.; Gurgul, E.; Biczysko, M.; Majewski, P.; Rewaj-Losyk, M.; Ruchala, M. Comparison of diagnostic value of conventional ultrasonography and shear wave elastography in the prediction of thyroid lesions malignancy. *PLoS ONE* **2013**, *8*, e81532. [CrossRef] [PubMed]
9. Brito, J.P.; Gionfriddo, M.R.; Al Nofal, A.; Boehmer, K.R.; Leppin, A.L.; Reading, C.; Callstrom, M.; Elraiyah, T.A.; Prokop, L.J.; Stan, M.N.; et al. The accuracy of thyroid nodule ultrasound to predict thyroid cancer: Systematic review and meta-analysis. *J. Clin. Endocrinol. Metab.* **2014**, *99*, 1253–1263. [CrossRef]
10. Campanella, P.; Ianni, F.; Rota, C.A.; Corsello, S.M.; Pontecorvi, A. Quantification of cancer risk of each clinical and ultrasonographic suspicious feature of thyroid nodules: A systematic review and meta-analysis. *Eur. J. Endocrinol.* **2014**, *170*, R203–R211. [CrossRef]
11. Wolinski, K.; Rewaj-Losyk, M.; Ruchala, M. Sonographic features of medullary thyroid carcinomas—A systematic review and meta-analysis. *Endokrynol. Pol.* **2014**, *65*, 314–318. [CrossRef]
12. Cordes, M.; Kondrat, P.; Uder, M.; Kuwert, T.; Sasiadek, M. Differential diagnostic ultrasound criteria of papillary and follicular carcinomas: A multivariate analysis. *Rofo* **2014**, *186*, 489–495. [CrossRef] [PubMed]
13. Sillery, J.C.; Reading, C.C.; Charboneau, J.W.; Henrichsen, T.L.; Hay, I.D.; Mandrekar, J.N. Thyroid follicular carcinoma: Sonographic features of 50 cases. *AJR Am. J. Roentgenol.* **2010**, *194*, 44–54. [CrossRef]
14. Zhang, J.Z.; Hu, B. Sonographic features of thyroid follicular carcinoma in comparison with thyroid follicular adenoma. *J. Ultrasound Med.* **2014**, *33*, 221–227. [CrossRef] [PubMed]
15. Seo, H.S.; Lee, D.H.; Park, S.H.; Min, H.S.; Na, D.G. Thyroid follicular neoplasms: Can sonography distinguish between adenomas and carcinomas? *J. Clin. Ultrasound* **2009**, *37*, 493–500. [CrossRef] [PubMed]
16. Koike, E.; Noguchi, S.; Yamashita, H.; Murakami, T.; Ohshima, A.; Kawamoto, H.; Yamashita, H. Ultrasonographic characteristics of thyroid nodules: Prediction of malignancy. *Arch. Surg.* **2001**, *136*, 334–337. [CrossRef]
17. Rago, T.; Di Coscio, G.; Basolo, F.; Scutari, M.; Elisei, R.; Berti, P.; Miccoli, P.; Romani, R.; Faviana, P.; Pinchera, A.; et al. Combined clinical, thyroid ultrasound and cytological features help to predict thyroid malignancy in follicular and Hupsilonrthle cell thyroid lesions: Results from a series of 505 consecutive patients. *Clin. Endocrinol. (Oxf.)* **2007**, *66*, 13–20. [CrossRef]
18. Raber, W.; Kaserer, K.; Niederle, B.; Vierhapper, H. Risk factors for malignancy of thyroid nodules initially identified as follicular neoplasia by fine-needle aspiration: Results of a prospective study of one hundred twenty patients. *Thyroid* **2000**, *10*, 709–712. [CrossRef] [PubMed]
19. Lin, J.D.; Hsueh, C.; Chao, T.C.; Weng, H.F.; Huang, B.Y. Thyroid follicular neoplasms diagnosed by high-resolution ultrasonography with fine needle aspiration cytology. *Acta Cytol.* **1997**, *41*, 687–691. [CrossRef]
20. Stoian, D.; Borcan, F.; Petre, I.; Mozos, I.; Varcus, F.; Ivan, V.; Cioca, A.; Apostol, A.; Dehelean, C.A. Strain Elastography as a Valuable Diagnosis Tool in Intermediate Cytology (Bethesda III) Thyroid Nodules. *Diagnostics* **2019**, *9*, 119. [CrossRef]
21. Asteria, C.; Giovanardi, A.; Pizzocaro, A.; Cozzaglio, L.; Morabito, A.; Somalvico, F.; Zoppo, A. US-elastography in the differential diagnosis of benign and malignant thyroid nodules. *Thyroid* **2008**, *18*, 523–531. [CrossRef] [PubMed]
22. Lee, E.K.; Chung, K.W.; Min, H.S.; Kim, T.S.; Kim, T.H.; Ryu, J.S.; Jung, Y.S.; Kim, S.K.; Lee, Y.J. Preoperative serum thyroglobulin as a useful predictive marker to differentiate follicular thyroid cancer from benign nodules in indeterminate nodules. *J. Korean Med. Sci.* **2012**, *27*, 1014–1018. [CrossRef] [PubMed]
23. Lai, X.J.; Zhang, B.; Jiang, Y.X.; Zhu, Q.L.; Yang, M.; Dai, Q.; Xia, Y.; Yang, X.; Zhao, R.N. Usefulness of ultrasonography in the differential diagnosis of thyroidal follicular tumor. *Zhongguo Yi Xue Ke Xue Yuan Xue Bao* **2013**, *35*, 483–487. [CrossRef] [PubMed]
24. Lee, K.H.; Shin, J.H.; Ko, E.S.; Hahn, S.Y.; Kim, J.S.; Kim, J.H.; Oh, Y.L. Predictive factors of malignancy in patients with cytologically suspicious for Hurthle cell neoplasm of thyroid nodules. *Int. J. Surg.* **2013**, *11*, 898–902. [CrossRef]
25. Lee, S.H.; Baek, J.S.; Lee, J.Y.; Lim, J.A.; Cho, S.Y.; Lee, T.H.; Ku, Y.H.; Kim, H.I.; Kim, M.J. Predictive factors of malignancy in thyroid nodules with a cytological diagnosis of follicular neoplasm. *Endocr. Pathol.* **2013**, *24*, 177–183. [CrossRef]
26. Pompili, G.; Tresoldi, S.; Primolevo, A.; De Pasquale, L.; Di Leo, G.; Cornalba, G. Management of thyroid follicular proliferation: An ultrasound-based malignancy score to opt for surgical or conservative treatment. *Ultrasound Med. Biol.* **2013**, *39*, 1350–1355. [CrossRef]
27. Kamran, S.C.; Marqusee, E.; Kim, M.I.; Frates, M.C.; Ritner, J.; Peters, H.; Benson, C.B.; Doubilet, P.M.; Cibas, E.S.; Barletta, J.; et al. Thyroid nodule size and prediction of cancer. *J. Clin. Endocrinol. Metab.* **2013**, *98*, 564–570. [CrossRef] [PubMed]
28. Tutuncu, Y.; Berker, D.; Isik, S.; Akbaba, G.; Ozuguz, U.; Kucukler, F.K.; Gocmen, E.; Yalcin, Y.; Aydin, Y.; Guler, S. The frequency of malignancy and the relationship between malignancy and ultrasonographic features of thyroid nodules with indeterminate cytology. *Endocrine* **2014**, *45*, 37–45. [CrossRef]

29. Yoon, J.H.; Kim, E.K.; Youk, J.H.; Moon, H.J.; Kwak, J.Y. Better understanding in the differentiation of thyroid follicular adenoma, follicular carcinoma, and follicular variant of papillary carcinoma: A retrospective study. *Int. J. Endocrinol.* **2014**, *2014*, 321595. [CrossRef]
30. Cordes, M.; Nagel, H.; Horstrup, K.; Sasiadek, M.; Kuwert, T. Ultrasound characteristics of thyroid nodules diagnosed as follicular neoplasms by fine-needle aspiration cytology. A prospective study with histological correlation. *Nuklearmedizin* **2016**, *55*, 93–98. [CrossRef]
31. Jeong, S.H.; Hong, H.S.; Lee, E.H. Can Nodular Hyperplasia of the Thyroid Gland be Differentiated From Follicular Adenoma and Follicular Carcinoma by Ultrasonography? *Ultrasound Q* **2016**, *32*, 349–355. [CrossRef]
32. Kobayashi, K.; Hirokawa, M.; Yabuta, T.; Masuoka, H.; Fukushima, M.; Kihara, M.; Higashiyama, T.; Ito, Y.; Miya, A.; Amino, N.; et al. Tumor protrusion with intensive blood signals on ultrasonography is a strongly suggestive finding of follicular thyroid carcinoma. *Med. Ultrason.* **2016**, *18*, 25–29. [CrossRef]
33. Yang, G.C.H.; Fried, K.O. Most Thyroid Cancers Detected by Sonography Lack Intranodular Vascularity on Color Doppler Imaging: Review of the Literature and Sonographic-Pathologic Correlations for 698 Thyroid Neoplasms. *J. Ultrasound Med.* **2017**, *36*, 89–94. [CrossRef]
34. Kuru, B.; Kefeli, M. Risk factors associated with malignancy and with triage to surgery in thyroid nodules classified as Bethesda category IV (FN/SFN). *Diagn. Cytopathol.* **2018**, *46*, 489–494. [CrossRef] [PubMed]
35. Kim, M.; Han, M.; Lee, J.H.; Song, D.E.; Kim, K.; Baek, J.H.; Shong, Y.K.; Kim, W.G. Tumour growth rate of follicular thyroid carcinoma is not different from that of follicular adenoma. *Clin. Endocrinol. (Oxf.)* **2018**, *88*, 936–942. [CrossRef] [PubMed]
36. Kuo, T.C.; Wu, M.H.; Chen, K.Y.; Hsieh, M.S.; Chen, A.; Chen, C.N. Ultrasonographic features for differentiating follicular thyroid carcinoma and follicular adenoma. *Asian J. Surg.* **2020**, *43*, 339–346. [CrossRef]
37. Liu, B.J.; Zhang, Y.F.; Zhao, C.K.; Wang, H.X.; Li, M.X.; Xu, H.X. Conventional ultrasound characteristics, TI-RADS category and shear wave speed measurement between follicular adenoma and follicular thyroid carcinoma. *Clin. Hemorheol. Microcirc.* **2020**, *75*, 291–301. [CrossRef]
38. Aschebrook-Kilfoy, B.; Grogan, R.H.; Ward, M.H.; Kaplan, E.; Devesa, S.S. Follicular thyroid cancer incidence patterns in the United States, 1980-2009. *Thyroid* **2013**, *23*, 1015–1021. [CrossRef] [PubMed]
39. Slowinska-Klencka, D.; Klencki, M.; Sporny, S.; Lewinski, A. Fine-needle aspiration biopsy of the thyroid in an area of endemic goitre. Influence of restored sufficient iodine supplementation on the clinical significance of cytological results. *Eur. J. Endocrinol.* **2002**, *146*, 19–26. [CrossRef] [PubMed]
40. Russ, G.; Bonnema, S.J.; Erdogan, M.F.; Durante, C.; Ngu, R.; Leenhardt, L. European Thyroid Association Guidelines for Ultrasound Malignancy Risk Stratification of Thyroid Nodules in Adults: The EU-TIRADS. *Eur. Thyroid J.* **2017**, *6*, 225–237. [CrossRef]
41. Kunt, M.; Cirit, E.; Eray, I.C.; Yalav, O.; Parsak, C.K.; Sakmann, G. Parameters predicting follicular carcinoma in thyroid nodules with indeterminate cytology. *Ann. Ital. Chir.* **2015**, *86*, 301–305; discussion 306. [PubMed]
42. Chng, C.L.; Kurzawinski, T.R.; Beale, T. Value of sonographic features in predicting malignancy in thyroid nodules diagnosed as follicular neoplasm on cytology. *Clin. Endocrinol. (Oxf.)* **2015**, *83*, 711–716. [CrossRef] [PubMed]
43. Maia, F.F.; Matos, P.S.; Pavin, E.J.; Vassallo, J.; Zantut-Wittmann, D.E. Value of ultrasound and cytological classification system to predict the malignancy of thyroid nodules with indeterminate cytology. *Endocr. Pathol.* **2011**, *22*, 66–73. [CrossRef]
44. Russ, G.; Bigorgne, C.; Royer, B.; Rouxel, A.; Bienvenu-Perrard, M. The Thyroid Imaging Reporting and Data System (TIRADS) for ultrasound of the thyroid. *J. Radiol.* **2011**, *92*, 701–713. [CrossRef] [PubMed]
45. Verburg, F.A.; Mäder, U.; Luster, M.; Reiners, C. Histology does not influence prognosis in differentiated thyroid carcinoma when accounting for age, tumour diameter, invasive growth and metastases. *Eur. J. Endocrinol.* **2009**, *160*, 619–624. [CrossRef] [PubMed]
46. Borowczyk, M.; Szczepanek-Parulska, E.; Debicki, S.; Budny, B.; Verburg, F.A.; Filipowicz, D.; Wieckowska, B.; Janicka-Jedynska, M.; Gil, L.; Ziemnicka, K.; et al. Differences in Mutational Profile between Follicular Thyroid Carcinoma and Follicular Thyroid Adenoma Identified Using Next Generation Sequencing. *Int. J. Mol. Sci.* **2019**, *20*, 3126. [CrossRef] [PubMed]
47. Frates, M.C.; Benson, C.B.; Doubilet, P.M.; Cibas, E.S.; Marqusee, E. Can color Doppler sonography aid in the prediction of malignancy of thyroid nodules? *J. Ultrasound Med.* **2003**, *22*, 127–131. [CrossRef]
48. Fukunari, N.; Nagahama, M.; Sugino, K.; Mimura, T.; Ito, K.; Ito, K. Clinical evaluation of color Doppler imaging for the differential diagnosis of thyroid follicular lesions. *World J. Surg.* **2004**, *28*, 1261–1265. [CrossRef]
49. Rago, T.; Scutari, M.; Santini, F.; Loiacono, V.; Piaggi, P.; Di Coscio, G.; Basolo, F.; Berti, P.; Pinchera, A.; Vitti, P. Real-time elastosonography: Useful tool for refining the presurgical diagnosis in thyroid nodules with indeterminate or nondiagnostic cytology. *J. Clin. Endocrinol. Metab.* **2010**, *95*, 5274–5280. [CrossRef]
50. Trimboli, P.; Castellana, M.; Piccardo, A.; Romanelli, F.; Grani, G.; Giovanella, L.; Durante, C. The ultrasound risk stratification systems for thyroid nodule have been evaluated against papillary carcinoma. A meta-analysis. *Rev. Endocr. Metab. Disord.* **2020**. [CrossRef] [PubMed]
51. Koc, A.M.; Adibelli, Z.H.; Erkul, Z.; Sahin, Y.; Dilek, I. Comparison of diagnostic accuracy of ACR-TIRADS, American Thyroid Association (ATA), and EU-TIRADS guidelines in detecting thyroid malignancy. *Eur. J. Radiol.* **2020**, *133*, 109390. [CrossRef]
52. Migda, B.; Migda, M.; Migda, A.M.; Bierca, J.; Slowniska-Srzednicka, J.; Jakubowski, W.; Slapa, R.Z. Evaluation of Four Variants of the Thyroid Imaging Reporting and Data System (TIRADS) Classification in Patients with Multinodular Goitre—Initial study. *Endokrynol. Pol.* **2018**, *69*, 156–162. [CrossRef]

53. Grant, E.G.; Tessler, F.N.; Hoang, J.K.; Langer, J.E.; Beland, M.D.; Berland, L.L.; Cronan, J.J.; Desser, T.S.; Frates, M.C.; Hamper, U.M.; et al. Thyroid Ultrasound Reporting Lexicon: White Paper of the ACR Thyroid Imaging, Reporting and Data System (TIRADS) Committee. *J. Am. Coll. Radiol.* **2015**, *12*, 1272–1279. [CrossRef]
54. Singaporewalla, R.M.; Hwee, J.; Lang, T.U.; Desai, V. Clinico-pathological Correlation of Thyroid Nodule Ultrasound and Cytology Using the TIRADS and Bethesda Classifications. *World J. Surg.* **2017**, *41*, 1807–1811. [CrossRef] [PubMed]
55. Shayganfar, A.; Hashemi, P.; Esfahani, M.M.; Ghanei, A.M.; Moghadam, N.A.; Ebrahimian, S. Prediction of thyroid nodule malignancy using thyroid imaging reporting and data system (TIRADS) and nodule size. *Clin. Imaging* **2020**, *60*, 222–227. [CrossRef] [PubMed]
56. Slowinska-Klencka, D.; Wysocka-Konieczna, K.; Klencki, M.; Popowicz, B. Diagnostic Value of Six Thyroid Imaging Reporting and Data Systems (TIRADS) in Cytologically Equivocal Thyroid Nodules. *J. Clin. Med.* **2020**, *9*, 2281. [CrossRef] [PubMed]
57. Chaigneau, E.; Russ, G.; Royer, B.; Bigorgne, C.; Bienvenu-Perrard, M.; Rouxel, A.; Leenhardt, L.; Belin, L.; Buffet, C. TIRADS score is of limited clinical value for risk stratification of indeterminate cytological results. *Eur. J. Endocrinol.* **2018**, *179*, 13–20. [CrossRef]
58. Shamseer, L.; Moher, D.; Clarke, M.; Ghersi, D.; Liberati, A.; Petticrew, M.; Shekelle, P.; Stewart, L.A.; Group, P.-P. Preferred reporting items for systematic review and meta-analysis protocols (PRISMA-P) 2015: Elaboration and explanation. *BMJ* **2015**, *350*, g7647. [CrossRef]
59. Lo, C.K.; Mertz, D.; Loeb, M. Newcastle-Ottawa Scale: Comparing reviewers' to authors' assessments. *BMC Med. Res. Methodol.* **2014**, *14*, 45. [CrossRef] [PubMed]
60. Egger, M.; Davey Smith, G.; Schneider, M.; Minder, C. Bias in meta-analysis detected by a simple, graphical test. *BMJ* **1997**, *315*, 629–634. [CrossRef]
61. Sterne, J.A.; Egger, M.; Smith, G.D. Systematic reviews in health care: Investigating and dealing with publication and other biases in meta-analysis. *BMJ* **2001**, *323*, 101–105. [CrossRef] [PubMed]
62. Newcombe, R.G. Two-sided confidence intervals for the single proportion: Comparison of seven methods. *Stat. Med.* **1998**, *17*, 857–872. [CrossRef]

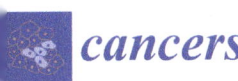

Editorial

Advancements in Ultrasound and Ultrasound-Based Risk Stratification Systems for the Assessment of Thyroid Nodule

Pierpaolo Trimboli [1,2]

1 Servizio di Endocrinologia e Diabetologia, Ente Ospedaliero Cantonale (EOC), 6500 Bellinzona, Switzerland; pierpaolo.trimboli@eoc.ch
2 Facoltà di Scienze Biomediche, Università della Svizzera Italiana (USI), 6900 Lugano, Switzerland

Citation: Trimboli, P. Advancements in Ultrasound and Ultrasound-Based Risk Stratification Systems for the Assessment of Thyroid Nodule. *Cancers* 2022, *14*, 1668. https://doi.org/10.3390/cancers14071668

Received: 22 March 2022
Accepted: 23 March 2022
Published: 25 March 2022

Publisher's Note: MDPI stays neutral with regard to jurisdictional claims in published maps and institutional affiliations.

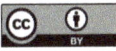

Copyright: © 2022 by the author. Licensee MDPI, Basel, Switzerland. This article is an open access article distributed under the terms and conditions of the Creative Commons Attribution (CC BY) license (https://creativecommons.org/licenses/by/4.0/).

Ultrasound (US) is an essential in-office imaging procedure used for evaluating thyroid nodules. This Special Issue entitled "Risk Stratification of Thyroid Nodule: From Ultrasound Features to TIRADS" published in *Cancers* allows us to improve the information about US and US-based risk stratification systems used for the assessment of thyroid nodules. Neck and thyroid US has been widely used during the last two to three decades and several significant developments have been reported in terms of the performance of US to detect thyroid cancer [1]. After an initial phase in which most clinicians used single US parameters in clinical practice, several international societies in the field of thyroid diseases have developed specific US-based systems (i.e., Thyroid Imaging Reporting And Data Systems, TIRADS) to improve the performance of US operators and standardize their terminology [2]. The latter represents a non-negligible advancement that eminent cytologists have also involved in the management of thyroid nodules [3]. Obviously, further efforts still are needed to achieve the optimal performance of US and TIRADSs, and the present Special Issue will contribute to these efforts. If how to discriminate benign from malignant lesions among the indeterminate nodules is still a matter of debate, the meta-analysis by Borowczyk et al. [4] reports interesting findings about the US differences between follicular adenoma and follicular carcinoma. The presence of Hashimoto's thyroiditis is a potential pitfall when assessing thyroid nodules with US and the paper by Słowińska-Klencka et al. [5] analyzes the impact of changes in the threshold for the nodule's shape criterion in four TIRADSs. Thermal ablation of benign thyroid nodules can represent another pitfall when we face previously treated patients and this was addressed by Bernardi et al. [6]. Other specific data have been reported about the role of contrast-enhanced US [7], grading of hypogenicity [8], assessment of neck lymph-nodes [9], and the potential future impacts of artificial intelligence on the thyroid field [10]. Moreover, how particular thyroid nodules, such as autonomously functioning nodules, may be put in the TIRADSs categories are reported by Seifert et al. [11]. Finally, the performance of TIRADSs in detecting thyroid cancer in a pediatric population was assessed by Scappaticcio et al. [12] and Piccardo et al. [13]. Overall, ultrasound is increasingly a necessary and essential tool in order to manage patients with thyroid nodules [14] and these new advancements can be useful in clinical practice.

Funding: This research received no external funding.

Acknowledgments: The author would like to say thank you to all of authors of the articles included in the present Special Issue, as well as all the reviewers who critically revised the papers to improve them.

Conflicts of Interest: The author declares no conflict of interest.

References

1. Rago, T.; Vitti, P. Risk Stratification of Thyroid Nodules: From Ultrasound Features to TIRADS. *Cancers* **2022**, *14*, 717. [CrossRef] [PubMed]
2. Russ, G.; Trimboli, P.; Buffet, C. The New Era of TIRADSs to Stratify the Risk of Malignancy of Thyroid Nodules: Strengths, Weaknesses and Pitfalls. *Cancers* **2021**, *13*, 4316. [CrossRef] [PubMed]
3. Rossi, E.D.; Pantanowitz, L.; Raffaelli, M.; Fadda, G. Overview of the Ultrasound Classification Systems in the Field of Thyroid Cytology. *Cancers* **2021**, *13*, 3133. [CrossRef] [PubMed]
4. Borowczyk, M.; Woliński, K.; Więckowska, B.; Jodłowska-Siewert, E.; Szczepanek-Parulska, E.; Verburg, F.A.; Ruchała, M. Sonographic Features Differentiating Follicular Thyroid Cancer from Follicular Adenoma–A Meta-Analysis. *Cancers* **2021**, *13*, 938. [CrossRef] [PubMed]
5. Słowińska-Klencka, D.; Klencki, M.; Wojtaszek-Nowicka, M.; Wysocka-Konieczna, K.; Woźniak-Oseła, E.; Popowicz, B. Validation of Four Thyroid Ultrasound Risk Stratification Systems in Patients with Hashimoto's Thyroiditis; Impact of Changes in the Threshold for Nodule's Shape Criterion. *Cancers* **2021**, *13*, 4900. [CrossRef] [PubMed]
6. Bernardi, S.; Palermo, A.; Grasso, R.F.; Fabris, B.; Stacul, F.; Cesareo, R. Current Status and Challenges of US-Guided Radiofrequency Ablation of Thyroid Nodules in the Long Term: A Systematic Review. *Cancers* **2021**, *13*, 2746. [CrossRef] [PubMed]
7. Radzina, M.; Ratniece, M.; Putrins, D.S.; Saule, L.; Cantisani, V. Performance of Contrast-Enhanced Ultrasound in Thyroid Nodules: Review of Current State and Future Perspectives. *Cancers* **2021**, *13*, 5469. [CrossRef] [PubMed]
8. Popova, N.M.; Radzina, M.; Prieditis, P.; Liepa, M.; Rauda, M.; Stepanovs, K. Impact of the Hypoechogenicity Criteria on Thyroid Nodule Malignancy Risk Stratification Performance by Different TIRADS Systems. *Cancers* **2021**, *13*, 5581. [CrossRef] [PubMed]
9. Chung, S.R.; Baek, J.H.; Choi, Y.J.; Sung, T.-Y.; Song, D.E.; Kim, T.Y.; Lee, J.H. Diagnostic Algorithm for Metastatic Lymph Nodes of Differentiated Thyroid Carcinoma. *Cancers* **2021**, *13*, 1338. [CrossRef] [PubMed]
10. Bini, F.; Pica, A.; Azzimonti, L.; Giusti, A.; Ruinelli, L.; Marinozzi, F.; Trimboli, P. Artificial Intelligence in Thyroid Field—A Comprehensive Review. *Cancers* **2021**, *13*, 4740. [CrossRef] [PubMed]
11. Seifert, P.; Schenke, S.; Zimny, M.; Stahl, A.; Grunert, M.; Klemenz, B.; Freesmeyer, M.; Kreissl, M.C.; Herrmann, K.; Görges, R. Diagnostic Performance of Kwak, EU, ACR, and Korean TIRADS as Well as ATA Guidelines for the Ultrasound Risk Stratification of Non-Autonomously Functioning Thyroid Nodules in a Region with Long History of Iodine Deficiency: A German Multicenter Trial. *Cancers* **2021**, *13*, 4467. [CrossRef] [PubMed]
12. Scappaticcio, L.; Maiorino, M.I.; Iorio, S.; Docimo, G.; Longo, M.; Grandone, A.; Luongo, C.; Cozzolino, I.; Piccardo, A.; Trimboli, P.; et al. Exploring the Performance of Ultrasound Risk Stratification Systems in Thyroid Nodules of Pediatric Patients. *Cancers* **2021**, *13*, 5304. [CrossRef] [PubMed]
13. Piccardo, A.; Fiz, F.; Bottoni, G.; De Luca, C.; Massollo, M.; Catrambone, U.; Foppiani, L.; Muraca, M.; Garaventa, A.; Trimboli, P. Facing Thyroid Nodules in Paediatric Patients Previously Treated with Radiotherapy for Non-Thyroidal Cancers: Are Adult Ultrasound Risk Stratification Systems Reliable? *Cancers* **2021**, *13*, 4692. [CrossRef] [PubMed]
14. Trimboli, P. Ultrasound: The Extension of Our Hands to Improve the Management of Thyroid Patients. *Cancers* **2021**, *13*, 567. [CrossRef] [PubMed]

MDPI
St. Alban-Anlage 66
4052 Basel
Switzerland
Tel. +41 61 683 77 34
Fax +41 61 302 89 18
www.mdpi.com

Cancers Editorial Office
E-mail: cancers@mdpi.com
www.mdpi.com/journal/cancers

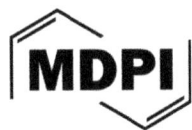

www.ingramcontent.com/pod-product-compliance
Lightning Source LLC
LaVergne TN
LVHW070747100526
838202LV00013B/1323